Understanding Post-COVID-19 Social and Cultural Realities

Sajal Roy · Debasish Nandy
Editors

Understanding Post-COVID-19 Social and Cultural Realities

Global Context

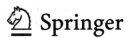

Editors
Sajal Roy
Centre for Social Impact UNSW
UNSW Business School
The University of New South Wales
Sydney, NSW, Australia

Debasish Nandy
Head of the Department, Political Science
Kazi Nazrul University
Asansol, India

ISBN 978-981-19-0808-8   ISBN 978-981-19-0809-5 (eBook)
https://doi.org/10.1007/978-981-19-0809-5

© The Editor(s) (if applicable) and The Author(s), under exclusive license to Springer Nature Singapore Pte Ltd. 2022
This work is subject to copyright. All rights are solely and exclusively licensed by the Publisher, whether the whole or part of the material is concerned, specifically the rights of translation, reprinting, reuse of illustrations, recitation, broadcasting, reproduction on microfilms or in any other physical way, and transmission or information storage and retrieval, electronic adaptation, computer software, or by similar or dissimilar methodology now known or hereafter developed.
The use of general descriptive names, registered names, trademarks, service marks, etc. in this publication does not imply, even in the absence of a specific statement, that such names are exempt from the relevant protective laws and regulations and therefore free for general use.
The publisher, the authors and the editors are safe to assume that the advice and information in this book are believed to be true and accurate at the date of publication. Neither the publisher nor the authors or the editors give a warranty, expressed or implied, with respect to the material contained herein or for any errors or omissions that may have been made. The publisher remains neutral with regard to jurisdictional claims in published maps and institutional affiliations.

This Springer imprint is published by the registered company Springer Nature Singapore Pte Ltd.
The registered company address is: 152 Beach Road, #21-01/04 Gateway East, Singapore 189721, Singapore

Dedicated to all unfortunate COVID victims

Preface

The idea of the edited volume entitled *Understanding Post-COVID-19: Social and Cultural Realities-Global Context* came into our mind considering the outbreak of the COVID-19. Since December 2019, pandemic COVID-19 has impacted the socio-cultural milieu of the globe. The impact of coronavirus on worldwide cultural, social relations, diplomatic relations, medication, tourism, and economy has been marked by chilling bitterness. Many people have lost their lives, and many of them have been severely affected and also have been psychologically depressed. Nation-states have been suffered from financial recession due to the decline in trade volume. The financial crisis created a high rate of unemployment. Due to the maintenance of social distance in social relations, psychological distance has been created among the common masses.

In the global political order, China has been pressurized by the Western countries led by the USA. The Chinese government has been alleged for hiding the information of coronavirus. To suppress the Chinese hegemonic economic presence in the global economic milieu, an informal alliance has been made. The pandemic COVID-19 has compelled the nation-states to think about self-reliance. The management of state authority in controlling COVID-19 has not only raised the questions of health security but also executing the directives of the government. The tourism sector, hotels, restaurants, and aviation sector have been vehemently affected by COVID-19. The flow of tourism has been restricted enormously. During the COVID-19, countries like India have sent medical equipment to many countries. Humanitarian diplomacy has taken a new shape during COVID-19. Vaccine diplomacy has been an additional tool for many countries. Due to the shortage of vaccines, many countries have failed to fight against the various strains of coronavirus, like alpha, beta, gamma, delta, etc. Many countries have supplied vaccines to those countries which are unable to produce vaccines free of cost or with cost. The key objective of this book is to understand the socio-cultural relations in the post-COVID-19 world which are based on several interrelated factors.

This book is the outcome of 12 chapters. Scholars across the globe have contributed chapters from different perspectives. The editors are grateful to all of them. We are thankful to all well-wishers and to those who have directly or indirectly helped up in many ways. We are also thankful to the publishing editor of this series and publishing house for giving us the opportunity in publishing this book. We anticipate that this book will endeavor a new revenue to the study of social science.

Sydney, Australia   Dr. Sajal Roy
Asansol, India   Dr. Debasish Nandy

Acknowledgments

The edited volume entitled *Understanding Post-COVID-19 Social and Cultural Realities: Global Context* consists of 12 chapters. We have interacted with a vast network of people: respondents, researchers, journalists, academicians, military personnel, police officers, administrators, and politicians to understand the dynamic of COVID-19. The contributors from different countries have shared their opinions and experiences through their writings. The editors are immensely grateful to all of them. Within this short space, it is impossible to mention the name of all individuals and institutions.

First, we are thankful to the University of Technology Sydney, Australia, and Honourable Vice Chancellor of Kazi Nazrul University, Asansol, West Bengal, for his continuous support in initiating this study. We are thankful to Professor Sanjay Kumar Bhardwaj, School of International Studies, Jawaharlal Nehru University, New Delhi, India, for his continuous guidance.

We are thankful to our colleagues and family members for their continuous support and encouragement. We are thankful to Professor Pranab Kumar Pandey, Department of Public Administration, University of Rajshahi, Bangladesh. We are thankful to Professor

During our study, we interacted with many dignitaries to collect data and obtain interpretation and understanding. Some people helped us to collect the relevant facts. Most of them did not agree to disclose their names. The authors are thankful to all of them. We are thankful to our family members for their continuous support and encouragement. The editors are thankful to the authority of Springer Nature, Singapore, for giving us the opportunity to publish this pertinent and timely edited volume. They are thankful to other dignitaries of Springer Nature for their assistance.

Sydney, Australia   Sajal Roy
Asansol, West Bengal, India   Debasish Nandy

About This Book

The edited volume entitled *Understanding Post-COVID-19 Social and Cultural Realities: Global Context* is a combination of 12 chapters. This volume attempted to address social and cultural realities of post-COVID-19 global order. This volume has projected a global scenario of the post-COVID-19 diplomatic scenario, administrative realities, gendered-violence, medication system, and human security-related issues. Through an interdisciplinary approach, this edited volume has been designed.

Contents

1 Understanding COVID-19: An Introduction of Social and Cultural Realities 1
Sajal Roy, Debasish Nandy, and Utsab Bhattarai

2 Role of Big and Emerging Powers in the Post-Covid World Order 13
Mahesh Ranjan Debata

3 COVID-19 Pandemic and Its Impact on Our Physical Environment: A Critical Analysis 27
Amir Mohammad Nasrullah

4 The Austrian State and the COVID-19 Crisis: Achievements and Failures of a Small European Country During the Pandemic Since 2020 49
Martin Malek

5 The Changing Dimensions of India's Foreign Relations During COVID-19 77
Debasish Nandy and Alik Naha

6 Pandemic and the Administrative Rationality: Understanding the Administrative Response to the Pandemic 103
Arindam Roy

7 Negotiating Access to Maternal Health Services During COVID-19 Pandemic in Kilifi County, Kenya: Rapid Qualitative Study 123
Stephen Okumu Ombere

8 #I Stay Home (If I Can): COVID-19 and Social Inequality in Peru: A View from Auto-Ethnography 137
Cristian Terry

9 *Koro ti Lo:* Popular Deconstruction of the COVID-19 Pandemic in Southwestern Nigeria 151

Mofeyisara Oluwatoyin Omobowale, Olugbenga Samuel Falase, Olufikayo Kunle Oyelade, and Ayokunle Olumuyiwa Omobowale

10 COVID-19 and Decline of Multilateralism 165

Khushnam P N

11 COVID-19 and Its Impact on Culture: The Experience of Nepal ... 181

Shree Prasad Devkota and Laxmi Paudyal

12 Pandemic Within a Pandemic: Gendered Impact of COVID-19 in Bangladesh with a Focus on Child Marriage and Domestic Violence 199

Nazmunnessa Mahtab and Tasnim Nowshin Fariha

Index 227

Editors and Contributors

About the Editors

Sajal Roy, Ph.D. is the Postdoctoral Fellow at Centre for livelihoods and Wellbeing, UTS Business School, Sydney, Australia. Dr. Roy was a Doctoral Fellow at Western Sydney University, Australia.

Debasish Nandy, Ph.D. is an Associate Professor and Head in the Department of Political Science, Kazi Nazrul University, Asansol, West Bengal, India. Dr. Nandy is the Coordinator of the Centre for Studies of South and Southeast Asian Societies at the same university. He is the Visiting Faculty Member in the Department of Foreign Area Studies at the National University of Tajikistan, Dushanbe, Tajikistan.

Contributors

Utsab Bhattarai Western Sydney University, Sydney, NSW, Australia

Mahesh Ranjan Debata Centre for Inner Asian Studies, School of International Studies, Jawaharlal Nehru University, New Delhi, India

Shree Prasad Devkota Tribhuvan University, Kathmandu, Nepal

Olugbenga Samuel Falase Department of Sociology, Lead City University, Ibadan, Nigeria

Tasnim Nowshin Fariha Department of Gender and Women Studies, University of Dhaka, Dhaka, Bangladesh

Khushnam P N Independent Researcher, Bangaluru, India

Nazmunnessa Mahtab Department of Gender and Women Studies, University of Dhaka, Dhaka, Bangladesh

Martin Malek Institute for Strategy and Security Policy, National Defence Academy, Vienna, Austria

Alik Naha Department of Political Science, Vidyasagar College, Kolkata, India

Debasish Nandy Head of the Department, Political Science, Kazi Nazrul University, Asansol, India

Amir Mohammad Nasrullah Department of Public Administration, University of Chittagong, Chittagong, Bangladesh

Stephen Okumu Ombere Department of Sociology and Anthropology, Maseno University, Kisumu, Kenya

Ayokunle Olumuyiwa Omobowale Department of Sociology, University of Ibadan, Ibadan, Nigeria

Mofeyisara Oluwatoyin Omobowale Social and Behavioural Health Unit, Institute of Child Health, College of Medicine, University of Ibadan, Ibadan, Nigeria

Olufikayo Kunle Oyelade Emmanuel College of Theology and Christian Education, Ibadan, Nigeria

Laxmi Paudyal Gandaki Medical College Teaching Hospital and Research Center, Pokhara, Nepal

Arindam Roy Department of Political Science, University of Burdwan, Burdwan, West Bengal, India

Sajal Roy Centre for Livelihood and Wellbeing, UTS Business School, University of Technology Sydney, Sydney, NSW, Australia

Cristian Terry Independent researcher, Lausanne, Switzerland

Abbreviations

ACFTA	African Continental Free Trade Area
ADB	Asian Development Bank
ASEAN	Association of South East Asian Nations
BOD	Biochemical Oxygen Demand
BRI	Belt and Road Initiative
BRICS	Brazil Russia India China South Africa
COD	Chemical Oxygen Demand
CPCB	Central Pollution Control Board
DO	Dissolved Oxygen
EC	Electric Conductivity
EEA	The European Environmental Agency
FMS	Free Maternity Services
GDP	Gross Domestic Production
GHS	Global Health Security
ICMR	Indian Council of Medical Research
JCPOA	Joint Comprehensive Plan of Action
KNBS	Kenya National Bureau of Statistics
MHS	Maternal Health Services
NATO	North Atlantic Treaty Organisation
PHIEC	Public Health Emergency of International Concern
RCEP	Regional Comprehensive Economic Programme
SCO	Shanghai Cooperation Organization
SDG	Sustainable Development Goal
SLOCs	Sea Lines of Communication
TBA	Traditional Birth Attendant
TPP	Trans Pacific Partnership
UNCTAD	United Nations Conference on Trade and Development
UNDP	United Nations Development Programme
UNESCO	United Nations Educational, Scientific and Cultural Organization
UNICEF	United Nations Children's Fund
UNWTO	United Nations World Tourism Organization

| UPCB | Uttarakhand Pollution Control Board |
| WHO | World Health Organization |

Chapter 1
Understanding COVID-19: An Introduction of Social and Cultural Realities

Sajal Roy, Debasish Nandy, and Utsab Bhattarai

Abstract COVID-19 (SARS-Cov-2) was declared a global pandemic by The World Health Organization (WHO) on March 11, 2020. The virus became a pandemic with initial small chains of spread followed by increasingly wider transmission across most countries of the world. As a result, within a short period, the virus has affected almost every continent. Even with a risk of fatality of 1%, it is now known to kill healthy adults and children as well as elderly people with underlying health problems. The virus has created fear, anxiety and panic among people everywhere. Months of living in isolation and lockdown have negatively affected the mental health of large numbers of people. Most developing and underdeveloped countries are facing severe economic crisis, together with significant societal problems. Even in developed countries, the negative outcomes are clear. Any contagious pandemic outbreak has lethal effects on individuals and society. However, the outcomes of COVID-19 have created a situation the world is unprepared for (Rashid, 2020). Not only has the virus identified the existing loopholes in our systems, it has also shown that our lives will never be the same again. This chapter intends to critically analyses on impact of COVID-19 on socio-economic and cultural milieu of global society.

Keywords COVID-19 · Healthcare · Socio-economic · Cultural · Environmental · Supply chain

The novel coronavirus disease (COVID-19), now known as the severe acute respiratory syndrome coronavirus 2 (SARS-CoV-2) was declared a global pandemic by the World Health Organization (WHO) on 11 March 2020. The virus became a pandemic with initial small chains of spread followed by increasingly wider

---

S. Roy (✉)
Centre for Social Impact, UNSW Business School, UNSW Sydney, The University of New South Wales, Sydney, NSW, Australia
e-mail: Sajal.Roy@unsw.edu.au

D. Nandy
Department of Political Science, Kazi Nazrul University, Asansol, India

U. Bhattarai
Western Sydney University, Sydney, NSW, Australia

© The Author(s), under exclusive license to Springer Nature Singapore Pte Ltd. 2022
S. Roy and D. Nandy (eds.), *Understanding Post-COVID-19 Social and Cultural Realities*, https://doi.org/10.1007/978-981-19-0809-5_1

transmission across most countries of the world. Its effects are now experienced by the people of every continent Even with a risk of fatality of 1%, it is now known to kill healthy adults and children as well as elderlies who are undergoing health problems. The virus has created fear, anxiety and panic among people everywhere. Months of living in isolation and lockdown has negatively affected the mental health of a large number of people. Most developing and underdeveloped countries are facing severe economic crisis, together with significant societal problems. The negative outcomes are evident even in developed nations. Any contagious pandemic outbreak has lethal effects on individuals and society. However, the outcomes of COVID-19 have created a situation about which the world was unprepared for (Rashid, 2020). The virus has identified not only the existing loopholes in our systems but also the reality that our lives will never be the same again. This chapter intends to critically analyse the impact of COVID-19 on the socio-economic and cultural milieu of the global society.

The consequences of COVID-19 go far beyond the contagious nature of the disease, with its quarantine requirements and social distancing. It also brings about serious social, political and economic consequences. For most countries, the virus has had the greatest impact on the economic and social sectors, taking into consideration population density, healthcare capacity, limited resources, existing poverty, environmental factors, social structure, and cultural norms. Work sectors have become increasingly pessimistic as the pandemic significantly affects all economies (Raihan, 2020). Consumer demand has plunged, affecting business revenues and margins. Supply chains have been disrupted, leaving retail shelves empty and production lines out of material. Stock markets are falling. Companies are concerned that they will be unable to obtain investors' funding. Business continuity plans have replaced business expansion plans. The worst affected industries have been the travel and tourism sectors (Kosteas, 2020).

The pandemic has also changed the global social order. It is having an impact on every aspect of life around the globe, from individual relationships to institutional operations and international collaborations. Societies are endeavoring to protect themselves despite severe restrictions, while the pandemic continues to upset family relations and overturn governance (Altman, 2020). The COVID-19 has made it clearer than ever before that where many strains on the social sector occur, the current global system, with its interconnectedness and vulnerabilities, is under threat. Due to the changing patterns of economic and societal elements caused by COVID-19, further research is urgently required to analyze these changing trends.

This study concentrates on the changing patterns of work and global social order as a result of COVID-19. There have been enough speculations that there will be a wide gap between the pre-COVID-19 and the post-COVID-19 scenarios. The world order would change massively with significant differences from an individual's private life to the society they live in, the economic factors, patterns of work, job markets, and global social systems. The pandemic of COVID-19 has brought socio-cultural changes which might be continued for a time being in interactive cultural relations. It is uncertain that things will turn normal in absence of effective strategies to adjust them to bring back to the new normal. The first step would be to properly examine the trends and characteristics of the changing patterns. This book attempts to suitably scrutinize the changes in the patterns of work and global social order to point out possible reasons behind the outbreak of the COVID-19. It will also shed light on the differences between the conditions of underdeveloped and developed countries, with evidence of how they have struggled and attempted to find the way outs for coping such dreadful situation.

This study attempts to portray what work and the global social order might look like in the future. The book will benefit people from all sectors as it works with both economic and social perspectives—notably, individuals involved in the business and commercial sectors including the fields within the social science discipline. It will not only contribute to the research and academic learning of both teachers and students but also does aim to educate many about the impacts of COVID-19 from distinct perspectives.

The pandemic of COVID-19 has influenced every aspect of human lives. The social scientists have made rationale of the study and its importance in the current situation. The two mostly influenced areas by this pandemic are economic and societal sectors. Work trends and the global social order have been massively crushed by COVID-19. As a result, we can see significant changes in their previous patterns. These changing patterns dictate the future trajectory of work and the global social order, that is why it is crucial to examine these altering patterns. This chapter focuses on this part.

The COVID-19 outbreak affects all segments of the population. It is particularly detrimental to the members' social groups undergoing most vulnerable situations such as the poor elderly and disable as well as youths, and indigenous communities. Early evidence indicates that the health and economic impacts of the virus are being borne disproportionately by poor people. For example, homeless people, who are unable to find safe shelters and, are thus highly exposed to the danger of the virus. People without access to running water, refugees, migrants, or displaced persons also stand to suffer disproportionately both from the pandemic as well as its aftermath— either due to limited movement and fewer employment opportunities or increased xenophobia and so on.

If not properly addressed through policy the social crisis created by the COVID-19 pandemic may also increase inequality, exclusion, discrimination and global unemployment in the medium as well as in the long term. Since comprehensive, universal social protection systems act as automatic stabilizers, they play a much durable role in protecting workers and in reducing the prevalence of poverty when they are in place. As such, they ever provide basic income security and thus enhancement in people's capacity to manage and overcome shocks.

The rapid spread of COVID-19 in Africa has generated perseverance. The economy of African countries has been severely affected due to the pandemic of COVID-19. African nations have sought to mitigate such crises by developing a coordinated framework. The UNESCO has played a special role in supporting African countries in this regard. Looking upon priority to Africa, the UNESCO has paid efforts to fight against the problems caused by COVID-19 in the short, medium and long terms. As a specialized agency of the UN family, it is inescapable that UNESCO's involvement is very crucial in both the fast reaction and the expedition for a post pandemic reclamation in Africa (UNESCO, 2020). With the outbreak of the pandemic in Africa, governments across the continent took very stringent measures to control the spread. Among others, these measures included a ban on all public gatherings and indefinite closure of public institutions such as schools and universities, halt domestic and international flights, shutdown of cities and towns across countries making strict rules to stop the movement of people, and the launch of testing programmes to identify, isolate and treat infected people. These measures have had huge immediate effects on the economies of countries in the continent, the worst since the 2008 global financial crisis. Economic growth is predicted to drop considerably in the short as well as long-term, as gains in the tourism, aviation and extractive sectors, among others, are completely wiped out. The WHO has taken necessary actions to maintain the health security in collaboration with the African governments. In additional, it has taken numerous preventive measures to mitigate the effects of COVID-19 on socio-cultural, political and economic aspects.

The virus gradually distorted into a hazardous pandemic leading the world to a cessation. The community transmission of coronavirus intensified with high contamination rates across the world. It also makes a massive problems different regions of the world. These narrative sheds light on many essential factors associated with large-scale infection, apart from the virus itself. There are so many structural factors in every society which can assist in intensifying or de-intensifying the infection rate. During the COVID-19, 'community responsibility' and 'community consciousness' to combat COVID-19 have found across the globe.

The overall impact of COVID-19 on human lives is multidimensional. The coronavirus has affected the lives of people all around the world. It has made a significant difference in every aspect of our lives, from our personal lives to broader societal relations. Many structural problems in societies have been highlighted because of the corona virus. Particularly, the governance systems of developing countries are facing immense difficulties as their economic sectors have been significantly ruined by due to the consequences of COVID-19. It has indeed changed the social behaviour and habits across the globe.

The economic impact of COVID-19 is very high. Almost the economy of every country has been immensely suffered due to lock downs, massive job losses, and cessation of nearly all travels both domestic and international. The rate of unemployment has risen sharply in poor and developing countries. Many companies are experiencing ongoing financial difficulties. Working from home may not be an option for everyone. COVID-19 has caused widespread uncertainty, proving work sectors the hardest hit.

The COVID-19 is responsible for the changing patterns of work-culture and occupation. The virus is a highly contagious disease, and for this reason, the former way of working and attending traditional workplaces is no longer the norm. COVID-19 has forced work patterns to change and adapt to survive, putting additional pressure on the labour market. Despite the efforts of many to find ways to adjust, millions remain helpless and without solutions. The pandemic has added many new dimensions to the work sector while eliminating many of its previous ones.

The impact of COVID-19 on organisations around the globe has alarmed very remarkably. While discussing the impacts to cause change on the work sectors, it is essential to consider the situation of many national and multinational organisations. CEOs of many organisations have faced overwhelming and competing challenges and unmapped situations as they are continuing to direct the impacts of COVID-19. Many organisations are already taking 'no regret' actions so as to emerge from the pandemic stronger. These leaders are facing the crisis with a spirit of reinvention by accelerating digital transformation, establishing variable cost structures, and implementing agile operations.

The COVID-19 has also affected the work environments of local sectors. It is crucial to evaluate the sectoral impact of work in all sectors for a proper assessment of the influence of the pandemic. The local sectors are especially essential to the economy of the poor and developing countries. The majority of the population in these countries is involved in local sectors for earning their livelihoods. The national, international and multinational organizations and companies are quick to combat the negative consequences as they have the skills and human resources. However, the scenario is different in the case of the local job sectors.

As a result of the pandemic of COVID-19, emerging challenges and changes in the workplace have been noticed around the globe. Since the virus is highly contagious people are required to maintain social distancing for their as well as others safety. In such context, the technology and the digital world have become greatly advantageous for the office workers as they are able to work from home. The only feasible option for moving forward with the 'new normal' is an increased utilization of technology. Most workplaces have become dependent on the use of technology, and meetings are held online along with the recruitment and other processes such as monetary transactions. The use of technology has also ushered in a new requirement for skilled human resources for workplaces. Major changes of procedure in the workplace have also created a digital divide. Emerging trends in work sectors have not only increased our dependence on technology, but also created a digital divide, together with inequality. It is overly—ambitious to expect that all workers will possess the same skill levels. This is especially the case in developing and poor countries. This is because the education of many people may not necessarily enhance their skills, creating a significant divide among employees. The financial situation of each person is closely related to this.

The social aspect of COVID-19 has been a key area of research for the social scientists. Along with the economy, societal elements have been significantly damaged by the pandemic. The new normal has created many structural problems in almost every society in the world. The situation is even worse in many developing and poor countries. Already existing social trends have been blamed for the larger community transmission of COVID-19 in these countries. However, social scenarios are going through their own major changes. The social order connects all regions of the globe.

The COVID-19 is influencing the global social order will leave a long-lasting impact even after the pandemic is over The crisis and the necessary public health response are causing the largest and fastest decline in the movement of people and goods all over the world. The collapse of international travel (stands out against a much steadier growth trend), and the damage to tourism is indisputable. Tourism contributes more to global output than automotive manufacturing, and business travel facilitates international trade and investment. There are currently strict restrictions on travel because of the pandemic, which is significantly affecting the global social economy. 2020 was a low point for many globalization metrics and this situation has continued to be so in 2021.

The global social order caused by COVID-19 has been dramatically changed. Humanity is now facing an unprecedented existential crisis due to tiny virus which is highly contagious and life-threatening. Globalization relies on complex links of global value chains (GVCs) which connect producers across multiple countries. These producers often use highly specialized intermediate goods, or inputs, produced by only one distant, overseas supplier. COVID-19 has severely disrupted these links. The long-term societal impacts include the exacerbation of inequality, changes in consumer behavior, and adjustments of work as well as the role of technology. Our lives, as individuals, workforce, and society will be changed forever at work and home.

The scientists, policy-makers, NGOs and INGOs will have to find-out possible solutions to overcome the new challenges posed by COVID-19. Undoubtedly, mental stress due to COVID-19 has been caused by massive lockdowns, enforced without ensuring the fundamental needs of the vulnerable. The weak governance of many healthcare systems and poor health facilities further exacerbates the anxiety of the general public. Henceforth, the primary undertaking is to ensure strong policy formulations. The future under this pandemic is uncertain without a vaccine. People need to learn to adjust to the new normal. Both economic and social aspects depend largely on the governments' decisions in any state. Even in the case of increasing use of technology, people must not be discriminated and undergo the fear of unemployment. Furthermore, a safe work environment must be ensured for them. The governments must be a responsible body for such safeguarding. Additionally, civil societies can also take part in this venture.

The pandemic of COVID-19 has dramatically changed the existing global order. The general pattern of global diplomatic equations has been altered due to this pandemic. The USA, some European countries, Japan, and India have formed an informal anti-Chinese forum to counter China. The growing dominance of China in the global political economy over the last few years has posed a threat to its global competitors. Some countries have already decided to reduce their dependency on particular countries and adopt a policy of self-reliance. The global supply chain has been interrupted. The nature of interaction among the nation-states is changing. The changing equations of diplomatic relations among the states in the post-COVID-19 period influences the multilateralism.

The outbreak of the COVID 19 pandemic has not only caught our napping but has also dashed our arrogance to enlightened scientific rationality. The entire humanity till now is literally clueless about the invisible enemy. The devastating pandemic has already taken a toll of more than five million lives around the globe. Neither doctors nor epidemiologist or virologist has become able to suggest the solution to the COVID pandemic. The beleaguered humanity is in a bid to put a tab on the contagion to break the so-called 'chain of the virus.' It has adopted a series of strict protocols like lockdown, quarantine, isolation, but, so far, to no avail. These strict protocols have bequeathed severe collateral damages, including disruption of normal socio-economic activities, political and civic engagements of the people. This book intends to explore the administrative responses to the pandemic of COVID-19 through the lens of administrative rationality. This chapter argues that administrative rationality seems to be the only wherewithal at our disposal. Yet it expresses the optimism that administrative rationality can find a bailout programme by partnering with the stakeholders like the civil society, market and the community people.

It mentions two of the most virus—affected aspects of human lives. The chapter addresses the economic and social sectors and the consequences they face because of this pandemic. The major focus has been on the area of work sectors and the changing global social order. The book seriously considers the changing nature of these sectors and the challenges they invite. The final chapter that reflects the whole book concludes with some recommendations.

This book consists of 12 chapters.

In the Chapter 2 entitled *Role of Big and Emerging Powers in the post-Covid World Order* Mahesh Ranjan Debata has argued that the outbreak of Novel Corona Virus (COVID-19) is one of the biggest dangers humanity has faced so far in the twenty-first century. Big international actors, militarily-powerful and economically-vibrant nations across the globe have fallen prey to an unprecedented human tragedy. The world community continues to be engaged in protecting its citizens as the top most priority using every possible means. In the meantime, the pandemic has added new dimensions, altering the international order both economically and strategically. This chapter foresees big power rivalry in the world stage. While the state of affairs during and following the pandemic will prompt USA to make earnest efforts in resurrecting its lost power, position and preponderance in the global corridor, the paper argues, Russia will not leave any stone unturned to regain its lost name, fame and glory.

In the Chapter 3 entitled *COVID-19 Pandemic and Its Impact on our Physical Environment: A Critical Analysis* Dr. Amir Mohammad Nasrullah has wanted to analysis that COVID-19 (Coronavirus Disease-2019) has created adverse effects globally on human lives in various ways, including the economy and the physical environment. Different national and international research reports confirmed that it has killed many people and many of them have been suffering seriously. Governments around the world have taken different measures to comprehend the spread of COVID-19 through human to human diffusion such as maintaining physical distance, avoiding public gathering and many other disciplinary actions. However, these measures have also created significant effects on the environment. Lockdown in many countries, along with minimal human movement has positively impacted the natural environment slightly. this chapter aim is to identify the environmental consequences due to COVID-19 pandemic, as well, recommend probable ways as future policy inputs for a sustainable environment. A number of published materials such as various research reports of different government, non-government and international organizations as well as internet sources were reviewed critically for the purpose.

The Chapter 4 entitled *The Austrian State and the COVID-19 Crisis:Achievements and Failures of a Small European Country During the Pandemic since 2020* has been written by Martin Malek. The prime argument of this chapter is the financial crisis from 2008 onwards had already led to a "return of the state" in many countries. This tendency intensified in the face of the COVID-19 pandemic from the beginning of 2020—as well as in Austria. This chapter asks several research questions on the Austrian state's handling of the pandemic in comparison with the other members of the European Union (EU). The most important are: What were the consequences of the pandemic in the areas of public health, the economy and the labour market. This chapter has presented a comparative survey of the state performance of the EU member.

In the Chapter 5 entitled *The Changing Dimensions of India's Foreign Relations During COVID-19* Debasish Nandy and Alik Naha have critically analyzed India's changing dimensions of foreign policy during COVID-19. India's strategy to counter China in association with Australia, the USA, Japan, and other democratic countries of the world has been highlighted in this chapter. India's policy of 'self-reliant' and financial challenges has been sequentially discussed in this chapter. The chapter has further delineated the relations between the domestic factors and external factors in the formulation of the new orientation-based foreign policy of India.

In Chapter 6, entitled *Pandemic and the Administrative Rationality: Understanding the Administrative Response to the Pandemic* Arindam Roy has argued that The outbreak of the COVID 19 pandemic has literally dashed our enlightened scientific rationality. It has claimed more than six million lives around the globe. The struggling humanity has adopted a series of strict legal-administrative protocols like lockdown, quarantine, isolation, to contain the spread of the virus. The strict adherence to the above—mentioned protocols have brought several collateral damages like disruption of normal socio-economic activities; suspension of political and civic engagements of the people. Further, given the nature of neoliberal governance, where delivery of services is a collective venture of all the stakeholders like state, civil society, market and community, administrative rationality is perhaps the most important means.

The Chapter 7 entitled *Negotiating Access to Maternal Health Services during COVID-19 Pandemic in Kilifi County, Kenya: Rapid Qualitative Study* is written by Stephen Okumu Ombere. In this chapter it has been argued that globally, women do a lot of unpaid work even before the onset of the COVID-19 pandemic. COVID-19 has delivered a blow to existing gender systems that could recalibrate gender roles, with beneficial effects on population health. Initial research suggests that the crisis and its consequent shutdown responses have resulted in an intense increase in this burden. There is a dearth of information on expectant mothers' negotiation mechanism to access maternal health services during COVID-19 in Kenya. This rapid qualitative study draws data from purposefully selected 12 mothers who were either pregnant or had new-born babies during the COVID-19 pandemic in Kilifi countyA variety of women's experiences with their husbands' presence or absence and how this impacted access to maternal health services is discussed. In this study, the household economic situation, in particular, emerged as a crucial gendered factor associated with negotiation for access to maternal health care.

In the Chapter 8 entitled ***I Stay Home (If I Can): COVID-19 and Social Inequality in Peru: A View from Auto-ethnography*** Cristian Terry has critically analyzed the COVID-19 pandemic from an auto-ethnography carried out in Cusco (Peru). This highlights the social differences and socioeconomic conditions that influence the way of living the pandemic and suffering its effects, which, in the Peruvian case, has more critically affected the most vulnerable populations. Thus, the privileged people can stay at home while the rest must go out to live/survive. This chapter lead us to think about a new social pact, more equitable and fairer, that divorces the pandemic-social inequality marriage, observed in different parts of the planet, particularly in the Americas. This is necessary to avoid future problems of equal or greater magnitude that tend to take their toll on vulnerable populations that often do not have the means to pay, or pay at the risk of their lives.

The Chapter 9 entitled ***Koro ti Lo: Popular Deconstruction of the COVID-19 Pandemic in Southwestern Nigeria*** have been written by Mofeyisara Oluwatoyin Omobowale, Olugbenga Samuel Falase, Olufikayo Kunle Oyelade and Ayokunle Olumuyiwa Omobowale. The authors have argued that emergence of the COVID-19 pandemic and its persistence are global phenomena, that greatly impact human life and existence. In Nigeria, the incidence and prevalence of the COVID-19 has attracted various interpretations and actions across cultures and spaces. While many people accept the reality of the deadly virus, many others still live in the denial of its existence and persistence. Many Nigerians have thrown caution to the wind celebrating the supposed decline of the pandemic with a popular slogan: Koro ti lo (COVID-19 has gone). Preventive measures were largely abandoned and interactions in public spaces returned to pre-COVID-19 social and spatial relations.

In the Chapter 10 entitled ***COVID-19 and Decline of Multilateralism*** Khushnam P has critically discussed on multilateralism and multilateral diplomacy for a peaceful and stable global system with capacity to deal with challenges and streamline the deviations as and when it comes on the way. The changes in the structure of international system must be reflected by the commensurate reforms in the multilateral institutions like United Nations Organizations. There is a growing concern about unilateral actions and withdrawal by powers in the recent years and the changing power landscape of the globe is not appropriately reflected in the existing multilateral institutions and mechanism. The COVID-19 with its global spread has impacted heavily on the multilateral institutions as never before. But is its very transnational implications impacting on the global supply chain and economic process have been pushing the nations for multilateral and global cooperation to deal with such impending pandemic. The mini-lateralism and regional multilateralism has shown greater pandemic outreach diplomacy and cooperation but their effective functioning needs an inclusive global multilateral structure. India with its global aspiration must work as an emerging world leader to shape a robust multilateral world with its pandemic measures, outreach and diplomacy.

The Chapter 11 entitled ***COVID-19 and its Impact on Culture: The Experience of Nepal*** have written by Shree Prasad Devkota Laxmi Paudyal. In this chapter they have given an outline of cultutural and phycycological impact of COVID-19 in Nepal. Nepal government has adopted a complete nationwide lockdown for almost six months with shut down of all cinema halls, gyms, health clubs, and museums as well as banned the gathering of people for cultural, social, and religious activities including temples, monasteries, churches, and mosques and partial lockdown for next two months. Still, yet many of the public places are not open. Although these measures have been taken to prevent this contagious disease, the fear, anxiety, panic situation, and uncertainty created in the people are in ruins. The psychological and sociocultural effects of the illness and its mitigation measures are significantly higher than the actual physical health effect due to COVID-19, which are in the shadow and not noticed. Moreover, the indirect impact on the economy, social harmony, religious and cultural beliefs, and processes, and others so many sectors are beyond the fact seen on the face of this pandemic.

The Chapter 12 entitled *Pandemic within a Pandemic: Gendered Impact of COVID-19 in Bangladesh with a focus on Child Marriage and Domestic Violence* is written by Nazmunnessa Mahtab and Tasnim Nowshin Fariha. In this chapter the authors have tried to explore how COVID 19 pandemic exacerbates the pre-existing gender inequalities in Bangladesh and expose women and girls to compounding forms of discrimination and maltreatment in home setting, including domestic violence, child marriage, abuse or exploitation. The findings underscore that the country's child marriage rate has increased by manifold as lockdowns exacerbate many of the complex factors that drive up under-aged marriages in emergency settings including poverty, lack of security of girls, risk of violence or early pregnancy. Similarly, for a significant portion of women and girls home became a site of conflict and violence due to factors like financial insecurities, disaster-related vulnerabilities, increased exposure to abusive relationships, and reduced options for external support.

References

Altman, S. A. (2020), Will Covid-19 have a lasting impact on globalization? *Harvard Business Review.* https://hbr.org/2020/05/will-covid-19-have-a-lasting-impact-on-globalization

Kosteas, B. (2020), How will COVID-19 change the way we work? *The Hill.* https://thehill.com/opinion/technology/495798-how-will-covid-19-change-the-way-we-work

Rashid, S. (2020), A pandemic of fear and changing social behaviour. *The Dhaka Tribune.* https://www.dhakatribune.com/opinion/op-ed/2020/05/11/a-pandemic-of-fear-and-changing-social-behaviour

Raihan, S. (2020), Covid-19 and employment challenges. *The Financial Express.* https://thefinancialexpress.com.bd/views/views/covid-19-and-employment-challenges-1595172556

UNESCO. (2020). *Socio-economic and cultural impacts of Covid-19 on Africa: UNESCO responses.* https://en.unesco.org/sites/default/files/stand_alone_executive_summary_fin.pdf. Accessed on 1 June 2021.

Sajal Roy, PhD is a Research Fellow at the Centre for Social Impact, UNSW Sydney.

Debasish Nandy, PhD is an Associate Professor and Head in the Department of Political Science, Kazi Nazrul University, Asansol, West Bengal, India. Dr. Nandy is the Coordinator of the Centre for Studies of South and South-East Asian Societies at the same University. He is a visiting faculty member in te Department of Foreign Area Studies at Tajik National University, Republic of Tajikistan.

Utsav Bhattarai, PhD Researcher Western Sydny University, Australia.

Chapter 2
Role of Big and Emerging Powers in the Post-Covid World Order

Mahesh Ranjan Debata

Abstract The outbreak of Novel Corona Virus (COVID-19) is one of the biggest dangers humanities has faced so far in the twenty-first century. Big international actors, militarily-powerful and economically-vibrant nations across the globe have fallen prey to an unprecedented human tragedy. The world community continues to be engaged in protecting its citizens as the top most priority using every possible means. In the meantime, the pandemic has added new dimensions, altering the international order both economically and strategically. The pandemic may well be remembered as the turning point of the end of an American-led global system that has paved way for the arrival of an Asian century with two Asian giants and emerging global powers, China and India, at the forefront. This chapter, at the outset, dilates upon various dimensions of the pandemic. This chapter foresees big power rivalry in the world stage. While the state of affairs during and following the pandemic will prompt USA to make earnest efforts in resurrecting its lost power, position and preponderance in the global corridor, the chapter argues, Russia will not leave any stone unturned to regain its lost name, fame and glory. Besides, China would make earnest efforts to position itself as a power to reckon with as it has done in the last one decade or so. The paper argues further that amidst struggle for power among big powers, traditional powers from Europe (Great Britain, France and Germany), Asia (India and Japan), Latin America (Brazil) and Australia will have leverage in the new global order that marks the beginning of a new saga of multipolar world. The chapter argues that with the North Atlantic Treaty Organisation (NATO) loosing its significance, important regional organizations like Association of South East Asian Nations (ASEAN), Shanghai Cooperation Organization (SCO), G-20 and BRICS will come forward for a far bigger role in international affairs. However, the paper ends with a positive note that competition among global and emerging powers will continue in a healthy manner, and in case of any conflict or confrontation, strong cooperation will be the only way to achieve peace and stability across the world. This chapter offers a balanced overview of the global order (some may call it disorder) before the

---

M. R. Debata (✉)
Centre for Inner Asian Studies, School of International Studies,
Jawaharlal Nehru University, New Delhi, India

© The Author(s), under exclusive license to Springer Nature Singapore Pte Ltd. 2022   13
S. Roy and D. Nandy (eds.), *Understanding Post-COVID-19 Social and Cultural Realities*, https://doi.org/10.1007/978-981-19-0809-5_2

pandemic occurred, during and the post-pandemic period, where many a factors and actors play their respective roles. Further, this qualitative study will add significantly and give a varied dimension to the existing researches on the international political and economic order.

Keywords Covid-19 · Pandemic · World order · Asian century · USA · Russia · India · China

2.1 Introduction

After the outbreak of the Novel Corona Virus (COVID-19), the world history has been divided into the era of "BC and AC"—"Before Corona" and "After Corona" (Friedman, 17 March 2020). The world community, in its "war against an elusive and invisible enemy" (Didili, 17 March 2020), is trying every possible means to safeguard human beings. The biggest fallout of the pandemic is the near end of American-led global system and the beginning of a new era where Asian powers i.e. India and China, aims at making a significant mark in the global corridor. The main objective of this paper is to dilate upon various dimensions of the pandemic, in addition to foreseeing big power rivalry in the world stage. While the state of affairs during and following the pandemic has prompted USA to make earnest efforts in resurrecting its lost power, position and preponderance in the global corridor, the paper argues, Russia will not leave any stone unturned to regain its lost name, fame and glory. Besides, China would make earnest efforts to position itself as a power to reckon with as it has done in the last one decade or so. The paper makes three arguments. Firstly, amidst struggle for power among big powers, few traditional and emerging powers from Europe (Great Britain, France and Germany), Asia (India and Japan), Latin America (Brazil) and Australia will have leverage in the new global order that marks the beginning of the age of multipolarity. Secondly, with the North Atlantic Treaty Organisation (NATO) loosing its sheen, important regional organizations like Association of South East Asian Nations (ASEAN), Shanghai Cooperation Organization (SCO) and Brazil Russia India China South Africa (BRICS) will come forward for a far bigger role in international affairs. And thirdly, competition among global and emerging powers will continue in a healthy manner, and in case of any conflict or confrontation, strong mutual cooperation will be the only way to achieve peace and stability across the world. The present study is qualitative in research and follows only secondary source materials such as books, newspaper and journal articles and web materials. The overall structure of this paper includes (a) Important Dimensions of the Covid-19; (b) Big Power Rivalry in the World Stage; (c) The Advent of Asian Century; (d) Multipolar World as the New Reality; (e) India, Covid-19 and the New World Order; and (g) Conclusion.

2.2 Important Dimensions of the COVID-19

The uniqueness of the COVID-19 pandemic stems from various dimensions it had during the last one year or so and it has right now. While there are "medical, socio-economic and epidemiological dimensions" (Misra, 30 December 2020) at the initial days of the pandemic, it has "psychological" (Paric et al., October–December 2020), "spatial" (RBI, 27 October 2020), "gender" (World Bank, 16 April 2020), "human rights" (UNDRR, 19 June 2020), territorial, political and governance (Dodds et al., 2020: 289) dimensions as well. It has resulted in, as summarized by Harsh Pant (4 January 2021), (a) changing global balance of power; (b) weakening of multilateral institutions; (c) growing disenchantment with the international economic order; and (d) challenges to the extant normative consensus. It is, therefore, imperative to discuss here with various dimensions of Covid-19 before embarking on the main arguments of the present study. The following section of this paper narrates the economic jolt due to the pandemic, during which the role of the state has expanded considerably.

First, on the economic sense, not only the small, poor and developing countries, but also the big, rich and developed, and emerging economies have suffered incalculable loss. Almost all the sectors of economy have been badly hit due to spread of Covid-19. It has deleterious effect on primary sectors (agriculture, and oil and petroleum), secondary sectors (manufacturing) and tertiary sectors (education and finance). The economic cost of the pandemic has been astronomical. According to the Asian Development Bank (ADB), the pandemic has cost the world a whopping 8.8 trillion USD, and even to prevent a pandemic of this scale, the world will need 30 billion USD a year or more (BBC, 15 May 2020). According to another estimate, the cumulative financial costs of the pandemic related to lost output and health reduction could be a whopping $16 trillion, some 90 per cent of America's annual GDP (Cutler & Summers, 2020: 1496). However, Avery Koop (14 January 2021) finds out the economic cost of the Covid-19 pandemic in US alone at $16.2 trillion, which includes $7.6 trillion loss of GDP, $4.4 trillion loss due to premature death, $2.2 trillion for long term health impairment and $1.6 trillion for mental health impairment.

Second, one of the main casualties due to the pandemic is the process of globalisation, which has been an integral part of global order in the last half a century or so. The Covid-19 has seriously affected all the four major components of globalisation (i) free movement of goods and elimination of trade obstructions; (ii) free flow of capital; (iii) transfer of technology; and (iv) free movement of people (Nayak, 2021). Globalized cities have suffered the most. Anyone, who passes or transacts through these cities, is in the high risk category (Zeeshan, 7 April 2020). Further, the "borderless world", one of the key facets of globalisation, becomes a myth amidst the closure of borders, be it national/international, and state/provincial borders.

Third, at this critical juncture, the role of state has expanded considerably. The states across the globe have taken up the critical role and responsibility to protect their citizens from the pandemic. It is important to highlight here some key state interventions during the Covid-19 that have enhanced the role of the State:

1. Complete lockdown in many countries including India; protection and prevention as the key; spreading awareness about the pandemic through various means;
2. Mobilizing resources (with Corona Warriors i.e. doctors, health workers, defence forces etc. at the vanguard), coordinating with the provincial administration to deal with the pandemic related issues, capacity build up
3. Economic packages to deal with the post-pandemic issues
4. Health is wealth, as the old adage goes, is understood not only by the State alone, but by one and all. Priority is given to the health sector; Vaccine has been manufactured by various countries including India;

Fourth, it is believed that the COVID-19 pandemic has changed the trajectory and dimension of an "undeclared Third World War" (Asthana, 26 May 2020), the world has been witnessing for the last so many years. The reason for the aforesaid argument stems from the fact that the world has experienced several horrific global wars in the last one century or so, such as First World War, Second World War, Cold War, Global War on Terrorism, and the latest War against Corona. However, it can be argued that the new paradigm, unlike earlier world wars, will not witness all countries simultaneously at war. Some countries could engage in actual conflict (such as Saudi Arabia and Yemen), some countries may restrict themselves to military posturing, and others will engage in economic, trade, diplomatic, technological and information warfare, including cyber warfare (Asthana, 26 May 2020).

Fifth, COVID-19 has exposed a substantial deficit in the Western liberal order. For example, lack of collaboration and leadership in fighting the pandemic has put an end to what Nath Aldalala'a (June 2020) dubs as the "triumphalism of liberalism" in the global order. Aldalala'a argues that "while liberalism still plays a role in global politics, triumphalism that dominated Western political rhetoric after the end of the Cold War is ending as a result of the impact of this (COVID-19) outbreak." Norloff (2020: 811) summarizes that the pandemic has not only imperilled the liberal order, but also complicated the implementation of policies consistent with liberal order. The pandemic compelled liberal democracies to curtail freedom (both political and economic), its most priceless possession, by means of border closures, discrimination and restrictions on the right to privacy. Similarly, Norloff argues, "international threats to global supply chains, employment and economic welfare gather economic security policies emphasizing self-sufficiency with protectionist impulses may crowd out policies consistent with the liberal international order, jeopardizing long-term prosperity."

The aforesaid analysis of facts, figures and sequence of events found out that the pandemic has exposed the proverbial chinks in the global political and socio-economic order. While the huge financial challenge it has posed for the humanity is beyond imagination, its impact on globalisation is immeasurable, especially in changing the contours, myths and dynamics of this astounding economic phenomenon of last half a century. Amidst this critical time, greater emphasis has been given on the role of state not only in protecting its citizens, but also taking care of their needs, demands and aspirations. The most important facet of the pandemic time has been the united efforts of everyone to fight a "global war on Corona". Conflicts among states have taken a back seat for over a year, even enemies of yesteryears are joining hands to stave off the pandemic. Similarly, the liberal democratic order, for which most of the Western nations have been basking in glory, is in disarray during the pandemic. This state of affairs too brings out power rivalry in the global corridor, which will be dealt with in details in the following section.

2.3 Big Power Rivalry in the World Stage

In this section, the paper argues that the pandemic, despite its widespread impact on all quarters of human life, has not been able to deter some global actors' insatiable quest for spreading their tentacles in the international power corridor. The struggle amongst big powers (USA and Russia) for global power and influence has been a continuous process in the last seven decades or so. Even before the pandemic broke out, there has been a conflict of interest amongst big powers. Three contemporary geopolitical constructs: (a) Indo-Pacific patronised by USA; (b) Greater Eurasia by Russia; and (c) Belt and Road Initiative (BRI) by China have influenced the global order in recent times. The pandemic has added a new dimension to the whole gamut of issues related to the power competition.

It is believed that important regions like the Middle East will turn out to be an important cog in the contest for power. In this context, it is important to highlight the observations made by Michnik (2021), who charts out five factors that remain crucial to the power rivalry in the region: (i) protracted conflicts in Syria, Libya and Yemen; (ii) ongoing rivalry between Saudi-led coalition and Iran and its proxies; (iii) the strained US-Iran dynamics; (iv) growing international agency of smaller Arab Gulf states (such as Qatar and UAE) and the intra-GCC crisis of 2017; and (v) economic fallout of the pandemic and its potential effect on the security of the Middle East. Similarly, the Black Sea, which is an important junction between Europe, Asia and the Middle East, and is home to important energy and transit routes, will serve as one of the "geopolitical fault lines in the competition between great powers such as Russia, the US and the Europeans" (Coffey, 6 December 2020).

The US's fall from grace as a great power is one of the important highlights of the Covid-19 crisis. The image of a hapless superpower with the world's greatest economy and military has been eroded after the US led the table of casualties due to the pandemic. Further, the US-China stand-off in recent times, often dubbed as a new Cold War, has already aggravated the situation and will have more far-reaching consequences. It is imperative to note herewith that the Russia-China bonhomie in the post-Soviet period, especially on regional and global issues such as Syria, Iran, North Korea, Venezuela—or even arms control, has prompted the US to devise new national security strategy against Russia and China.

The beleaguered Russia, which had lost its superpower status after the disintegration of erstwhile Soviet Union, has making strategic moves through its idea of "Greater Eurasia" (Malle et al., 2020). This Russian move has two important objectives: (a) to regain its lost glory in the global corridor; and (b) to thwart the worldwide influence of USA, its inveterate enemy. David Lewis (2019) summarizes how foreign policy thinkers in the pro-Kremlin Valdai Club, led by Sergei Karaganov, Timofey Bordachev etc., talked about the concept of "Greater Eurasia" in 2015 as Russia's first genuine strategic concept since the end of the Soviet Union. He added that while rejecting the idea of a "China threat" concocted by the United States, the foreign policy thinkers considered that China should be a key ally for Russia in the development of a new "greater Eurasian community." Russian leadership was convinced to embrace new Chinese investment in transport and other infrastructure projects, using the Belt and Road Initiative as a way of shifting the focus of Russia's development from the European part of Russia to Siberia and the Far East. David Lewis gave examples of a couple of official announcements in this context. For example, Sergei Naryshkin, then Speaker of the State Duma, began talking of a "Greater Eurasia" stretching from Murmansk to Shanghai. Further, in June 2016, Russian President Vladimir Putin, at the plenary session of the Petersburg International Economic Forum, talked about the creation of a greater Eurasian partnership with the participation of the Eurasian Economic Community, and also countries such as China, India, Pakistan, and Iran. Similarly, at the Belt and Road Forum in Beijing in May 2017, Putin argued that "One Belt, One Road, the Shanghai Cooperation Organization, the Association of South East Asian Nations (ASEAN) are capable of becoming the basis for the formation of a Greater Eurasian partnership." He reiterated the same at Belt and Road Initiative meeting in 2019, claiming that the "the PRC president's Belt and Road initiative echoes the Russian idea of creating a "Greater Eurasian Partnership," which would involve an "integration of integrations" or "a close linking of various ongoing bilateral and multilateral integration processes in Eurasia. It is, therefore, apprehended that the above state of affairs will result in the continuance of US-Russia rivalry of Cold War days in the coming years.

At this juncture, China, the talk of the world, in the last one decade or so, is making all-out efforts to strengthen position as a global power. China's credibility, both internally and externally, as an alternative to the USA, at least on economic terms, has been eroded. Internally, the communist giant is plagued by COVID-19 crisis, economic uncertainty and a demographic precipice, and issues like Uyghurs, Tibet, Taiwan, Hong Kong etc. The pandemic has caused a massive disruption of the Chinese economy. For example, the industrial output fell, for the first time in last three decades, by 13.5% by January–February 2020 compared to the same period in 2019 (CNBC, 15 March 2020). The manufacturing Purchasing Managers' Index (PMI) published by the National Bureau of Statistics (NBS) and the China Federation of Logistics and Purchasing (CFLP) fell from 51.9% in December 2020 to 51.3% in January 2021 (Focus-Economics, 1 February 2021). Externally, China is accused of leveraging the distraction caused by the pandemic to "coerce its neighbors" in the region, continuing aggressive designs in the South China Sea, especially against Taiwan, and a failed gambit in India's Union Territory of Ladakh.

China has been successful in using the Corona crisis as an opportunity to expand her geopolitical footprint across the world—from the South and East China Seas to the Himalayas, from Europe to the Middle East. Beijing is upgrading relations with Moscow to form a pro-China power bloc in Asia (Ranade, 19 December 2020). China claims to have recovered from the pandemic by (i) showcasing a "Health Silk Road" (Belt & Road News, 18 August 2020); and (ii) activating a much-needed supply chain of medical equipment and medicines as an attempt to earn maximum profit out of the pandemic. Chinese President Xi Jinping proposed building a "Health Silk Road" in 2017, a concept under the Belt and Road Initiative, which has been given a new meaning and mission amid the global COVID-19 pandemic, namely, to build a global community of health for all and protect the life and health of people in all countries. However, the future of its twenty-first century signature strategy, Belt and Road initiative (BRI), is at stake. To corroborate the aforesaid argument, it is important to highlight the Chinese Foreign Ministry announcement in June 2020, which states that about 20% projects under the BRI had been affected by the pandemic, which was some 30 to 40% according to another estimate (Hui, 28 September 2020). However, the signing of Regional Comprehensive Economic Partnership (RECP) during the pandemic period (in November 2020), brings out a win–win situation for China on one hand, and will have major impact on the future of Asian order on the other (Mie, 30 December 2020).

It is found from the above analysis that the quest for wielding power in the world has been a common and continuous process in the contemporary times. Even pandemic of such intensity and impacts could not stop countries like USA and Russia being involved in global power game. Their agendas, designs and intentions are crystal clear and their ultimate goal is to grab world headlines, and they find opportunity in a pandemic to nurture their ambitions. Amidst such power rivalry, the vistas for a new groundbreaking "Asian century" are opened up putting Asian continent as the new hub of global power and economy.

2.4 The Advent of Asian Century

This section discusses the beginning of Asia as the world's new power centre following the paradigm shift due to Corona virus pandemic. This is a fact that the pandemic may well be remembered for important international events such as: (i) the beginning of the end of an American-led global system, which prevailed throughout the twentieth century; and (ii) the arrival of an Asian century (Loong, 4 June 2020) making the Asian continent a hub of all global activity, be it political, strategic or economic. In this context, it is important to cite European Union Foreign Policy Chief, Josep Borrell's remarkable observations. In a landmark speech on 25 May 2020, while addressing the annual German Ambassadors' Conference 2020 in Berlin, Josep Borrell stated: "First, we live in a leaderless world, where Asia will be increasingly important—in economic, security and technological terms" (European Union External Action, 25 May 2020).

Further, the Asian Development Bank (ADB) has given a fascinating account in this context. As per ADB estimates, by the year 2050, three billion Asian people could have living standards similar to those of Europe, and Asia could account for over half of global output. Three important points are noteworthy in this connection. Firstly, to quote the late economic historian, Angus Maddison, "Asia accounted for more than half of the world's economic output for 18 of the last 20 centuries, and the region's growing clout in the world economy is a "restoration, not a revolution." It took the massive concentration of capital in the West, the result of the Industrial Revolution and colonialism, for Europe to usurp the centre of economic power in the nineteenth century. And it took two world wars for the US to supplant the latter. Secondly, at present, Asia's vast population, having more than half the world's total population, is wielding economic predominance once again. For example, "in the eighteenth and nineteenth centuries, when economic might began to swing in Europe's favour, political and cultural influence followed. The same happened when the US surged ahead in the twentieth century. Political power and cultural influence followed economic production. Asia is in the same position right now as the US at the beginning of the twentieth century, an economic giant, but a political dwarf." Thirdly and lastly, global leadership is dwindling at the moment, with the failure of US to upkeep the liberal world order. For instance, there are many vacuums created, from Covid-19 vaccines to trade deals to climate change. Few Asian countries want to see China dominate their region so also the world. Asia remains fractured politically, but grows amidst great-power rivalry, exactly the way Europe did in the nineteenth century (Nikkei Asia, 30 September 2020).

It is imperative to highlight herewith a beautiful analysis by South Korean philosopher Byung-Chul Han, who argues that the victors in the war against Corona pandemic are the "Asian states like Japan, Korea, China, Hong Kong, Taiwan or Singapore that have an authoritarian mentality which comes from their cultural tradition [of] Confucianism. People (in the aforesaid Asian nations) are less rebellious and more obedient than in Europe. They trust the state more. Daily life is much more organised. Above all, to confront the virus, Asians are strongly committed to digital surveillance. The epidemics in Asia are fought not only by virologists and epidemiologists, but also computer scientists and big data specialists" (Wintour, 11 April 2020). It is, therefore, believed, and even proved, that the Asian nations will dominate world affairs in the next few years.

2.5 Multipolar World as the New Reality

The pandemic has opened up many chinks in US's armour that have led to the decline of her position as a global hegemon, which will perhaps result in, what Amitav Acharya (18 April 2020) puts in, "a multiplex world." According to him, the "multiplex world" stresses issue-oriented governance by multiple actors over traditional great powers status in defining the emerging world order. Multipolarity will continue to be the order of the day in this penultimate decade of the present century with traditional and rising powers from Europe (UK, Germany and France), Asia (India and Japan), Latin America (Brazil) and Australia at the forefront. The clarion call by Britain for D-10 to club India, South Korea and Australia along with G7 countries—UK, US, Italy, Germany, France, Japan and Canada could be a pointer in this regard. The aim of the D-10 is to create alternative suppliers of 5G equipment and other technologies to avoid dependence on China for vital technologies. The Atlantic Council think tank in Washington has been promoting it for years with regular working-level meetings between officials (Brattberg & Judah, 10 June 2020).

Further, a study by Jayant Sinha and Samir Saran (29 December 2020) summarizes those three factors, in addition to multipolarity, which will influence the new global order: (a) national interest; (b) reliability of partners; and (c) economic issues. In early June 2020, an Inter-Parliamentary Alliance of senior lawmakers from world's eight democracies, including the US, Germany, the UK, Japan, Australia, Canada, Sweden and Norway, was set up to "construct appropriate and coordinated responses, and to help craft a proactive and strategic approach on issues related to China. This group is calling upon democratic countries "to unite in a common defence of shared values" (Indian Express, 7 June 2020).

Meanwhile, conflict and confrontation have opened up avenues for realignment of friends, at the bilateral, trilateral and multilateral levels, against adversaries of humanity, for example, US-Japan-Australia-India "Quad" (Sajjanhar, 15 October 2020). Similarly, 'Quad-Plus' engagements with South Korea, Vietnam, New Zealand, Philippines, Singapore, etc., is testament to the growing security, and more importantly, intra-region interactions. Further, regional actors deepen networks with middle powers and on the other, strengthen institutional frameworks. The most vital regional actor in this context will be Association of South East Asian Nations (ASEAN), which has signalled its intent to maintain what it perceives as its "centrality" in the Indo-Pacific (Parpiani & Basu, 10 January 2021). In addition, regional cooperation mechanisms such as Shanghai Cooperation Organisation (SCO), Brazil Russia India China and South Africa (BRICS) and Eurasian Economic Union will form the core of the new international order. For example, expanding ties between the SCO and the Conference on Interaction and Confidence-Building Measures in Asia (CICA) can provide a viable framework for seeking Asian stability and security, which will further contribute to world security and stability (Mukerji, 2020).

The UN Committee for Development Policy (July 2020), in a policy note, describes how the pandemic has evoked a strong and "bold multilateral response." India's advocacy for "reformed multilateralism" (Mukerji, 8 December 2020) as an integral part of her new age foreign policy in order to strengthen its position as an important world power in twenty-first century seems significant in this context. This was highlighted in the international fora by none other than the Prime Minister of India, Shri Narendra Modi, first at the high level meeting of the United Nations Economic and Social Council (ECOSOC) on 17 July 2020. Prime Minister Modi stated that "reformed multilateralism", that has become the quintessential part of India's external affairs policy, "reflects today's realities, gives voice to all the stakeholders, addresses contemporary challenges, and focuses on human welfare."

2.6 India, Covid-19 and the New World Order

Keeping in view the argument that India has not only handled the Covid-19 crisis in a more mature way, both internally and internationally, but also exhibited resilience, world leadership and generosity during the pandemic, this section of this research work examines India's future role in the new global order. Notwithstanding the year-long ordeal due to the pandemic, India has emerged as the most favoured nation around the world. There is a huge number of confirmed Covid cases (42,975,883), out of which 42,413,566 have recovered, and 5,15,355 people have lost their lives by the first week of March 2022 (Aarogya Setu, 2022). After the indigenously manufactured make-in-India vaccine, more than 1800 million doses have been administered, justifying India's claim as the "pharmacy of the world."

The Narendra Modi government handled the crisis efficiently, and the evacuation of Indian citizens stranded abroad under Vande Bharat Mission was highly appreciated. Further, the crisis provided Indian government an opportunity to make India a manufacturing base for pharmaceutical products for local consumption and exports. Indian government's stress on "Atmanirvar Bharat", even after 70 years of its independence, is a unique step towards the world of self-dependence. On the external front, India not only supplied medicines and medical equipment (85 million hydroxy-chloroquine tablets and 500 million Paracetamol tablet to 108 countries), but also has exported 163 million Make-in-India Covid vaccine to 98 countries. In addition, India launched a regional cooperation program in South Asia pledging $10 million towards an emergency SAARC fund. India explored an information exchange platform (IEP) to facilitate exchange of expertise among South Asian health professionals.

Suddenly, the number of the buyers and takers of Indian democratic values has risen. New Delhi has long been emphasizing its democratic credentials to underscore the point that it is different from an aggressive and expansionist China. These democratic values have emerged as crucial variables in the way Indian foreign policy trajectory has evolved in the last few years, be it in its engagement with the West or other small and big international actors. Despite domestic problems, India has stood out for its globalism and international stature during the ongoing pandemic.

India's importance as a benign power with loads of soft power, as a no-nonsense actor, and always helpful nation, its economic potential, social, political and intellectual capital, and abundant human resources could be a boon for this ascendance in the global stage. The possibility of India's entry into G-7 nations, as was hinted by the American President Donald Trump, is a clear signal in this regard. In the 'AC (after Corona) world', New Delhi has many more miles to go. There is a need to expand its cooperation programs into a global effort; engage in the multilateral development of solutions to global policy challenges; and share lessons and experiences to progressively strengthen public systems and state institutions worldwide.

2.7 Conclusion

The present study under research has found many interesting facts. First, the "order" of the day is no doubt in a state of disorder, but as there is always light at the end of tunnel, this state of disorder, is slowly and steadily bringing back "order" in the world system. Nations have come closer to combat their country, people, and the entire world from the scourge of the Covid-19 pandemic, as they had done in the past in fighting the menace of terrorism. Several countries have manufactured vaccines to save teeming millions from the recurrence of the pandemic.

Second, there are claims that the process of globalisation is at the receiving end. However, the pandemic will not do away with the process of globalization, as Amitava Acharya (18 April 2020) puts in on an optimistic note, will rather "increase demands for making it more humane and regulated." In addition, to negotiate changes following the end of the pandemic, the possibility of "gated globalisation or re-globalisation" (Singh, 25 June 2020) cannot be ruled out.

Third, the competition for power, conflict of interest, confrontation and rivalry among big powers to wield influence in the global power theatre has been one of the grim realities before, during and after the pandemic. As seen in the past, competition and conflict have bred cooperation among nations and integration of their interests, this state of affairs will usher in a new era of cooperation. The US President Joe Biden has hinted his preference for "talks" and "dialogues" to "confrontation" (Ranade, 29 December 2020). Even earlier prognosis about the possibility of another World War remains bleak, because the world community understands the huge cost involved in case of a war and the irreparable loss of innocent lives due to it.

Fourth, a multipolar international order has ushered in with new powers emerging in the world stage. The last three quarters of century have witnessed bipolar power system (during the Cold War) and unipolar world (in the post-Soviet period), and many believe the future lies in multipolarity. Even Chinese President, Xi Jinping, while addressing the World Economic Forum on 25 January 2021, announced "let the torch of multilateralism light up humanity's way forward" (Xinhua, 25 January 2021).

Fifth, though economic resilience, political values and identities of democracies are put to test during the pandemic, democracy has not lost its sight, rather emerged as the central pivot around which the future global order is being sought to be constructed by several stakeholders. Democratic values continue to upkeep their vitality and sublimity during the global order rejig (Jacob, 28 December 2020).

Sixth, the age of digital consciousness has ushered in with digitisation, robotisation and artificial intelligence becoming the new buzzwords. Work from home, online webinars via Zoom, Google, Webex etc. and digital payments have been the regular features during the pandemic. Besides, creativity and performing arts have become a hope against despair during the pandemic. Social media platforms such as YouTube, Twitter, Instagram, Face Book and Whatsapp were flooded with so many creativities to keep the public in good mood and humour during the pandemic.

The paper wraps up with a few major policy recommendations: (i) to build stronger and more effective public systems across countries. It needs cooperation and coordination amongst nations at all levels—bilateral, trilateral, multilateral, regional and global—which have become key to fight such pandemics in future. It has been done in the past and it will be done in future as well; (ii) Exchange of information and multilateral collaboration would be crucial—not just in resisting a relapse of the virus, but also in preventing a future pandemic; (iii) international organizations must receive strong support from all global powers in drawing up and implementing policies to strengthen public systems, especially healthcare, worldwide; (iv) countries must be more transparent about their shortcomings and needs—and other countries must be more willing to support them in fixing those gaps; (v) stronger trade links must make healthcare cheaper and more accessible around the world; (vi) international laws must be enforced to ensure the transparency and accountability of governments, collectively by the world community (Zeeshan, 7 April 2020). Many sane human beings, and responsible powers, who made exemplary efforts to deal with the pandemic, believe in world peace, not war, and on an optimistic note, the world community will strive for peace at any cost in the post-Covid period, despite the changes or shifts in the global order.

References

Acharya, A. (2020, April 18). How corona virus may reshape the world order. *The National Interest*. https://nationalinterest.org/feature/how-coronavirus-may-reshape-world-order-145972

Aldalala'a, N. (2020, June). End of liberal triumphalism: A perspective on china in the post-covid global order. *Strategic Trends*, 1.

Asthana, Major General S. B. (2020, May 26). *Covid-19 adds a new dimension to an undeclared third world war*. www.futuredirections.org.au

Belt & Road News. (2020, August 18). *Health Silk Road: Building sustainable healthcare infrastructure*. https://www.beltandroad.news/2020/08/18/way-to-well-being-building-sustainable-healthcare-infrastructure/

Brattberg, E., & Judah, B. (2020, June 10). *Forget the G-7, build the D-10*. https://foreignpolicy.com/2020/06/10/g7-d10-democracy-trump-europe/

British Broadcasting Corporation. (BBC). (2020, May 15). *Corona virus could cost global economy $8.8 trillion, says ADB*. https://www.bbc.com/news/business-52671992

CNBC. (2020, March 15). *China January-February industrial output shrinks 13.5%; investment plunges 24.5%*. https://www.cnbc.com

Coffey, L. (2020, December 6). *Major Power Rivalry in the Black Sea*. Arab News. https://www.arabnews.com/node/1773371

Cutler, D. M., & Summers, L. H. (2020, October 20). The Covid-19 pandemic and the $16 trillion loss. *Jama, 324*(15), 1495–1496.

Didili, Z.(2020, March 17). *Macron says France is "at war" with coronavirus. New Europe*. https://www.neweurope.eu/article/macron-says-france-is-at-war-with-coronavirus/

Dodds, K., et al. (2020). The Covid-19 pandemic: Territorial, political and governance dimensions of the crisis. *Territory, Politics, Governance, 8*(3), 289–298.

European Union External Action. (2020, May 25). *Opening remarks to the annual German ambassadors' conference 2020 in Berlin*. https://www.eeas.europa.eu

Focus Economics. (2021, February 1). *China: Manufacturing and non-manufacturing PMIs decline in January.* https://www.focus-economics.com/countries/china/news/pmi/manufacturing-and-non-manufacturing-pmis-decline-in-january

Friedman, T. L. (2020, March 17). Our new historical divide: B.C. and A.C.—The world before corona and the world after. *The New York Times.*

Hui, L. Y. (28 September 2020). Covid-19: The nail in the coffin of china's belt and road initiative? *The Diplomat.* https://thediplomat.com/2020/09/covid-19-the-nail-in-the-coffin-of-chinas-belt-and-road-initiative/

Indian Express. (2020, June 7). *Senior lawmakers in eight countries form new alliance to counter China.*

Jacob, J. T. (2020, December 28). *China in post-covid 19 era—How will the CCP tackle its image problem?* Observer Research Foundation. https://www.orfonline.org

Koop, A. (2021, January 14). *Putting the cost of Covid-19 in perspective.* https://www.visualcapitalist.com/putting-the-cost-of-covid-19-in-perspective/

Lewis, D. (2019, July). *Strategic culture and Russia's "Pivot to the East": Russia, China, and "Greater Eurasia"* (George C. Marshall Centre European Centre for Security Studies, No. 34). https://www.marshallcenter.org

Loong, L. H. (2020, June 4). *The endangered Asian century: America, China and the perils of confrontation.* https://www.foreignaffairs.com/print/node/1126085

Malle, S., Cooper, J., & Connolly, R. (2020). Greater Eurasia: More than a vision? *Post-Communist Economies, 32*(5), 561–590.

Michnik, W. (2021, January 18). *Great power rivalry in the Middle East.* http://www.realinstitutoelcano.org

Mie, O. (2020, December 30). Signing of the RCEP and the future of Asian order. *The Diplomat.* https://thediplomat.com/2020/12/signing-of-the-rcep-and-the-future-asian-order/

Ministry of External Affairs. Government of India. Vande Bharat Mission.

Ministry of Health. Government of India. (2022, February 7). AarogyaSetu.

Misra, S. (2020, December 30). Pandemic has pushed back process of wealth generation, poverty reduction. *Indian Express.*

Mukerji, A. (2020, December 8). *India and the Shanghai Cooperation Organisation.* Observer Research Foundation. https://www.orfonline.org

Mukerji, A. K. (2020). Call for reformed multilateralism at the UN. *India Perspectives*, 05. Ministry of External Affairs, Government of India. https://www.indiaperspectives.gov.in

Nayak, P. (2021, January 21). Globalisation in the time of a pandemic. *The Hindu.*

Norloff, C. (2020). Is Covid-19 a liberal democratic curse? Risks for liberal international order. *Cambridge Review of International Affairs, 33*(5), 799–813.

Nikkei A. (2020, September 30). *This is the Asian century: Seven reasons to be optimistic about it.* https://asia.nikkei.com/Spotlight/The-Big-Story/This-is-the-Asian-Century-Seven-reasons-to-be-optimistic-about-it

Pant, H. (2021, January 4). *From turmoil to clarity: International relations in the new decade.* Observer Research Foundation. https://www.orfonline.org

Paric, A., Ravindran, L., & Ravindran, A. (2020, October–December). Psychological dimensions of Covid-19: Perspectives for the practicing clinician. *International Journal of Noncommunicable Diseases, 5*(4), 83–89.

Parpiani, K., & Basu, P. (2021, January 10). *Biden and the Indo-Pacific will regional powers shape America's approach?* Observer Research Foundation. https://www.orfonline.org

Ranade, J. (2020, December 29). 2021 strategic outlook, India must not yield any ground to China. *Hindustan Times.*

Reserve Bank of India (RBI). (2020, October 24). *Covid-19 and its spatial dimensions.* www.rbi.org.in

Sajjanhar, A. (2020, October 15). *Institutionalisation of the Quad.* Observer Research Foundation. https://www.orfonline.org

Singh, R. (2020, June 25). *'Gated Globalization' or re-globalization: What India should aim for?* www.marketexpress.in

Sinha, J., & Saran, S. (2020, December 29). Gated globalisation. *The Indian Express.*

The United Nations Committee for Development Policy. (2020, July). *Development policy and multilateralism after Covid-19.* www.un.org

United Nations Office for Disaster Risk Reduction (UNDRR). (2020, June 19). *The human rights dimensions of the Covid-19 pandemic.* UNDRR Asia Pacific Covid-19 Brief. www.undrr.org

Wintour, P. (2020, April 11). Coronavirus: Who will be winners and losers in new world order. *The Guardian.* www.theguardian.com

World Bank. (2020, April 16). *Gender dimensions of the Covid-19 pandemic.* www.worldbank.org

Xinhua. (2021, January 25). *Let the torch of multilateralism light up humanity's way forward.* http://www.xinhuanet.com/english/2021-01/25/c_139696610.htmv

Zeeshan, M. (2020, April 7). Can India organize post-covid-19 global action. *The Diplomat.* https://thediplomat.com/2020/04/can-india-organize-post-covid-19-global-action/

Dr. Mahesh Ranjan Debata, Centre for Innar Asian Studies, School of International Studies, Jawharlal Nehru University, New Delhi, India.

Chapter 3
COVID-19 Pandemic and Its Impact on Our Physical Environment: A Critical Analysis

Amir Mohammad Nasrullah

Abstract Coronavirus Disease-2019 (COVID-19) has created adverse effects globally on human lives in various ways, including the economy and the physical environment. Different national and international research reports confirmed that it has killed many people and many of them have been suffering seriously. Governments around the world have taken different measures to comprehend the spread of COVID-19 through human-to-human transmission such as maintaining physical distance, avoiding public gathering and many other disciplinary actions. However, these measures have also created significant effects on the environment. Lockdown in many countries, along with minimal human movement has positively impacted the physical environment slightly. It has steered to a perfection in the overall air quality and a reduction in water pollution in many places, overall carbon emissions have dropped and also reduces the pressure on the tourist places around the world. These may support to restore our ecological system. Conversely, some researches argue that due to COVID-19 outbreak significant environmental damages wait for us, that include increase of medical waste, random use and disposal of sanitizers, masks and gloves, and burden of unprocessed wastes incessantly jeopardizing the physical environment. Researchers also argued that economic events will be normal as soon as the pandemic is over, or somehow during pandemic, and the situation might be changing. In these backdrop, it is necessary to think of possible ways to attain enduring environmental advantages. However, the aim of this chapter is to identify the environmental consequences due to COVID-19 pandemic, as well, recommend possible ways as future policy inputs for a sustainable environment. A number of published materials such as various research reports of different government, non-government and international organizations as well as internet sources were collected and reviewed critically for the purpose. It is hoped that the findings and suggestions would be contributory to the academia as well as to the policy makers.

Keywords COVID-19 pandemic · Impact · Physical environment · Sustainability

---

A. M. Nasrullah (✉)
Department of Public Administration, University of Chittagong, Chittagong, Bangladesh
e-mail: amir.nasrullah@cu.ac.bd

© The Author(s), under exclusive license to Springer Nature Singapore Pte Ltd. 2022
S. Roy and D. Nandy (eds.), *Understanding Post-COVID-19 Social and Cultural Realities*, https://doi.org/10.1007/978-981-19-0809-5_3

3.1 Introduction

The Coronavirus Disease-2019 (COVID-19) first appeared from the Hunan Seafood Market in the city of Wuhan, China at the end of December 2019. As the disease was spreading rapidly, the World Health Organization (WHO) declared an international public health emergency in a couple of weeks (WHO, 2020a, b). It is such a worldwide health catastrophe of the present time and the utmost challenge that the world has confronted since World War II. Since it appeared in Asia in late 2019, the COVID-19 has blowout to every part of the world except Antarctica continent. Cases have been increasing day by day in Africa, America, the Europe as well as in Asia. There was a worldwide influenza pandemic earlier in the year 1918. The exact number of deaths due to that influenza pandemic is still unknown. But some researchers believe that the death toll would have been about 50–100 million people during that influenza pandemic (Karunathilake, 2020). However, globally, as of 13 December 2021, there have been nearly 270 million confirmed cases of COVID-19, among which 98,690,724 in Americas, 91,903,122 in Europe, 44,748,558 in South-East Asia, 16,947,823 in Eastern Mediterranean, 10,612,501 in Western Pacific and 6,564,819 in Africa. It is also reported that there are more than 5 million deaths across almost 200 countries around the globe due to COVID-19, among which 2,373,674 in Americas, 1,601,656 in Europe, 714,546 in South-East Asia, 312,514 in Eastern Mediterranean, 148,037 in Western Pacific and 153,808 in Africa (https://covid19.who.int/) and the number is increasing day by day. The USA, India and Brazil are the countries with the highest number of confirmed COVID-19 cases in the world. They are closely followed by a number of European countries such as the UK, Germany, Italy, France, Russia, Turkey etc. Countries have been trying to slow down the spread of the disease by testing and treating patients, carrying out contact tracing, limiting travel, quarantining citizens, and cancelling large gatherings such as social events, sporting events, concerts, and all types of academic institutions. However, the things are changing now as vaccination started worldwide. As of 12 December 2021, a total of 8,200,642,671 vaccine doses have been administered to the people around the globe (https://covid19.who.int/). But, the virus has surged across the world and very few places have managed to avoid it. Nonetheless, the COVID-19 pandemic is moving like a wave, one that may yet crash on those least able to cope. It is much more than a health crisis. It has been affecting different people in different ways. Some people have lost their jobs due to COVID-19 crisis, others experienced loneliness and loss, yet, others discovered new things about themselves. It has led to a dramatic loss of human life worldwide and boons an unprecedented challenge to public health, food systems, the world of work and also to the environment. The socio-economic disturbance caused by the pandemic is overwhelming. Tens of millions of people are at risk of falling into extreme poverty. On the other hand, the number of under-nourished and starving people could increase by up to 132 million by the end of the year 2020, currently which are estimated at nearly 690 million (ILO, FAO, IFAD & WHO, 2020).

The United Nations (UN) report shows that the pandemic will push 96 million people into extreme poverty by 2021 (Azcona et al., 2020). Experts from the United Nations Development Program (UNDP), and the World Health Organization (WHO) have stressed deep concern about the long-term impact the pandemic could have on these nations. Developing countries tend to be poorer. They have been working to become more advanced economically and socially, but their infrastructures are not as established as those found in the developed countries such as Europe and the USA. They also rely on primary sector roles, all activities that consist of exploiting natural resources, like agriculture, mining, and forestry. Therefore, they are particularly impacted by disrupted supply chains and lower demand for their goods due to COVID-19 crisis.

However, COVID-19 has severe impacts on the global economy, society and also the physical environment. In these context, this chapter especially tries to explore the impact of COVID-19 pandemic on our physical environment. This chapter also tries to suggest some possible recommendations to face the challenges of COVID-19 pandemic, that may lead towards a sustainable environment.

3.2 Method Followed

In achieving the objectives of the study, a qualitative research method was followed. Mainly secondary data were collected for the purpose of the study. A number of research articles, as well as, reports both printed and e-resources of different government, non-government and international organizations were collected, and different web sources were visited. All the collected materials were thoroughly reviewed and analyzed by using content analysis technique to attain the aim of the study. All the materials are acknowledged dully.

3.3 COVID-19 Pandemic

COVID-19 is an infectious disease. Though it was first originated in China, but spread widely in the developed countries, especially in Europe and some parts of the America. This infectious disease caused by Severe Acute Respiratory Syndrome Coronavirus-2 (SARS-CoV-2), which is phylogenetically associated with SARS viruses, and bats could be the possible primary source (Chakraborty & Maity, 2020). Although the transitional source of origin and transfer to humans is not clearly known, it has been recognized and proven that human to human transmission capability of the virus is very fast (Hui et al., 2020). The spread of the virus is mainly happening through person to person by direct interaction or droplets created by sneezing, coughing and talking (Islam et al., 2020; Li et al., 2020; Wang et al., 2020).

3.4 Physical Environment

Environment is our surrounds where we live that includes both the biotic and abiotic elements around us. These are the surrounding settings where humans, plants, and animals live. Every individual has an impact on environment, because environment also effects behavior of individual. Thus, individuals and the environment are related and complementary to each other. The existence of the environment is very significant. Because human life and any other living being cannot survive without it. Environment provides natural beauty, maintains the balance of life, supports the food chain and benefits living lives and their various activities (Johnson et al., 1997).

Environment may be categorized into two: physical and social. Physical environment is the surrounding settings and components with which a living object interacts with. In fact, the physical environment is where individuals live, learn, work, and play that includes the air, water bodies, land, and living organisms etc. The water bodies include the ponds, streams, rivers, lakes, lagoons, sea, and oceans etc. People interact with their physical environment through the air they breathe, water they drink, houses they live in, and the transportation they access to travel to work and school. However, poor physical environment can affect our ability and that of our families and neighbors to live long and healthy lives (https://www.countyhealthran kings.org).

Social environment is human made. Human cannot live directly in the physical environment. Therefore, they create some of their environmental settings to adjust to it. Social environment consists of people, their interpersonal relationship, religion, political beliefs and practices, buildings, machines, languages and so on (Barnett & Casper, 2001). Indeed, it includes all human things that directly or indirectly affect the individuals in their day to day activities. It is an important aspect for humankind to exist, live and rise that entirely depends on human social influence. It sustains as long as society values.

Nonetheless, physical environment affects social environment in many ways, such as physical environment determines the soil, climate and vegetation of an area which tends to affect the type of crops to plant and eat by the human. Clean air and safe water are necessary for good health. Air pollution is associated with increased asthma rates and lung diseases, and an increase in the risk of premature death from heart or lung disease. Water contaminated with chemicals, pesticides, or other contaminants can lead to illness, infection, and increased risks of cancer. Therefore, it is very important to protect our physical environment.

3.5 Sustainability

The concept of sustainability focuses on the capacity to sustain in a relatively ongoing way across various domains of human life (James et al., 2015). Generally, it refers to the ability to co-exist for Earth's biosphere and human civilization. It has also been termed as "meeting the needs of the present generation without compromising the ability of future generations to meet their needs" (Kono, 2014). For many scholars, sustainability is the interconnected domains of environment, economy and society (James & Magee, 2016). Despite the increased popularity and usage of the term "sustainability", the possibility that human societies will achieve environmental sustainability has been, and continues to be, questioned, in the light of environmental degradation, biodiversity loss, climate change, overconsumption, population growth and quest for unlimited economic growth by the societies (Kuhlman & Farrington, 2010; James & Magee, 2016).

However, there is a good link between physical and social environment. Sustainability in physical environment is very important for the survival of social environment and continuation of our human race. Therefore, this chapter tries to identify the nature of the impact of COVID-19 on our physical environment so that we may understand it and take necessary steps in future.

3.6 COVID-19 Pandemic and the Nature of Its Impact

It has now been resulting in a global economic and financial recession that may be deeper and wider than the great downturn which followed the global financial crisis in 2008/2009 (UNCTAD, 2020). The crisis has spread into the developing countries. The UN's Framework for the Immediate Socio-Economic Response to the COVID-19 crisis warns that "the COVID-19 pandemic is far more than a health crisis". It has seriously distressed the global economy with serious consequences impacting all the societies and entities. It has been affecting our social and economic environment as well as the physical environment at the core. Moving rapidly across the countries, along with the major channels of the global economy, the spread of COVID-19 has benefited from the underlying interconnectedness and maladies of globalization, projecting a global health crisis into a global economic shock that has hit the most vulnerable the toughest (UNCTAD, 2020).

COVID-19 has emerged from the natural environment and later paralyzed our societies. However, it validates the interdependence contained in the Sustainable Development Goals (SDGs), but has been disrupting the worldwide efforts to achieve them. It has created a psychosocial impact on the global people, specifically it creates a global human disaster with disturbing mental health of the world population. Nonetheless, while the impact of the COVID-19 pandemic varies from country to country, it is most likely to increase poverty and inequalities at a global scale, making achievement of SDGs even more urgent. It has been intensifying the inequalities faced by individuals and families in humanitarian crises.

Moreover, the impact of COVID-19 on the physical environment is also enormous and a matter of serious concern. Therefore, assessing the impacts of the COVID-19 crisis on societies, economies, environment and vulnerable groups is fundamental to update and adapt the responses of the governments and their cohorts to recover from the crisis and ensure that no one is left behind in this effort. Nonetheless, this chapter tried to analyze the overall impact of COVID-19 on the physical environment. The global reduction in contemporary human activity such as the considerable deterioration in scheduled travel has caused many places to experience a large drop in air and water pollution. In China, lockdowns and other disciplinary measures resulted in a 25% reduction in carbon emissions and 50% reduction in nitrogen oxides emissions. The earth scientists estimated that this reduction in emissions in China may have saved at least 77,000 lives over two months (UNCTAD, 2020).

Up to 2020, increases in the amount of Greenhouse gases produced since the beginning of the industrialization era caused average global temperatures on the earth to rise, causing effects including the melting of glaciers and sea level rise. In various forms, human activity caused environmental degradation and an anthropogenic effect. Independently, also prior to the COVID-19 pandemic, researchers argued that reduced economic activity would help decrease global warming, as well as, air and marine pollution, allowing the environment to slowly flourish. This effect has been observed following the past pandemics in fourteenth century Eurasia and sixteenth-seventeenth century North and South America. However, we will focus on the impact of COVD-19 on our physical environment in this chapter.

3.7 Impact of COVID-19 on Physical Environment

Elements of physical environment, such as, clean air and good quality drinking water are vital for the maintenance of people's physical health. Some other environmental factors, such as, noise pollution can cause both physical harm and psychological stress. However, the cleanliness and beauty of the physical environment is vital for the sense of wellbeing of the people. A healthy physical environment provides recreational opportunities, allowing people to take part in activities they value. The COVID-19 outbreak have impacted our physical environment seriously and the impact is enormous. In this context, it is very important to investigate the impacts of COVID-19 on our physical environment, as because the problems of physical environment increasingly impact our whole society and nature. Various national and international reports show that the crisis has created both positive (affirmative) and negative (harmful) impact on our physical environment. The following sections discusses about the impacts in details.

3.7.1 Positive Impact of COVID-19 on the Physical Environment

There are some positive and affirmative impacts of COVID-19 on our physical environment. They are discussed below:

3.7.1.1 Decrease of Air Pollution and Green House Gas (GHG) Emission

To face COVID-19 crisis all over the world many industries, transportation and many companies have closed down. It has brought an impulsive drop of the emission of Green House Gases (GHGs). Comparing with this time of last year, the levels of air pollution in New York, USA has condensed by nearly 50%, because of the measures taken to control the spread of the virus. In China, it was projected that nearly 50% reduction of Nitrous Oxide (N_2O) and Carbon Monoxide (CO) occurred due to the shutdown of heavy industries (Caine, 2020). Similarly, emission of Nitrogen Dioxide (NO_2) is one of the key indicators of global economic activities. In many countries around the globe, such as, USA, Canada, China, India, Italy, and Brazil etc., due to the recent shut down, a sign of reduction of NO_2 is noticed. Usually, NO_2 is emitted from the burning of fossil fuels, 80% of which comes from transportation sector, mainly motor vehicle exhaust (Ghosh, 2020; Saadat et al., 2020; Somani et al., 2020).

Researchers (Adams, 2020; Berman & Edisu, 2020; Nakada, 2020) show that NO_2 causes acid rain with the interaction of Oxygen (O_2) and water (H_2O), and several respiratory diseases suffered by humans. The European Environmental Agency (EEA) projected that, because of the COVID-19 lockdown, NO_2 emission dropped from 30–60% in many European cities that includes Barcelona, Madrid, Milan, Rome and Paris (EEA, 2020). In the USA, NO_2 deteriorated 25.5% during the COVID-19 period compared to previous years (Berman & Edisu, 2020). The level of NO_2 demonstrated a decrease across Ontario (Canada) and found to be reduced from 4.5 ppb to 1 ppb (parts per billion) (Adams, 2020). Up to 54.3% reduction of NO_2 was observed in Sao Paulo, Brazil (Nakada, 2020). It was also specified that, the levels of NO_2 and PM2.5 (inhalable particles with span 2.5 μm and remain deferred for longer) reduced by almost 70% in New Delhi, India. Overall, 46% and 50% decrease of PM2.5, and PM10 (inhalable particles, with span 10 μm and remain deferred for longer) respectively, which are formed due to fuel burning and chemical reactions in the atmosphere, was reported in India during the nationwide lockdown (IEP, 2020; Thiessen, 2020).

Zogopoulos (2020) reported that, automobiles and aeronautics are the key contributors of emissions and contribute almost 72% and 11% of the GHGs emission of transportation sector respectively. The global measures taken for the control of COVID-19 are also having a dramatic impact on the aviation sector. Many countries restricted worldwide travelers from entrance and departure. As a result of the reduced passengers and restrictions, international flights are being cancelled by the commercial aircraft companies. For example, in China almost 50–90% capacity of departing and 70% domestic flights are reduced due to the pandemic, compared to January 20, 2020, which ultimately deducted nearly 17% of national Carbon Dioxide (CO_2) emissions. Additionally, it is reported that 96% of air travel fallen globally from a similar time last year, due to the COVID-19 pandemic, which has ultimate effects on the environment (Wallace, 2020).

Largely, far less consumption of fossil fuels decreases the GHGs emission, that helps to fight against global climate change. International Energy Agency (IEA,

2020) reported that oil demand has fallen 435,000 barrels worldwide in the first three months of 2020, compared to the same period of last year. Besides, worldwide coal consumption is also reduced because of less energy demand during the lockdown period. It is also informed that, coal-based power generation reduced 26% in India with 19% decrease of total power generation after lockdown. Again, in China, the highest coal consumer in the world, the consumption of coal has dropped 36% compared to same time of the preceding year (early February to mid-march) (CREA, 2020; Ghosh, 2020). UK based Climate Science and Policy Website Carbon Brief reported that recent crisis of COVID-19 reduces 25% CO_2 emission in China, and nonetheless below the normal limit more than two months after the country entered lockdown. They also estimated that, the pandemic could cut 1,600 metric tons of CO_2, equivalent to above 4% of the global total in 2019 (Evans, 2020). As a result, air pollution is decreased worldwide.

3.7.1.2 Decrease of Water Pollution

Water pollution is a common phenomenon of the developing countries like India, and Bangladesh, where domestic and industrial wastes are dumped into rivers without any treatment. During the lockdown period, the major industrial sources of pollution have shrunk or completely stopped, that helped to reduce the pollution load (Bodrud-Doza et al., 2020; Yunus et al., 2020). For example, in India, the river Ganga and Yamuna have reached a momentous level of purity as a result of the absence of industrial pollution during lockdown. Researchers also observed that, among the 36 real-time monitoring stations of river Ganga, water from 27 stations met the acceptable limit (Singhal & Matto, 2020). This perfection of the water quality was also recognized at Haridwar and Rishikesh in India due to the sudden drop of the number of visitors and 500% reduction of dirt and industrial wastes (Singhal & Matto, 2020; Somani et al., 2020).

Uttarakhand Pollution Control Board (UPCB) of India, based on real-time water quality monitoring data reported that, Physicochemical Parameters (pH) (7.4–7.8), Dissolved Oxygen (DO) (9.4–10.6 mg/L), Biochemical Oxygen Demand (BOD) (0.6–1.2 mg/L) and Total Coliform (TC) (40–90 MPN/100 mL) of the river Ganga was found within the surface water quality standard of India. Except TC in some monitoring stations, all others parameters even meet the national standard of drinking water quality, that can be used without conventional treatment but after disinfection (UPCB, 2020). It is also observed that, the concentration of pH, Electric Conductivity (EC), DO, BOD and Chemical Oxygen Demand (COD) has reduced almost 1–10%, 33–66%, 45–90%, and 33–82% respectively in different monitoring stations during the lockdown in comparison to the pre-lockdown period in India. Furthermore, due to obligatory ban of public gathering, number of tourists and water activities were reduced in many places (Cripps, 2020; Zambrano-Monserrate et al., 2020). Researchers (Kundu, 2020; Rahman, 2020) also indicated that, as a result of lockdown during COVID-19 crisis, in Italy the Grand Canal turned clear, and many aquatic species reappeared (Clifford, 2020). Water pollution decreased in the sea beaches of Bangladesh, Malaysia, Thailand, Maldives, and Indonesia and many more.

In Tunisia the amount of food waste is reduced as a result of the lockdown during COVID-19, that ultimately lessens the soil and water pollution (Jirbi et al., 2020). Cooper (2020) mentioned that the amount of industrial water consumption is also reduced globally, especially in the textile sector. Generally, vast number of solid wastes is generated from construction and manufacturing sectors that are accountable for water and soil pollution. It is also reduced. Furthermore, due to the decrease of export and import business, the movement of commercial ships and other vessels are reduced globally, that also diminishes carbon emissions as well as marine contamination. As a result, water pollution worldwide is decreased.

3.7.1.3 Decrease of Noise Pollution

Noise pollution is the preeminent levels of sound that is created from diverse human activities such as machineries, automobiles, and construction work etc. It may lead to adverse effects in human and other living creatures (Zambrano-Monserrate et al., 2020). Generally, noise creates negative effects on our physical health, along with cardiac disorders, hypertension, and sleep disruptions etc. In a recent report Sims (2020) shows that worldwide around 360 million people are inclined to hearing loss due to the noise pollution. It is also projected that in Europe, over 100 million people are exposed to high noise levels, above the endorsed limit (WHO, 2020a, b). Furthermore, anthropogenic noise pollution has also adverse effects on wildlife through the fluctuating balance in predator and prey detection and avoidance. Undesirable noise also has negative effects on the invertebrates. It helps to control environmental processes that are vital for balancing the ecological system (Solan et al., 2016). Nonetheless, the measures, such as quarantine and lockdown during COVID-19 indicate that if people stay at home, reduce their economic activities and unimportant global communication, ultimately helps reducing the noise level in the world (Zambrano-Monserrate et al., 2020). For example, noise level of New Delhi, India is decreased considerably around 40–50% in the recent lockdown period (Somani et al., 2020). During the lockdown period, the noise levels of Govindpuri metro station, New Delhi, India is reduced 50–60 dB (Decibel) (Decibel is a relative measurement unit corresponding to one tenth of a bel) from 100 dB as a result of reduced automobile movement (Gandhiok & Ibra, 2020).

It is also reported by Central Pollution Control Board of India that, noise level of Delhi residential area in India is reduced 55 dB in day time and 45 dB in night time to 40 dB in day time and 30 dB in night time respectively (CPCB, 2020). As a result, inhabitants of the city are now enjoying the chirping of birds, that generally ranges from 40–50 dB (Gandhiok & Ibra, 2020). Furthermore, as a result of travel restrictions, the number of flights and vehicular movements have drastically reduced around the world that ultimately have decreased the noise pollution level.

For instance, in Germany, inside air travel has been reduced by over 90%, car traffic has dropped by >50% and trains are running <25% than the normal rates. Largely, lockdown during COVID-19 and reduced socio-economic activities of people have decreased the level of noise pollution worldwide (Sims, 2020).

3.7.1.4 Ecological Restoration and Adaptation of Tourist Places

As a result of technological advancements and transport networks the tourism sector has observed an outstanding growth over the past few years. It has been contributing meaningfully to the worldwide Gross Domestic Product (GDP). However, it is estimated that the tourism industry is responsible for 8% of global GHGs emissions. The places of natural beauty such as sea beaches, islands, national parks, mountains, deserts and mangroves have generally attracted the tourists, and make a massive harsh. A lot of hotels, motels, restaurants, bars and markets are built in order to expedite and accommodate them, which consume a lot of energy and other natural resources. Such as, in calculating the carbon footprint of coastland hotel services in Spain, it is observed that electricity and fuels consumption take a key role. It is also found that 2-star hotels have the highest carbon emissions (Puig et al., 2017).

Furthermore, tourists dump numerous wastes that damage natural beauty and generate ecological disparity. As a result of the outburst of COVID-19 pandemic and local restrictions, the number of tourists have decreased in the tourist places around the globe (Zambrano-Monserrate et al., 2020). Such as, due to COVID-19 Thailand's most popular tourist's destination, Phuket goes into lockdown on April 9, 2020. There is an average of 5,452 tourists visit per day (Cripps, 2020). Likewise, local administration imposed a ban on public gathering and tourist arrivals at Cox's Bazar Sea beach in Bangladesh. It is recognized as the longest unbroken natural sandy sea beach in the world. However, due to the restrictions, the color of sea water is found changed, which usually remain muddled because of swimming, bathing, playing and riding motorized boats in the sea (Rahman, 2020). It seems that nature has got a time to integrate human annoyance. Moreover, due to decreased water pollution during these restrictions returning of dolphins is observed in the coast of Bay of Bengal in Bangladesh. It is also observed in the canals, waterways, and ports of Venice in Italy after a long period of time (Kundu, 2020; Rahman, 2020). As a result, we see ecological restoration around the globe.

3.7.2 Harmful Impact of COVID-19 on the Physical Environment

There are some harmful impacts of COVID-19 on the physical environment. They are discussed below:

3.7.2.1 Increased Generation of Biomedical Waste

Since the outbreak of COVID-19, medical waste generation is increased worldwide. It is a big threat to our environment and public health. For collecting sample of the suspected COVID-19 patients, diagnosis, treatment of a vast number of COVID-19 patients, and also for the purpose of disinfection a lot of transmissible and biomedical wastes are being generated in different hospitals around the world (Somani et al., 2020; Zambrano-Monserrate et al., 2020). It is reported that, Wuhan in China produced more than 240 metric tons of medical wastes every day during the time of the COVID-19 outbreak. It is almost 190 metric tons higher than that of the usual time. It is also observed that in Ahmedabad, India, the amount of the generation of biomedical waste is increased from 550–600 kg per day to around 1000 kg per day during the first phase of lockdown (Saadat et al., 2020). In case of Bangladesh, it is found that around 206 metric tons of biomedical waste are generated per day in Dhaka, the capital city of Bangladesh during COVID-19 (Rahman et al., 2020).

On the other hand, cities like Manila, Kuala Lumpur, Hanoi, and Bangkok experienced similar types of increases. These cities on an average have been producing 154–280 metric tons more medical waste per day than before the pandemic situation. Such an unexpected increase of hazardous medical wastes and their appropriate management has become a significant challenge to the local waste management authorities in these cities (ADB, 2020). Van-Doremalen et al. (2020) shows that the SARS-CoV-2 virus can exist a day on cardboard, and up to 3 days on plastics and stainless steels. Therefore, medical wastes that are generated mainly from the hospitals and medical clinics, such as, needles, syringes, bandages, masks, gloves, used tissues, and discarded medicines etc. should be managed in an appropriate manner. Otherwise, it will not be possible to lessen further contamination and environmental pollution. Now it is a matter of global concern.

3.7.2.2 Haphazard Disposal of Safety Equipment

People currently are using face masks, hand gloves and other safety equipment to protect from themselves from COVID-19 contamination, which have been increasing the amount of healthcare waste. Researchers (Calma, 2020; Singh et al., 2020) show that in the USA, trash amount has been increasing due to increased PPE (Personal Protective Equipment) use at the domestic level. Since the outbreak of COVID-19, the production and use of plastic-based PPE is increased globally. For instance, China increased the daily production of medical masks to 14.8 million since February 2020, which is much higher than before (Fadare & Okoffo, 2020).

Due to lack of sufficient knowledge about contagious waste management, people mostly have been dumping these wastes especially face masks and hand gloves in open spaces and in some cases with household wastes. This disorganized dumping of these wastes creates congestion in water ways and aggravates environmental pollution (Rahman et al., 2020; Singh, et al., 2020; Zambrano-Monserrate et al., 2020). Likewise, face masks, hand gloves and other plastic based PPE are the potential sources of micro plastic fibers in the environment. Generally, polypropylene is used to make N-95 masks (N-95 means that it may blocks about 95% of particles which are of 0.3 microns in size or larger), on the other hand, Tyvek is used for making protective suits, gloves, and medical face shields both of which can persist for a long time and release dioxin and toxic elements to the environment. Though, experts and responsible authorities suggest for the appropriate dumping and segregation of household organic waste and plastic based protective equipment, i.e., hazardous medical waste, but mixing up these wastes increases the risk of disease transmission, and exposure to the virus of waste workers (Fadare & Okoffo, 2020; Ma et al., 2020; Somani et al., 2020; Singh et al., 2020).

3.7.2.3 Generation of Municipal Solid Waste

During COVID-19, in the municipal areas there is an increase of both organic and inorganic municipal solid wastes. These municipal wastes have direct and indirect effects on environment. These may pollute adversely the air, water and soil (Islam et al., 2016). Due to the COVID-19 pandemic, many countries around the globe, have formulated quarantine and lockdown policies. It has led to an increase in the demand of online shopping for home delivery, which has eventually increased the volume of domestic wastes from dispatched package materials (Somani et al., 2020; Zambrano-Monserrate et al., 2020).

3.7.2.4 Decrease in Recycling

Now-a-days, recycling of different wastes is an effective means to prevent pollution. It benefits us to save energy, and conserve natural resources. But, due to COVID-19 pandemic many countries around the world have adjourned the waste recycling activities to lessen the spread of viral contamination. For example, as government of the USA is worried about the risk of spreading COVID-19 in recycling services, nearly 46% of recycling programs in many cities in the USA are controlled (Somani et al., 2020). The United Kingdom, Italy, and many other European countries also forbidden diseased inhabitants from sorting their waste (Zambrano-Monserrate et al., 2020). Largely, due to interruption of scheduled municipal waste management in many cities, waste retrieval and recycling events, increasing the landfilling and environmental contaminants worldwide.

3.7.2.5 Formation of Ecological Disparity

Currently, vast quantity of sanitizers is applied into roads, commercial, and residential areas to annihilate SARS-CoV-2 virus. However, extensive use such sanitizers may kill non-targeted beneficial species. It may create ecological disparity (Islam & Bhuiyan, 2016). Furthermore, SARS-CoV-2 virus was identified in the COVID-19 patient's faces and also from municipal wastewater in many countries including Australia, India, Sweden, Netherlands and the USA (Ahmed et al., 2020; Mallapaty, 2020; Nghiem et al., 2020). Thus, some extra measures in wastewater treatment are indispensable. But it is a big challenge for the developing nations like Bangladesh, where municipal wastewater is drained into the nearby water bodies, canals and rivers without any treatment (Islam & Azam, 2015; Rahman & Islam, 2016). In China, it is observed that they have strengthened the disinfection process by increasing the use of chlorine to prevent SARS-CoV-2 virus which are spreading through the wastewater. But it is to be mentionable that excessive use of chlorine in water could generate harmful by-product (Zambrano-Monserrate et al., 2020).

3.7.3 Towards Sustainable Environment: Some Policy Recommendations

All the environmental consequences listed above due to COVID-19 are assumed temporary. Therefore, it is important to take necessary steps to make an appropriate strategy for getting long-term extensive benefit. This would be supportive to sustainable environmental management as well. However, this COVID-19 pandemic has stimulated a worldwide response. It has made the world nations to work together so that they can win against the virus. Likewise, to safeguard this lovely planet, united efforts of all the nations around the world should be vital (Somani et al., 2020). Consequently, based on the analyses this chapter proposes some possible recommendations for global environmental sustainability, which are listed below:

3.7.3.1 Awareness on Environmental Sustainability

Awareness on environmental sustainability should be a priority for all the nations both developed and developing to adhere to existing and new environmental legislations. If people are not aware it is not possible for the governments to have a sustainable environment. If people are aware they will think of renewable fuel sources, reducing carbon emissions, protecting the physical environment and a way of keeping the delicate ecosystems of our planet in balance. They will look for protecting our natural environment, human and ecological systems, while driving innovations and not compromising the way of life.

3.7.3.2 Behavioral Change in Daily Life

Our lifestyle and behavior sometimes also responsible for carbon emissions. If we want to reduce the carbon footprint and global carbon emission, it is very significant to have a modification in our daily life styles and behavior. We should change our behavior in consumption, such as avoiding processed food and taking locally grown food. We can promote making fertilizer from food waste. We must switch off or unplug our electronic devices when they are not in use. These type of behavioral change may support reducing emissions and help protecting our environment.

3.7.3.3 Strong Leadership and Political Commitment

Strong leadership and political commitment of each and every country around the globe is a must for ensuring a sustainable environment for our next generation. If governments are not committed to ensure a sustainable environment all the strategies taken by the national and international organizations and respective governments will be in vain. World leaders should work together in this regard.

3.7.3.4 International Cooperation

World leaders are committed to safeguard the global environmental properties, such as the global climate and biodiversity. In order to ensure that it is necessary to achieve the goals of sustainable environment. However, without a combined global effort it is impossible to safeguard our planet (ICIMOD, 2020). Hence, responsible international authorities, especially United Nations Environment Program (UN Environment) as well as world leaders should take appropriate steps and active role to make policies, and coordinate for their effective execution.

3.7.3.5 Promote Sustainable Industrialization

Industrialization is considered vital for the growth and development of world economies. During earlier period of COVID-19 industrial sector was affected seriously. However, to reduce harmful effects of COVID-19 pandemic it is important to think about sustainable industrialization. For sustainable industrialization, Pan (2016) mentions that it is necessary to shift from heavy to less energy-intensive industries. We should use cleaner fuels and advanced technologies, as well as, should formulate appropriate energy efficient policies. Furthermore, governments should create specific industrial zones for industries. It is also necessary to build backward linkage industries, so that waste from one industry can be used as raw materials of another industry (Hysa et al., 2020). In order to decrease carbon emissions, it is important to shut down industrial zones in a circular way after certain period of time without hampering the national economy. Moreover, labor intensive industries, especially readymade garments (RMG) and others similar industries where a large number of people work, appropriate physical distance, and a safe and hygienic working environment should be maintained in order to decrease the spread of any type of transmittable contagious disease, such as COVID-19.

3.7.3.6 Encourage Green Public Transportation System

Green public transportation system is a new concept that refers to the suitable, safe, less-pollution, humanized and diversified transportation system. It adapts to the environmental development trends and coordinates with ecological environment. Green transportation vehicles include various less-pollution vehicles, such as dual-energy vehicle, natural gas vehicle, electric vehicle, hydrogen power vehicle and solar energy vehicle. It helps returning to healthy and leisure lifestyle. The green transportation system decreases energy consumption, reduce carbon emission and decrease greenhouse effect that improve air quality (Li, 2016). Therefore, we must promote and encourage green transportation system and encourage people to use green public transport, rather private vehicles.

3.7.3.7 Encourage Using Renewable Energy

Renewable energy is composed of some natural renewable sources. They are naturally refilled on a human span from carbon neutral sources such as sunlight, wind, hydropower, rain, tides, waves, biomass, and geothermal heat etc. We can lower the demand of fossil fuels like coal, oil, and natural gas etc. by using these renewable energies. They can play a vital role in decreasing GHGs emissions. During this COVID-19 pandemic situation, it is observed that the demand for global energy is decreased. This results in the reduction of carbon emissions, hence the air quality in many areas is improved. However, to continue and sustain the global economic growth of the nations around the globe it is impossible to cut-off the demand for energies. Hence, use of renewable energy can meet the energy demand and reduces the GHGs emission globally (Zambrano-Monserrate et al., 2020).

3.7.3.8 Wastewater Treatment

Wastewater treatment is such a process applied to take away pollutants from wastewater. It transforms the pollutants into sewages that can be returned to the water cycle and can be reused for different purposes. To face the challenges of water contamination, both industrial and municipal wastewater might be treated appropriately before discharge. Furthermore, suitably treated wastewater may be reused in different nonproduction processes such as flushing toilets, cleaning roads etc. It will reduce the burden of additional water withdrawal globally.

3.7.3.9 Waste Recycling

Waste recycling is such a process that alter wastes into new stuffs. It can prevent the waste of possible valuable resources and decrease the consumption of new raw materials. As a result, it is helpful to decrease energy usage, air and water pollution etc. Thus, to reduce waste burden and environmental pollution, recycling and reuse of both industrial and municipal wastes is recommended. Consequently, circular economy system should be implemented to minimize the use of raw materials and wastes generation in the manufacturing process (Hysa et al., 2020). Furthermore, harmful and contagious medical waste management should be appropriate and follow related guidelines (WHO, 2020a, b). It is observed that people, particularly in developing countries lack awareness and knowledge about waste separation and dumping matters (Rahman et al., 2020). Therefore, government around the world should implement extensive awareness campaign programs about the appropriate method of waste segregation, handling and disposal.

3.7.3.10 Restoration of Ecology and Promoting Ecotourism

Restoration of ecology is the process of supporting the retrieval of an ecosystem which has been despoiled, broken, or demolished. Ecosystems are demolished due to some events such as tourism, urbanization, erosion of coastal areas and mining etc. On the other hand, ecotourism involves responsible travel to nature. It usually encompasses traveling to such places where flora and fauna, and cultural traditions are the principal attractions. Closure of tourist places periodically after a certain period of time may help restoring our ecological systems. Furthermore, practice of ecotourism worldwide should be promoted that may support sustainable livelihoods, preservation of local culture, and protection of biodiversity (Islam & Bhuiyan, 2020).

3.8 Concluding Remarks

Covid-19 pandemic has brought the world to an oppressive end. It has left for the whole world a trajectory of tears and uncertainty. On an individual level, many families around the globe have lost their loved ones. Their lonely passing without final farewells were tough to tolerate. Despite this, people started to continue to step on the path of realistic optimism and positive resilience. However, Department of Economic and Social Affairs of the United Nations cautions that COVID-19 pandemic threatens to remove the advancement that has been made since the introduction of current Sustainable Development Goals (SDGs).

This chapter identified some positive and harmful impacts of COVID-19 on our physical environment. Positive impact listed above like decrease of air pollution and Green House Gas (GHG) emission, decrease of water pollution, decrease of noise pollution and ecological restoration and adaptation of tourist places and harmful impacts like increased generation of biomedical waste, haphazard disposal of safety equipment, generation of municipal solid waste, decrease in recycling and formation of ecological disparity are all temporary. Once we have control over COVID-19 in future, all the restrictions will be withdrawn and automatically these impacts will go to the opposite direction again. Therefore, we need to think of seriously.

Notwithstanding, the COVID-19 pandemic has been affecting our human life and the global economy as a whole. Especially, it has extremely been affecting our natural environment. It reminds us that we have seriously ignored our environment. The global response of COVID-19 also teaches us that we must work together to fight against the threat to humanity and civilization. Though the impacts of COVID-19 on the natural environment are short-term and temporary, a united and time-oriented effort is necessary that can strengthen environmental sustainability. Only then we can save the earth from the effects of environmental disaster.

Nonetheless, this chapter based on the review and analysis suggested some potential recommendations to combat the negative and harmful impacts on our physical environment due to COVID-19 pandemic. These may be helpful for the countries as well as people concerned around the globe. But which is very important here is to aware people and others concerned about the sustainability of our physical environment. If concerned people are aware and acquire the sustainability skills, they will be able to protect this lovely planet and get the ecological balance. They will also be able to apply innovations without hampering the ways of life. To make this happen strong commitment and political leadership of the concerned governments are necessary as well as international cooperation is a must. It is hoped that the findings and potential strategies proposed here in this chapter may contribute to the concerned to maintain our environment during pandemic as well as after the pandemic in the new normal world. It is to remind that COVID-19 pandemic is a common problem to all of us. It is not a personal problem of any country or anybody. We must consider that; it is our common global issue. We, the nations around the globe need to fight with it efficiently and effectively as citizens of the global village. Otherwise, it will be impossible for us to combat the challenges and problems of sustainable environment and save our lovely planet.

References

Adams, M.D. (2020). Air pollution in Ontario, Canada during the COVID-19 state of emergency. *Science of the Total Environment, 742*, 140516.

Ahmed, W., Angel, N., Edson, J., Bibby, K., Bivins, A., & O'Brier, J.W. (2020). First confirmed detection of SARS-CoV-2 in untreated wastewater in Australia: A proof of concept for the wastewater surveillance of COVID-19 in the community. *Science of the Total Environment, 728*, 138764.

Asian Development Bank (ADB). (2020, October). *Managing infectious medical waste during the COVID-19 pandemic.* https://www.adb.org/publications/managing-medical-waste-covid19

Azcona, G., Bhatt, A., Encarnacion, J., Plazaola-Castaño, J., Seck, P., Staab, S., & Turquet, L., (2020, December). *From insights to action: Gender equality in the wake of COVID-19.* https://www.unwomen.org

Barnett, E., & Casper, M. (2001). A definition of social environment. *American Journal of Public Health, 91*(3), 465. https://doi.org/10.2105/ajph.91.3.465a

Berman, J. D., & Edisu, K. (2020). Changes in U.S. air pollution during the COVID-19 pandemic. *Science Total Environment, 739*, 139864.

Bodrud-Doza, M., Islam, S. M. D., Rume, T., Quraishi, S. B., Rahman, M. S., & Bhuiyan, M. A. H. (2020). Groundwater quality and human health risk assessment for safe and sustainable water supply of Dhaka City dwellers in Bangladesh. *Groundwater for Sustainable Development, 10*, 100374.

Caine, P. (2020, April 2). Environmental impact of COVID-19 lockdowns seen from space. *Science of Nature.* https://news.wttw.com/2020/04/02/environmental-impact-covid-19-lockdowns-seen-space

Calma, J. (2020). The COVID-19 pandemic is generating tons of medical waste. *The Verge.* https://www.theverge.com/2020/3/26/21194647/the-covid-19-pandemic-is-generating-tons-of-medical-waste

Chakraborty, I., & Maity, P. (2020). COVID-19 outbreak: Migration, effects on society, global environment and prevention. *Science Total Environment, 728*, 138882.

Clifford, C. (2020). *The water in Venice, Italy's canals is running clear amid the COVID-19 lockdown.* https://www.cnbc.com/2020/03/18/photos-water-in-venice-italys-canals-clear-amid-covid-19-lockdown.html

Cooper, R. (2020). Institute of Development Studies; Brighton, UK: 2020. Water Security beyond Covid-19. *K4D Helpdesk Report 803*, https://opendocs.ids.ac.uk/opendocs/handle/20.500.12413/15240

CPCB. (2020). Central Pollution Control Board, Ministry of Environment, Forest and Climate Change, Government of India. Daily River Water Quality Monitoring Data.

CREA, (2020, April). Air quality improvements due to COVID-19 lockdown in India. *Centre for Research on Energy and Clean Air.* https://energyandcleanair.org/air-qualityimprovements-due-to-covid-19-lock-down-in-india/

Cripps, K. (2020, April 10). Thailand's most popular island goes into lockdown as Covid-19 cases surge. *CNN Travel, CNN.* https://edition.cnn.com/travel/article/phuket-thailand-lockdown/index.html

EEA (European Environmental Agency). (2020). Air pollution goes down as Europe takes hard measures to combat Coronavirus. *Copenhagen*, https://www.eea.europa.eu/highlights/air-pollution-goes-downas

Evans, S. (2020, September 4). Global emissions analysis: Coronavirus set to cause largest ever annual fall in CO2 emissions. *Carbon Brief*, https://www.carbonbrief.org/analysis-coronavirus-set-to-cause-largest-everannual-fall-in-co2-emissions

Fadare, O. O., & Okoffo, E. D. (2020). Covid-19 face masks: A potential source of microplastic fibers in the environment. *Science Total Environment, 37*, 140279.

Gandhiok, J., & Ibra, M. (2020, April 23). *The Times of India; 2020. Covid-19: Noise pollution falls as lockdown rings in sound of silence.* https://timesofindia.indiatimes.com/india/covid-19-noise-pollution-falls-as-lockdown-rings-in-sound-of-silence/articleshow/75309318.cms

Ghosh, I. (2020). The emissions impact of coronavirus lockdowns, as shown by satellites. https://www.visualcapitalist.com/coronavirus-lockdowns-emissions

Hysa, E., Kruja, A., Rehman, N. U., & Laurenti, R. (2020). Circular economy innovation and environmental sustainability impact on economic growth: An integrated model for sustainable development. *Sustainability, 12*, 4831.

ICIMOD. (2020). Annual Report 2020, ICIMOD.

ILO, FAO, IFAD, & WHO. (2020, October 13). Impact of COVID-19 on people's livelihoods, their health and our food systems", a Joint statement by ILO, FAO, IFAD and WHO.

India Environment Portal (IEP). (2020). *Impact of lockdown (25th March to 15th April) on air quality.* http://www.indiaenvironmentportal.org.in/content/467415/impact-of-lockdown-25th-march-to-15th-april-on-air-quality/

Islam S.M.D., Azam G. (2015). Seasonal variation of physicochemical and toxic properties in three major rivers: Shitalakhya, Buriganga, and Turag around Dhaka city, Bangladesh. *Journal of Biodiversity and Environmental Science, 7*(3), 120–131.

Islam, S.M.D., Bhuiyan, M.A.H. (2016). Impact scenarios of shrimp farming in coastal region of Bangladesh: An approach of an ecological model for sustainable management. *Aquaculture International, 24*(4), 1163–1190.

Islam, S. M. D., Bodrud-Doza, M., Khan, R. M., Haque, M. A., & Mamun, M. A. (2020). Exploring COVID-19 stress and its factors in Bangladesh: A perception-based study. *Heliyon, 6*(7), e04399.

Islam S.M.D., Rahman S.H., Hassan M., Azam G. (2016). Municipal solid waste management using GIS application in Mirpur area of Dhaka city, Bangladesh. *Pollution, 2*(2), 141–151.

James, P., Magee, L., Scerri, A., & Steger, M. B. (2015). *Urban sustainability in theory and practice: Circles of sustainability*. Routledge.

James, P., & Magee, L. (2016). Domains of sustainability. In A. Farazmand (Ed.), *Global encyclopaedia of public administration, public policy, and governance*. Springer.

Johnson, D. L., Ambrose, S. H., Bassett, T. J., Bowen, M. L., Crummey, D. E., Isaacson, J. S., Johnson, D. N., Lamb, P., Saul, M., & Winter-Nelson, A. E. (1997). Meanings of environmental terms. *Journal of Environmental Quality, 26*(3), 581–589. https://doi.org/10.2134/jeq1997.004 72425002600030002x

Jribi, S., Ismail, H. B., Doggui, D., & Debbabi, H. (2020). COVID-19 virus outbreak lockdown: What impacts on household food wastage? *Environmental Development and Sustainability, 22*, 3939–3955.

Karunathilake, K. (2020). Positive and negative impacts of COVID-19, an analysis with special reference to challenges on the supply chain in South Asian countries. *Journal of Social and Economic Development, 23*, 568–581.

Kono, N. (2014). Brundtland Commission (World Commission on Environment and Development). In A. C. Michalos (Eds.), *Encyclopedia of quality of life and well-being research*. Springer. https://doi.org/10.1007/978-94-007-0753-5_441

Kuhlman, T., & Farrington, J. (2010). What is sustainability? *Sustainability, 2*(11), 3436–3448. https://doi.org/10.3390/su2113436

Kundu, C. (2020). Has the Covid-19 lockdown returned dolphins and swans to Italian waterways? *The India Today*. https://www.indiatoday.in/fact-check/story/has-covid19-lockdownreturned-dolphins-swans-italian-waterways-1658457

Li, Han-ru. (2016). Study on green transportation system of international metropolises. *Procedia Engineering, 137*. Available online at www.sciencedirect.com

Li, Q., Guan, X., Wu, P., Wang, X., Zhou, L., Tong, Y., Ren, R., Leung, K. S., Lau, E. H., & Wong, J. Y. (2020). Early transmission dynamics in Wuhan, China, of novel coronavirus–infected pneumonia. *National English Journal of Medicine, 382*, 1199–1207.

Ma, Y., Lin, X., Wu, A., Huang, Q., Li, X., & Yan, J. (2020). Suggested guidelines for emergency treatment of medical waste during COVID-19: Chinese experience. *Waste Disposal and Sustainable Energy, 2*, 81–84.

Mallapaty, S. (2020). How sewage could reveal true scale of coronavirus outbreak. *Nature, 580*

Nakada, L. Y. K. (2020). Urban R.C. COVID-19 pandemic: Impacts on the air quality during the partial lockdown in São Paulo state, Brazil. *Science Total Environment, 730*, 139087.

Nghiem, L. D., Morgan, B., & Donner, E. (2020). Short M.D. The COVID-19 pandemic: considerations for the waste and wastewater services sector. Case Study, *Chemical and Environmental Engineering, 1*, 100006.

Pan, J. (2016). *China's Environmental Governing and Ecological Civilization*. China Insights. Springer Berlin Heidelberg.

Puig, R., Kiliç, E., Navarro, A., Albertí, J., Chacón, L., & Fullana-i-Palmer, P. (2017). Inventory analysis and carbon footprint of coastland-hotel services: A Spanish case study. *Science Total Environment, 595*, 244–254.

Rahman, M. (2020). *Rare dolphin sighting as Cox's Bazar lockdown under COVID-19 coronavirus*. https://www.youtube.com/watch?v=gjw8ZllIlbQ

Rahman, M. M., Bodrud-Doza, M., Griffiths, M. D., & Mamun, M. A. (2020). Biomedical waste amid COVID-19: Perspectives from Bangladesh. *The Lancet Global Health, 8*, 1262.

Rahman, S.H., & Islam, S.M.D. (2016). Degrading riverine ecology of Bangladesh and options for management. *SUB Journal of Sustainable Environmental Development, 1*, 11–27.

Saadat, S., Rawtani, D., & Hussain, C. M. (2020). Environmental perspective of COVID-19. *Science of the Total Environment, 728*, 138870

Sims, J. (2020). *Will the world be quieter after the pandemic?* https://www.bbc.com/future/article/20200616-will-the-world-be-quieter-after-the-pandemic

Singh, N., Tang, Y., & Ogunseitan, O. A. (2020). Environmentally sustainable management of used personal protective equipment. *Environmental Science Technology, 54*, 8500–8502.

Singhal, S., & Matto, M. (2020). COVID-19 lockdown: A ventilator for rivers. In M. Somani (ed.), *DownToEarth. 11*, 100491. https://www.downtoearth.org.in/blog/covid-19-lockdown-aventilator-for-rivers-70771

Solan, M., Hauton, C., Godbold, J. A., Wood, C. L., & Leighton, T. G. (2016). White P anthropogenic sources of underwater sound can modify how sediment-dwelling invertebrates mediate ecosystem properties. *Science Report, 6*(1), 20540.

Somani, M., Srivastava, A. N., Gummadivalli, S. K., & Sharma, A. (2020). Indirect implications of COVID-19 towards sustainable environment: An investigation in Indian context. *Bioresearch Technological Report, 11*, 100491.

Thiessen, T. (2020). *How clean air cities could outlast COVID-19 lockdowns.* https://www.forbes.com/sites/tamarathiessen/2020/04/10/how-clean-air-cities-could-outlast-covid-19lockdowns/#292a5e866bb5

UNCTAD, (2020, April). *The COVID-19 pandemic and the blue economy: New challenges and prospects for recovery and resilience.* UNCTAD Publication, UN.

Uttarakhand Pollution Control Board (UPCB). (2020). Water quality during lockdown period, Government of Uttarakhand: India. https://ueppcb.uk.gov.in/pages/display/96-water-quality-data

Van-Doremalen, N., Bushmaker, T., Morris, D. H., Holbrook, M. G., Gamble, A., Williamson, B. N., & Lloyd-Smith, J. O. (2020). Aerosol and surface stability of SARSCoV-2 as compared with SARS-CoV-1. *English Journal of Medicine, 382*(16), 1564–1567.

Wallace, G. (2020, April 9). Airlines and TSA report 96% drop in air travel as pandemic continues. *CNN.* https://edition.cnn.com/2020/04/09/politics/airline-passengers-decline/index.html

Wang, C., Pan, R., Wan, X., Tan, Y., Xu, L., Ho, C. S., & Ho, R. C. (2020). Immediate psychological responses and associated factors during the initial stage of the 2019 coronavirus disease (COVID-19) epidemic among the general population in China. *International Journal of Environmental Research and Public Health, 17*, 1729.

WHO. (2020a). *Coronavirus disease (COVID-19) pandemic.* https://www.who.int/emergencies/diseases/novel-coronavirus-2019

WHO. (2020b). *Rational use of personal protective equipment (PPE) for coronavirus disease (COVID-19).* https://apps.who.int/iris/bitstream/handle/10665/331498/WHO-2019-nCoV-IPCPPE_use-2020.2-eng.pdf

Yunus, A. P., Masago, Y., & Hijioka, Y. (2020). COVID-19 and surface water quality: Improved lake water quality during the lockdown. *Science Total Environment, 731*, 139012.

Zambrano-Monserrate, M. A., Ruanob, M. A., & Sanchez-Alcalde, L. (2020). Indirect effects of COVID-19 on the environment. *Science Total Environment, 728*, 138813.

Zogopoulos, E. (2020, April 17). *COVID-19: The curious case of a green virus.* https://energyindustryreview.com/analysis/covid-19-the-curious-case-of-a-green-virus/

Web Sources

https://www.corona.gov.bd/
https://www.covid19.who.int/
https://www.fao.org/2019-ncov/en/

https://www.icimod.org/reports/ar2020/
https://www.ilo.org/global/topics/coronavirus/
https://www.undp.org/coronavirus
https://www.un.org/en/coronavirus
https://www.unicef.org/coronavirus/covid-19
https://www.unctad.org/programme/covid-19-response
https://www.weforum.org/platforms/covid-action-platform/
https://www.who.int/emergencies/diseases/novel-coronavirus-2019

Dr. Amir Mohammad Nasrullah is a Professor in the Department of Public Administration, University of Chittagong, Bangladesh.

Chapter 4
The Austrian State and the COVID-19 Crisis: Achievements and Failures of a Small European Country During the Pandemic Since 2020

Martin Malek

Abstract The financial crisis from 2008 onwards had already led to a "return of the state" in many countries. This tendency intensified in the face of the COVID-19 pandemic from the beginning of 2020—as well as in Austria. This chapter asks several research questions on the Austrian state's handling of the pandemic in comparison with the other members of the European Union (EU). The most important are: What were the consequences of the pandemic in the areas of public health, the economy and the labour market; and what successes and failures were achieved in combating the pandemic? It is clear, however, that only an interim assessment can be made; a "definitive" comparative survey of the state performance of the EU members will be possible only in the years to come.

Keywords Eurpean Union · Public health · Pandemic · Financial Crisis · Spanish flu · COVID-19

4.1 Introduction and Research Questions

In 2020, the world, Europe and Austria were confronted with the biggest health crisis since the Spanish flu, which, according to very different estimates, claimed between 20 and 100 million lives worldwide in 1918–1920 (and thus at any rate more than the First World War). The Spanish flu hit Austria-Hungary when the monarchy was on the verge of collapse anyway after almost four and a half years of war. Historians speak of a total of 6,500 deaths from influenza in the capital Vienna between 1918 and 1920. But exact numbers cannot be determined even retrospectively. Doctors at the time were often unable to distinguish between different diseases with similar symptoms, such as pneumonia and influenza. The Spanish flu contributed to further undermining the legitimacy of the Imperial Government: The secession of the nationalities and

---

All translations from German were made personally by the author.—Many of the figures mentioned for 2020 are provisional and may still change.

M. Malek (✉)
Institute for Strategy and Security Policy, National Defence Academy, Vienna, Austria

© The Author(s), under exclusive license to Springer Nature Singapore Pte Ltd. 2022
S. Roy and D. Nandy (eds.), *Understanding Post-COVID-19 Social and Cultural Realities*, https://doi.org/10.1007/978-981-19-0809-5_4

the disintegration of the armed forces were now joined by an intensification of the chaos that had long reigned in the hinterland as well. Inevitably, there was a shortage of doctors, nursing staff and medicines, etc. On November 6, 1918, just a few days before the proclamation of the Republic in Austria, the newspapers reported that, although the flu had not completely disappeared from Vienna, the mortality rate had fallen sharply.

In the 75 years since the end of the Second World War in 1945, there had been no interstate wars, civil wars, revolutions, etc. in Central, Northern and Western Europe (but "only" home-grown left-wing and right-wing terrorism as well as terrorism "imported" from the Near and Middle East in particular). The residents of the region "knew" pandemics, if at all, only from media reports about distant countries (e.g. SARS outbreak 2002–2004, Western African Ebola virus epidemic 2013–2016). But this does not mean that the possibility of a pandemic outbreak has been completely ignored. In 2019, only a few months before the start of COVID-19, an article by a military doctor on this topic appeared in a publication of the Austrian Ministry of Defense. However, it only after the start of the pandemic attracted considerable attention and made the author a sought-after interview partner for many media. In places, the article read like a forecast of the very health crisis that was soon to hit the world, Europe and Austria. It stated that a pandemic can also be triggered by a pathogen that is currently completely unknown. Furthermore, influenza viruses, smallpox and plague are considered pathogens that can pose the greatest challenges to the public health system and consequently to the state structure. There is no question that Austria can also be affected by all these pathogens … Pandemics can have devastating consequences on society as a whole.

Admittedly, the article considered much more far-reaching consequences of a pandemic possible than those that the year 2020 actually brought—namely a collapse of the health system, the economy and services; bottlenecks in food supply; massive problems in transport and foreign trade etc., which could lead to "unmanageable burdens on the domestic state structure and its insecure society". Possibilities for preparedness were described here only in very general terms: "… one must strengthen the resilience of state and society; especially in poorer and thus more vulnerable states, outbreaks spread faster and stronger." The article also suggested a role for the Austrian Armed Forces (Speranido, 2019, pp. 220, 221–222, 221, 222–223), which was then actually called upon in 2020 to support the measures against the pandemic.

The financial crisis from 2008 onwards already led to a partial "return of the state" in Western Europe and North America, which in particular rescued banks that had come under massive pressure and increasingly regulated financial markets. In the media, politics and political science of many Western countries, complaints about "neoliberal globalization" and its disastrous effects had been common for many years. In fact, however, nowhere in the Western Europe and North America had the share of national income generated, managed and distributed by the state been significantly reduced. And the countries that participate most intensively in global interactions are often also those with the highest state share. With the outbreak of the financial crisis, the role of the Austrian state was pushed almost "unnoticed" by the public above the mark of 50% of economic output and distribution. This made the state by far the largest economic factor in the country. In this context, it was sometimes remarked that Austria did not have "a truly free market economy", but a "managed state economy with with semi-market components" (Schellhorn, 2016). Even decidedly left-wing authors then conceded that—although what they call "neoliberal globalization" is questioning the nation state and its ability to act—in view of the state interventions in many countries due to the financial crisis, "there can be no talk of an erosion of the (nation) state or of its overall lack of function" (Sauer, 2004/2011, p. 341).

In Austria, a new coalition Government, consisting of the Christian Democratic Austrian People's Party and the Greens, had only been inaugurated in January 2020, only a few weeks before the arrival of the pandemic in Central Europe. In Austria—as in all other countries affected by COVID-19—far-reaching decisions had to be made for state and society without being able to rely on any experience: As Health Minister Rudolf Anschober (Greens) put it, it is an "ongoing learning process" for the Government, the authorities, and the society. Even public health experts, epidemologists and virologists (not to mention lawyers, political scientists and public intellectuals) often expressed very different to mutually exclusive opinions in the mainstream media, in their political advisory activities and in (allegedly or actually) scientific publications about what to do now.

Against this backdrop, the state as an institution became one of the topics (also) increasingly discussed by social science again, as in the face of the global COVID-19 crisis it suddenly imposed things on citizens in the interest of public health that had been completely unthinkable only a short time before: curfews, closing or drastically reducing the activity of numerous educational institutions, shops, restaurants, cultural institutions, businesses and government agencies, etc. Some observers seemed to rejoice at the "return of the nation state" through the COVID-19 crisis (Schuster, 2020), but many others warned of exactly that.

Various voices—some with regret or even alarm, others with hope—in Austria and around the world also raised the question of whether this "return" meant the end of globalization and renationalization respectively. Stephen M. Walt (Harvard Kennedy School) suggested that the COVID-19 crisis would strengthen the state as well as nationalism. "Hyperglobalization" would end because more people would turn to their respective governments for protection (2020). Robin Niblett, Director of Chatham House, even spoke of an "end of globalization as we know it" (2020). Some observers also saw a reactualization of state sovereignty (which until then had been "talked down" for many years, portrayed as less and less relevant or already absent altogether, especially by a broad current in political science) through "biopolitics" because of the pandemic (Sommavilla, 2020).

This paper poses the following research questions on the Austrian state's handling of the pandemic in comparison with the other members of the European Union (EU):

- What were the initial conditions at the beginning of the pandemic (i.e. early 2020)?
- What measures did the state take, particularly in public health, the economy and the labour market, to limit the impact of the pandemic, and which criticism was voiced by the public?

- What were the consequences of the pandemic in the areas of public health, the economy and the labour market (the education sector must be left out of consideration here for reasons of space)?
- What successes and failures were achieved in combating the pandemic?
- What are the prospects for the near future?

When this article was completed, vaccination was still ongoing in Austria and all other EU countries. Therefore, of course, no "final" assessment of their effects and consequences can yet be made. This will only be possible in a few years' time, taking into account the possible or probable long-term consequences of the pandemic and the measures to combat it.

4.2 The Initial Concditions: Austria and the Other EU Member States in the Global Health Security Index of 2019

In 2019, the Global Health Security (GHS) Index presented the results of a worldwide survey of the state of preparedness to deal with epidemics and pandemics in 195 countries. This Index relied on open source information—data that a country has published on its own or has reported to or been reported by an international entity which then made such data public. The Index features six categories: Prevention of the emergence or release of pathogens, early detection and reporting for epidemics of potential international concern, rapid response to and mitigation of the spread of an epidemic, sufficient and robust health system to treat the sick & protect health workers, commitments to improving national capacity, financing and adherence to norms, overall risk environment and country vulnerability to biological threats.

The scale of the scoring is 0 (worst) to 100 (best). Aggregate scores are divided into three tiers, with countries scoring between 0 and 33.3 in the "bottom" tier ("low scores"), countries scoring between 33.4 and 66.6 in the middle tier ("moderate scores"), and countries scoring between 66.7 and 100 in the upper or "top" tier ("high scores"). The general result was that collectively, international preparedness for epidemics and pandemics was unsatisfactory: The average overall GHS Index score among all 195 countries assessed was 40.2. Among the 60 high-income countries, the average GHS Index score was 51.9 (Table 4.1).

However, the question arises as to whether this Index is sufficient to clearly assess the situation before the global outbreak of the pandemic. The sixth place for Thailand (score 73.2) is surprising, but above all the first place for the United States: There alone—at least according to the official figures (which are admittedly very implausible for China, among others)—about a quarter of the worldwide deaths of the pandemic occurred.

Table 4.1 The EU member states in the Global Health Security Index

Country	Rank in the index	Overall score
Netherlands	3	75.6
Sweden	7	72.1
Denmark	8	70.4
Finland	10	68.7
France	11	68.2
Slovenia	12	67.2
Germany	14	66
Spain	15	65.9
Latvia	17	62.9
Belgium	19	61
Portugal	20	60.3
Ireland	23	59
Austria	**26**	**58.5**
Estonia	29	57
Italy	31	56.2
Poland	32	55.4
Lithuania	33	55
Hungary	35	54
Greece	37	53.8
Croatia	38	53.3
Czech Republic	42	52
Slovakia	52	47.9
Romania	60	45.8
Bulgaria	61	45.6
Luxembourg	67	43.8
Cyprus	77	43
Malta	98	37.3

Source GHS Index (2019)

4.3 A Brief Chronology of the Events in Austria

On February 25, 2020, the first two COVID-19 cases were reported in Austria, namely from Innsbruck (capital of the province Tyrol). They were two 24-year-old Italians, a woman and a man, both from Lombardy. In March 2020, events in the winter sports resort of Ischgl (also in Tyrol) contributed decisively to the Europe-wide spread of COVID-19: Several thousand infections worldwide traced back to Ischgl; people from 45 countries were affected.

The Austrian Government decided to take far-reaching measures from March 2020 to slow down the spread of the virus and thereby protect known risk groups—especially the elderly and people with certain pre-existing and underlying diseases. The Austrian health system had a total of about 2,500 intensive care beds in normal operation. Their long-term average occupancy rate is about 80%; about 500 beds are normally free for emergencies. This figure was the pivotal point of the measures taken by the Ministry of Health: Model calculations were used to estimate how high the utilization of the intensive care units would be under different spread scenarios. If all beds were occupied, the attending physicians would have to resort to so-called triage measures, i.e. make a selection on the basis of a certain catalogue of criteria, for which patients (further) intensive care measures would be carried out and for which not. After this selection, some of the latter would only receive palliative care. The Austrian Government wanted to avoid this situation which prevailed for several weeks in Northern Italy and other European regions, especially in the spring of 2020. On March 12, 2020, researchers from the Complexity Science Hub Vienna calculated that if growth had remained constant, the capacity limit of intensive care units would have been reached by the end of the same month. In the course of the Government's countermeasures, additional beds were created and normal hospital operations were reduced in parallel. The stock of intensive care beds was then 3,000 at the beginning of April 2020, of which 1,300 were available at that time.

In a press conference on March 10, it was announced that events in enclosed spaces with 100 or more people and those outdoors with 500 or more people would be temporarily banned. This should also apply to cinemas and theatres. The Government additionally asked the population to reduce social life for a few weeks to reduce the risk of infection for the elderly.

Public transport was not cancelled so as not to make it difficult or impossible to travel to the workplace. On March 11, 2020, it was announced that as of March 16, face-to-face teaching at all Austrian universities, universities of applied sciences (in German: *Fachhochschulen*) and teacher training colleges would be cancelled and, if possible, replaced by distance learning. Schools were also closed. The upper classes (i.e. from the 9th grade onwards) were to be closed from March 16, and from March 18, the other schools (elementary schools and lower classes of high schools) were to be closed as well. Childcare facilities were created in the schools for pupils whose parents had to work outside the home. The children who stayed at home received their assignments from the teachers by e-mail or via learning platforms. The kindergartens were also open to children whose parents were unavailable for work. The measures were initially limited until Easter 2020.

On March 12, 2020, the first Austrian COVID-19 death was confirmed in Vienna: A 69-year-old man died in hospital after returning from Italy. On March 13, the Government announced that most shops would close from March 16, with the exception of grocery shops, pharmacies and drugstores. It was also announced that bars, restaurants and coffee houses would only be allowed to open until 3 p.m. from March 16. On March 14, 655 infected persons were registered in Austria. Soon after, the Government ordered these establishments to close completely from March 17, 2020. The restrictions in public spaces were controlled by the police, and there were administrative fines of up to €3,600, and in certain cases up to €30,000, under the COVID-19 law. This law, which also provided for a €4 billion crisis management fund, was fast-tracked on March 15, 2020: Resolutions were passed in both chambers of Parliament, namely the National Council (Lower House) and the Federal Council (Upper House), the bill was certified by the Head of State, Federal President Alexander Van der Bellen, and published in the *Federal Law Gazette* on a single day.

With effect from March 20, the exit restriction was extended. On March 30, Federal Chancellor (= Prime Minister) Sebastian Kurz (also leader of the Austrian People's Party) expressed fears in a press conference that intensive care could be overstretched as early as mid-April 2020. He also announced that protective mouth-nose masks must be worn in shops.

On April 6, the Government announced at a press conference that the obligation to wear protective mouth-nose masks would be extended to public transport and to the commercial and craft enterprises that would then reopen from April 14. After the Easter weekend (April 10–13), however, businesses were to reopen gradually.

On April 30, 2020, the previously existing exit restrictions expired, whereupon a new regulation by the Minister of Health came into force on May 1. This COVID-19 relaxation regulation (German: *Lockerungsverordnung*) imposed a general obligation to wear mouth-nose protection when entering public places indoors, at outdoor markets, in taxis and carpools. The previously existing obligation to wear it on public transport was retained.

On May 15, the catering industry reopened, accommodation establishments, fitness studios, outdoor swimming pools as well as thermal spas followed on May 29, 2020—in each case with certain protective measures. From June 15, the mask requirement only applied in public transport, in health care facilities such as pharmacies or when services were used where the minimum distance could not be maintained (e.g. at the hairdresser's). The obligation to wear masks in trade, in schools and for guests in restaurants or cafés was dropped.

On July 21, 2020, the Government announced at a press conference the reintroduction of a nationwide mask requirement in supermarkets, bank and post office branches as of July 24. In August, rising infection figures were noted, which were mainly attributed to people returning from holiday. As a result, travel warnings and testing obligations were intensified. Conversely, some other states declared Austria a risk area: returnees from Austria had to observe a quarantine of 14 days in Great Britain and ten days in Norway from August 22.

As of September 14, measures were tightened again in Austria in view of the rising infection figures, especially with regard to the use of masks. Thus, a mask had to be worn again in trade and gastronomy in closed rooms. The consumption of food and drinks was only permitted while sitting at tables.

On October 31, 2020, Chancellor Kurz announced that there would be a "lockdown light" from November 3, 2020 on. This meant that curfew restrictions applied nationwide between 8 p.m. and 6 a.m. During this time, leaving private living quarters was only permitted for certain reasons, in particular to "avert an immediate danger to life, limb or property", to "provide assistance to persons in need of support", to "exercise family rights and fulfil family duties", for "professional and educational purposes" and—outdoors—"for physical and mental recreation". Cultural and recreational facilities had to close, and with the exception of funerals and individual other exceptions, no more events took place. The ban also applied to private events, as long as they did not take place in "private living quarters". The hotel and restaurant industry also closed, although takeaway and delivery were allowed. Trade and service providers such as hairdressers initially remained open, subject to conditions. Upper high school classes and universities had to be converted to distance learning.

In autumn 2020, the Austrian business journalist Franz Schellhorn (2020) took stock of the situation as follows:

After the tough handling of the first lockdown, just about everything has gone off the rails. Austria has lost control of contact tracing (an epidemiological mortal sin), in old people's and nursing homes the second Corona wave is raging worse than the first, tens of thousands of schoolchildren are back at home in front of their TV sets, and large parts of the public sector are cut off from the digitalised world because they work with outdated IT systems. All this is happening in a state whose public spending is among the highest in the world.

On November 14, the Government announced another "hard" lockdown from November 17, to initially December 6, 2020. In the first half of December 2020, mass tests were to be carried out in Austria. Overall, however, only 22.6% of Austrians participated, with 4,200 people testing positive for the virus (Rosner, 2020). On December 18, the Government announced a third lockdown for the period between December 26, 2020 and January 24, 2021. On December 27, the first people in Austria were vaccinated against COVID-19. By January 2, 2021, only 6,000 people had been vaccinated, which led to criticism in the quality media (Ultsch, 2021).

4.4 Fatalities in Austria and the EU Due to COVID-19

As the statistics agency Statistik Austria announced at the end of February 2021, 90,517 people died in the country in 2020. Of these, 6,477 (i.e. 7%) deaths were related to COVID-19, which was thus the second most common cause of death (the undisputed leader was "chronic heart disease" with 15,582 cases, and in third place was stroke with 4,734 deaths) (Rosner, 2021).

Men (7.6%) died slightly more frequently in connection with COVID-19 than women (6.7%). In Austria, however, there are significantly more older women than men. Therefore, taking into account the different age structure of the sexes in the population, it can be assumed that the virus-related mortality among men is about one and a half times higher than among women. The majority of those who died were older people: 97% were older than 60 years. Overall, COVID-19 was the determining cause of death in 8.4% of all those who died aged 80 and more, but only in 0.9% of those who died under the age of 40.

Differences were also seen by provinces. A particularly high number of deaths was attributable to COVID-19 in Carinthia (9.4%), Tyrol (8.8%) and Styria (8.4%).

In Lower Austria (5.1%), Burgenland (5.4%) and Vienna (6.4%), however, the share of deaths due to COVID-19 was somewhat lower.

In 2020, 7,131 more people or 9% more died in Austria than in 2019 with 83,386 deaths. At the time of the second wave in Austria, COVID-19 mortality even surpassed mortality due to cardiovascular diseases.

According to Statistik Austria, the figure of 7,131 roughly corresponded to the number of deaths in an average month. If the increased population and changes in the age structure are taken into account, a slight increase in deaths would have been expected in 2020 even without the pandemic. Within the framework of the population forecast prepared by Statistik Austria in autumn 2019—i.e. before the start of the pandemic—a total of 85,075 deaths were predicted for 2020. This figure has now been exceeded by 5,442 deaths or 6.4% (Sieben Prozent der Toten, 2021).

There were also a few positive news items: suicides hardly increased because of the pandemic. And there was hardly anyone falling ill with influenza in 2020/21, which usually claims many lives, especially in the winter months (the peak in the recent past was in 2016/17, when 4,400 people died; in 2019/20 it had been 834) (Erstmals seit Jahrzehnten, 2021) (Table 4.2).

4.5 The Financial Burden of the Lockdowns

Martin Kocher, one of Austria's best-known living economists (specialising in behavioural economics), who became Minister of Labour in January 2021, estimated the costs of the lockdown in November 2020 at an average of €1 to 1.5 billion per week, compared to 2 billion during the lockdown in spring 2020. Without a lockdown, however, Kocher said the damage would have been even greater: Economic activity would probably have declined for months if infection rates had remained high. According to Kocher, the school closures were also associated with long-term economic consequences. The costs were high for both the students and the parents—for the latter, because the lockdown could make it difficult for them to reconcile work and childcare, thus reducing productivity ("IHS: Lockdown", 2020).

In January 2021, the damages of a one-week lockdown in Austria were specified as follows: €1.1 billion direct loss of sales (retail 500 million, hotel industry 255 million, gastronomy 200 million, arts/entertainment/recreation 100 million, personal services 40 million) plus 660 million indirect effects (of which 400 million alone for suppliers of retail, gastronomy, hotel industry) ("Kosten: Wer wird", 2021).

Table 4.2 Reported COVID-19 cases and deaths in the EU, December 5, 2021, at 5:45 a.m. ET, According to the Johns Hopkins University Center for Systems Science and Engineering

Country	Cases	...per 100 K people	Deaths	...per 100 K people
France	7,685,153	11,460	117,065	175
Germany	6,177,992	7,431	103,043	124
Spain	5,202,958	11,052	88,159	187
Italy	5,094,072	8,448	134,152	222
Poland	3,671,421	9,669	85,675	226
Netherlands	2,728,876	15,744	19,642	113
Czech Rep	2,240,721	21,001	33,665	316
Belgium	1,827,467	15,913	27,167	237
Romania	1,785,120	9,222	57,021	295
Slovakia	1,230,343	22,558	14,826	272
Sweden	1,212,145	11,785	15,170	147
Austria	1,198,478	13,501	12,796	144
Portugal	1,163,001	11,325	18,514	180
Hungary	1,134,869	11,616	35,122	359
Greece	962,695	8,983	18,516	173
Bulgaria	702,454	10,070	28,805	413
Croatia	628,241	15,445	11,150	274
Ireland	589,094	11,921	5,707	115
Denmark	506,085	8,698	2,939	51
Lithuania	479,839	17,218	6,847	246
Slovenia	430,064	20,597	5,303	254
Latvia	257,329	13,453	4,267	223
Estonia	224,993	16,960	1,823	137
Finland	191,226	3,464	1,360	25
Cyprus	136,525	11,391	601	50
Luxembourg	90,774	14,643	880	142
Malta	39,865	7,931	468	93

Source Tracking Covid-19's global spread (2021)

4.6 State Support for Companies

The Austrian Government reached an agreement with the banks that in 2020 a good part of the loans, especially to private individuals and small businesses, would not be called in, even if there were defaults. The deferrals initially ran until the end of January 2021.

Without the massive state support, tens of thousands of companies would already have been insolvent in 2020 and unemployment would be much higher; "rebuilding" after the virus would be even more difficult. But the state measures meant that in 2020 there were even far fewer corporate and personal insolvencies than in a "normal" year, specifically 3,155 corporate insolvencies (of which the largest item was "financial services/other services" with 667 companies), which was 37.6% less than in 2019 with 5,059 insolvencies (of which the largest item was "financial services/other services" with 1,003) (Bachner, 2021).

At the end of February 2021, the Government announced a reform of insolvency law, the central point of which is that the debt relief period for companies will drop from five to three years. This is a reaction to the fear expressed by many politicians, stakeholders and entrepreneurs that there will be a wave of insolvencies in 2021. In contrast, at the beginning of January 2021, the head oft he Economic Chamber, Harald Mahrer (People's Party), a confidant of Chancellor Kurz, said that one could "not say at all" that "there will be a wave of insolvencies" (Novak & Hofer, 2021) However, Mahr is a lobbyist who has already been wrong about many things—also and precisely because he believes he has to put himself before his clientele (i.e. the entrepreneurs) or "reassure" them.

Willibald Cernko, management board member for corporate clients at Austria's largest bank, Die Erste, pointed out at the beginning of January 2021 that the Government measures to save businesses from the effects of the pandemic would inevitably end. However, these initiatives had also helped companies that were not financially healthy even before the crisis. Therefore, it is, according to Cernko, only necessary to continue to support companies with promising business models. But then, of course, the question arises as to how this should be decided. Cernko proposed to have accountants assess the respective business model at the behest of the company's creditors—with a view to whether the company has a chance to get back on its feet later on; and only then should it be financed by the state through the crisis. In general, Cernko criticised that the equity capitalization of many companies in Austria was too low (Kleedorfer, 2021)—a problem that has been known for many years, but which has admittedly become even more acute under the conditions of the pandemic-induced economic slump.

4.7 Overstretching the Welfare State?

In a modern society and economy based on the division of labour, even minor disruptions in the function of one subsystem can have a massive impact on other subsystems and lead to far-reaching consequences. However, the pandemic does not damage "only" one subsystem, but several at the same time. Pandemics have massive economic effects that can be very long-term. During a pandemic, for example, the health system incurs considerable costs and hospital capacities have to be expanded. Medicines, tests, medical equipment etc. are often scarce and expensive. Normal economic activity is inevitably disrupted or partially interrupted. Many companies produce less or have to close down altogether because workers are ill or stay at home to protect themselves from infection. Thus, supply chains are delayed, interrupted or disrupted. In addition, activities where large numbers of people gather in relatively small spaces have to be cancelled or at least curtailed. This financially damages event organisers, hotels and other businesses, and eventually public transport, etc.

The decline in economic activity reduces the tax revenues of the state, which also faces the problem of massively increasing public expenditure (for health care and support for the economy and the unemployed). For all these reasons, the welfare state is in danger of being overstretched—also in Austria with its GDP of €397,575 billion (GDP per capita €44,780) in 2019. Total social expenditure had amounted to €113,668 billion in that year (Sozialausgaben, 2020). The majority of expenditure on social benefits in Austria is in the area of old age: in 2019, €51.2 billion was spent on old-age benefits, which was 45% of total expenditure on social benefits (1980: 34%, 1990: 39, 2000: 40 and 2010: 43). In second place with a share of 27% (1980: 29%, 1990 and 2000: 26, 2010: 25) was expenditure on sickness/health care amounting to €30.3 billion. More than 70% of social expenditure thus went to old-age and health care benefits. Significantly lower shares of expenditure went to social benefits in other functions (families/children: 9%, disability and surviving dependants: 6% each, unemployment: 5%, housing/social exclusion: 2%) (Sozialausgaben, 2021).

In an intra-EU comparison, Austria is one of the countries with the highest social expenditure. In 2018, it spent 29.1% of GDP on social affairs; this share was higher only in Germany (29.6), Finland (30.1) and France (33.7). The EU-27 average (i.e. excluding the United Kingdom) was 27.9% (Sozialausgaben in % des BIP, 2020). Given the expansion of benefits in the COVID-19 crisis, such as for families or the unemployed, a further increase in the welfare ratio across the EU is expected in 2021.

4.8 Developments on the Labour Market

At the end of April 2020, 522,253 people were unemployed and 49,224 were in training, which meant that a total of 571,477 people were looking for jobs; this was compared to only 53,846 "immediately available" vacancies (Übersicht über den Arbeitsmarkt, 2020). Many factories and production facilities came to a standstill, offices remained closed, employees were either on holiday or in home office. Only the employees of "system-relevant" sectors such as health care, energy supply, etc. were working "normally" for the most part. According to Austria's Ministry of Labour, 392,000 people were registered as unemployed at the end of November 2020, 66,000 in training and 276,400 in short-time work (Sempelmann, 2020, p. 101). At the end of December 2020, 459,700 people were unemployed (which was 31.4% more than in December 2019), in addition to 61,200 training participants (which was 5.4% more than in December 2019); thus, in total, 521,000 people were jobless in December 2020 (which was 27.7% more than in December 2019) (Winterer, 2021, p. 18). This was the highest level since 1945.

400,000 people were on short-time work in December 2020. The proportion of long-term unemployed rose to a record 171,000 in mid-December 2020 (by then the highest level had been in 2017 with 164,000) ("Langzeitarbeitslose: Rekord", 2021).

People with low levels of education suffer disproportionately from any crisis, and the situation caused by COVID-19 was, of course, no exception.

At the beginning of January 2021, 469,772 people were unemployed, and another 62,979 were undergoing training (in total, this was 532,751 and thus about 112,000 or 26% more than a year earlier). In addition, 414,773 people were on short-time work. Until January 2021, €5.6 billion were paid out to support short-time work. For this third phase of short-time work, which runs until the end of March 2021, €4 billion had been approved (Knapp 533.000 Menschen, 2021).

Short-time work is considered the most important instrument for job preservation in Austria. From the perspective of the Ministry of Labour, it has secured more than 1 million jobs by the beginning of January 2021, half of them in goods production and trade. 94.5% of the people who were on short-time work in April 2020 were still in employment at the end of October 2020.

Towards the end of February 2021, around 485,000 people were on short-time work. In addition, there were 441,482 unemployed and 71,416 training participants (Coronakrise hat Wirtschaft, 2021). At the same time, Labour Minister Kocher said that the easing of the lockdown had brought relief to the labour market: In the three weeks before, about 120,000 people had been able to take up regular jobs again. Due to the opening steps in trade, almost 20,000 people have found their way back into employment (Zahrer, 2021).

4.9 Government Support Schemes for the Economy

To an initial rescue package of €38 billion by the Austrian Government, another €12 billion was added in June 2020 for new measures as well as climate protection investments. The agreed package should primarily benefit businesses, but also provide relief for private individuals. According to Finance Minister Gernot Blümel (People's Party), just under €29 billion of the total €50 billion had been committed or already paid out as of the end of December 2020 (Staatliche Hilfszahlungen, 2021).

After the rebound in the third quarter of, 2020 (plus 12% compared to the previous quarter), domestic economic output declined again as a result of the measures taken in the second lockdown: in the fourth quarter, Austria's GDP fell by 4.3% compared to the third. Year-on-year, this meant a decline of 7.8% compared to the fourth quarter of 2019 (this comparable figure was 4.8% for the EU as a whole).

Renewed restrictive measures to contain the COVID-19 pandemic in the fourth quarter of 2020 mainly affected the consumer-related service sectors. Value added in trade, accommodation, food services and transport fell by 19.7%; in other services, which include personal services (e.g. hairdressers), arts, entertainment and recreation, the decline in value added was 25.2% (both compared to the previous quarter). In unison, household consumption demand (including non-profit institutions serving households) also fell sharply again (down 8.3% from the third quarter of 2020). Industrial and construction activity, on the other hand, was more stable, with value added in industry rising by 1% in the fourth quarter. A decline of 1.6% was recorded in the construction industry. Foreign trade dynamics continued to be marked by the global downturn, with exports falling by 1.1% and imports by 0.7%. Investment demand, on the other hand, developed stably—gross fixed capital formation hardly changed in comparison to the previous month (plus 0.1%) (BIP sank im IV. Quartal, 2020, 2021).

At the end of January 2021, the Ministry of Finance reported that the COVID-19 crisis had torn a hole of €22.5 billion in the budget in 2020: Government revenues of €73.6 billion were offset by expenditures of €96.1 billion. Or in other words, revenues collapsed by a full 8.4% in 2020 compared to 2019, while expenditure rose by 22% in parallel. In 2020, the Government budgeted a total of €28 billion to deal with the effects of the pandemic, of which €20.8 billion was paid out or granted as tax relief. By the end of January 2021, more than €31 billion had been paid out or legally committed (Krise lässt Budgetloch, 2021).

For 2021, economists from the Vienna-based think tank Agenda Austria calculated several scenarios for the development of the Austrian economy. In the best case, there is economic growth of 4.4, in the worst of 0.4%. In the first case, GDP would be €28.2 billion lower than without the crisis, with 2.8% growth the loss would be €34 billion, and with 0.4% it would be €42.7 billion. In addition, there will be additional federal expenditure, which according to the Government's budget decisions in autumn 2020 will amount to €14.4 billion. This means that the years 2020 and 2021 together will cost €101.2 billion in the best case; if things go less well (which is to be expected), it could be over €115 billion. And on top of that, there will be additional COVID-19-related expenditure in subsequent years (Schweiger, 2020, pp. 28–29).

Very popular in the EU and also in Austria in view of the pandemic is the idea that one must or can "invest one's way out of the crisis" or "take out strong economic stimulus packages": of course, only the state can do this on a large scale. Supporters of this policy like to point out that interest rates on these loans have been low for a long time and that all alternatives are much worse. Critics hardly spoke out; Stefan Aust, a well-known journalist in Germany, represented an absolute minority opinion when he remarked that "tomorrow's tax money" was currently being spent. And: "This is not really social, because future generations are left out in the cold" (Lauterbach, 2020).

According to the mainstream opinion, the interests of future generations have to take a back seat when it comes to the present and (which, of course, no one says openly) the next elections, which are always coming up somewhere.

Very popular is the demand to "invest one's way out of the crisis" primarily by investing in "green technologies" to combat climate change. Here, of course, fundamental contradictions arise, also and especially in Austria and Germany: on the one hand, they want to switch to renewable energy as far as possible; on the other hand, majority or largely state-owned energy companies, including Austria's OMV, are also and especially building infrastructure projects such as the Nord Stream II gas pipeline running along the bottom of the Baltic Sea, which will make the EU and many of its member states (even) more dependent on unreliable Russian supplies; and fossil fuels are driving climate change: It is demonstrably false that—as oil and gas companies (including, of course, OMV) claim—natural gas is "particularly environmentally friendly" (Borunda, 2020). And the discussions in Austria's politics, media and public largely ignore the fact that the country accounts for only about 0.2% of global CO2 emissions: Even if it were to disappear from the map without a trace from one day to the next, the effect would hardly be reflected in the statistics.

4.10 Criticism of the Government's Actions Against the Pandemic

In many, if not all, EU countries—and therefore also in Austria—there were registered and unregistered rallies against the lockdowns, masking, a feared compulsory vaccination, etc. But sometimes tens of thousands showed up. Some demonstrations against the pandemic measures were banned by the authorities and took place anyway, without then being broken up by the police (although this had actually been threatened). This concerned, for example, a rally (described by the organisers as a "walk") with several thousand participants, including the extreme right-wing "Identitarian" Martin Sellner and the convicted neo-Nazi Gottfried Küssel, on January 31, 2021, at which social distancing and the obligation to wear a mask were demonstratively disregarded. Four police officers were injured, ten people arrested and 800 charges filed. Minister of the Interior Karl Nehammer (People's Party) condemned—not for the first and not for the last time—the alleged or actual role of his predecessor in office Herbert Kickl (Freedom Party) in the incidents. According to Nehammer, it is "completely absurd that a former interior minister is adding fuel to the flames and forging unholy alliances with right-wing radicals" (Verletzte, Festnahmen, 2021).

Of course, by no means all demonstrators were radical and/or conspiracy theorists: among them were also supporters of the Social Democrats, environmental activists, people without recognisable or clear political sympathies and people who had lost their jobs or were afraid for them. However, Austria's Federal Office for the Protection of the Constitution and Counterterrorism warned against "extremists and radicals" among the demonstrators: such would "consciously and deliberately" carry out agitation against democracy and the rule of law under the pretext of a protest against the measures to combat the pandemic. According to the Federal Office's findings, there were calls on social networks for attacks on police stations, for arson in Parliament, the Federal Chancellery and other Government buildings, for the assault on Parliament (which, of course, immediately brought to mind the "capture" of the Capitol in Washington, D.C. by supporters of outgoing U.S. President Donald Trump on January 6, 2021) and the Austrian Broadcasting Corporation as well as for "civil war" in general ("Nehammer: Rechtsextreme", 2021). It was revealing, however, that nobody had the idea of demonstrating in front of the Viennese embassy of the country—China—from which the COVID-19-pandemic had originated.

For many months, the Freedom Party played the "background music" in the National Council to the activities of its sympathisers and functionaries on the streets.

For example, its MP Axel Kassegger said: "The Corona crisis is being exploited to strengthen multilateral sectors. The UN, NGOs and the so-called 'civil society' are to be given more power. Nation states are to be weakened, if not dissolved, which we strictly reject" (FPÖ setzt in Nationalrats-Debatten, 2020). Kickl, known for his brute rhetoric, but also other Freedom Party functionaries warned of a "corona dictatorship" (Pressekonferenz mit Herbert Kickl, 2020), a "new epidemic dictatorship", an "all-powerful state", a "paternalistic state", etc. as well as of compulsory vaccination (which the Government has admittedly always ruled out). However, the liberal opposition party Neos also—much more rarely, but nevertheless—hit the wrong tone e.g. when its chairwoman Beate Meinl-Reisinger accused the Government of "police state methods" (Bauer, 2020, p. 30).

On the internet, and especially in the social networks, anger about the state restrictions was expressed, with some resorting to conspiracy theories. Here, too, Austria was no different from other comparable countries. In any case, as the Viennese weekly *Profil* put it at the beginning of December 2020, "forces are at work in the networks that are fuelling these emotions and steering them in one direction: against the Governments, against their measures and against all recognised scientific findings. There is a disinformation campaign underway." The EU's East StratCom Task Force, which was in 2015 created as part of the European External Action Service to detect disinformation on the internet and combat it with objective information, found out that during the COVID-19 crisis "a large part of the senders of the curly messages are pro-Kremlin". The aim of this disinformation is to stir up tensions and incite conflicts among the population or between the population and the Governments in the Western countries in order to undermine the political capacity of the states (Geets & Treichler, 2020, p. 46). Certainly, Austria is much too small to be a "special target" of this disinformation about public health; it is only on the periphery of the attention of international troll factories. But this does not mean that this disinformation disguised as "critical information" does not find its recipients in Austria at all. And it is also difficult even for a large organization like the EU to counter this disinformation: brittle fact-checks almost inevitably generate far fewer clicks to simple and crude propaganda that may serve long-standing prejudices in the imaginations of many people.

Criticism of the Austrian Government's handling of the pandemic did not come from the radical right alone but also from the radical left, and the terminology was at times indistinguishable: for example, two left-wing Austrian authors said that the measures to combat the pandemic were "worse than the virus itself"; "politics" was pursuing a "panic course" (Hofbauer & Kraft, 2020, pp. 7–8). Several political "camps" (i.e. not only radicals) shared the fear that the pandemic was a pretext for the Austrian Government to gain as much information as possible about the citizens and their state of health. And that, in turn, was—according to this opinion—a (further) step towards a "surveillance state" and a "transparent citizen" whose privacy is becoming increasingly restricted *vis-à-vis* the state. Another relevant theory is that "those in power" could use the virus crisis to "stifle democracy and establish a form of authoritarian rule" (Krastev, 2020, p. 47). However, this is not yet emerging in any EU country; authoritarian tendencies, especially in Hungary and Poland, had already existed long before 2020.

4.11 The Role of the EU: Comparisons of Austria with Other EU Members

Health policy was always within the competence of the member states and thus not of the EU. Thus, the EU members declared their respective lockdowns completely independently of each other, which, however, is difficult to criticise: the conditions in the member states were objectively very different, why should Portugal have "coordinated" with Finland, Ireland with Greece? The EU members among the countries bordering the Alps in the 2020–2021 season also practised different approaches to winter tourism: France, Italy and Germany kept their ski lifts closed, while Austria opened them. And all EU members issued travel warnings for other EU countries.

In the face of the pandemic, the EU's role was small at first, but increased over the course of 2020—it became involved in jointly promoting research and development, funding, procurement and distribution of vaccine. In July 2020 the European Council agreed to a recovery fund of €750 billion branded Next Generation EU (NGEU) in order to support member states hit by the COVID-19 pandemic. The NGEU fund goes over the years 2021–2023 and will be tied to the 2021–2027 budget of the EU (MFF). The comprehensive packages of NGEU and MFF will reach the size of €1,824.3 billion (Special European Council, 2020).

The EU's COVID-19 aid fund of €750 billion is to go primarily to southern European countries. This first opportunity for the EU Commission to take on debt was celebrated by some media as an "amazingly far-reaching step towards integration" (Krupa, 2020)—but de facto it will amount to the richer states in the north of the EU having to pay for the poorer states in the south.

Under the NGEU, €312.5 billion will be given as non-repayable grants to EU members. Spain will receive the most—almost €70 billion, followed by Italy with €69 billion, France with €40 billion and Germany with €25.6 billion. Austria is promised €3.3 billion (in total, as of the beginning of February 2021, it is paying in about 12 billion, i.e. 8.7 billion is, as Finance Minister Blümel said, a "solidarity contribution for countries that are economically worse off" [Salomon & Bachner, 2021, p. 7]).

At the beginning of February 2021, the EU Parliament voted with a broad majority in favour of the Reconstruction and Resilience Facility, the core of the CoV reconstruction fund, which is endowed with a total of €672.5 billion, of which €312.5 billion is to flow into member states as grants and €360 billion as loans for reforms and investments. The EU Commission is to raise the necessary money on the financial markets. For this, the national parliaments of the member states still have to ratify separate resolutions. In the next step, the national governments submit spending plans to Brussels to request the release of the funds. These plans are to be submitted by the end of April 2021 and must be examined by the Commission and then adopted by the Council of Member States (Parlament segnet CoV-Aufbaufonds, 2021).

The EU's crisis management was judged sceptically to critically practically from the beginning of the pandemic—even by its own senior officials. The Bulgarian-born public intellectual Ivan Krastev (2020), who is anything but an "anti-European", opined in a volume published relatively early after the outbreak of the pandemic (also) in Europe that the EU proved to be "structurally unsuited to mitigate the unfolding [COVID-19] catastrophe, an irrelevant actor at the very moment when people were seeking shelter" (p. 77).

The European Commissioner for Budget and Administration, Austria's Johannes Hahn (People's Party), openly admitted (probably also because it would have been pointless to deny it) that the EU was not prepared for the pandemic (Lampl, 2020, p. 49). And European Commission President Ursula von der Leyen (by the way, a medical doctor) admitted in early February 2021 that the EU was late to authorise COVID-19 vaccines and "we're still not where we want to be". She also acknowledged the EU had been overconfident about production targets being met amid delays at factories (Covid: EU's von der Leyen admits, 2021). In addition, the EU was still dealing with the consequences of the United Kingdom's exit from the EU; the negotiations to avoid a "hard" Brexit were concluded just in time at the end of December 2020.

As to Austria, the economic slump in 2020 was bigger than the average for Eurozone members. And unemployment in Austria increased more than in the Eurozone and the average of the entire EU compared to the initial level.

The following picture prevailed for government debt in the EU countries in relation to the GDP in the third quarter of, 2020: Greece had the highest government debt ratio within the EU in the third quarter of, 2020 at around 199.9% of GDP. Italy had the second highest debt at 154.2% of GDP, followed by Portugal at 130.8%. At the other end of the list was Estonia with a debt ratio of around 18.5% of GDP. All 27 EU countries had an average debt of around 89.8% of economic output, the members of the Eurozone an average of around 97.3% of GDP. Austria was comparatively well off at 79.1%, but Germany was even better at 70% (Third quarter of 2020, 2021, p. 4).

In the pandemic year 2020, Austria's economic performance recorded the most striking decline since 1945 with a minus of 6.6%. GDP thus fell by 2.8 per centage points more than in 2009 due to the financial crisis. At minus 5.7%, the decline in the fourth quarter of 2020 compared to the fourth quarter of 2019 was smaller than originally feared. Only in Portugal (6.1%), Italy (6.6%), Croatia (7.1%) and Spain (9.1%) this decline was greater (Österreichs Wirtschaftsleistung im 4. Quartal 2020, 2021).

The aforementioned 4.3% quarter-on-quarter contraction in Austria's GDP in the fourth quarter of 2020 was the largest relevant figure in the entire EU (where the average figure was only 0.5%) (Schnauder & Laufer, 2021). The reasons for this were controversially discussed in Austria. The Government endeavoured to put this decline into perspective on the one hand and to explain it with tourism on the other. Finance

Minister Blümel pointed out that tourism, with a share of more than 5% of Austria's economic output, was almost twice as big as the EU average. However, economists argued that tourism could not be the only explanation: the sector that slumped the most towards the end of 2020 was "other services" (as called in the statistics). Here, there was a minus of 25% compared to the previous quarter. This includes personal services such as beauty salons and hairdressers, but also sports, culture and entertainment, which is particularly large in Austria. According to a study by Oxford University, Austria is one of the countries that have taken particularly rigorous measures since the outbreak of the pandemic: As of February 2021, the number of days in "hard lockdowns" was comparatively high at 79 ("Studie: Versammlungsverbot", 2020; Schnauder, 2021) (Table 4.3).

Before the COVID-19 crisis, Austria in 2020 was predicted to have an economic growth rate of 1.2%.

Table 4.3 GDP decline in 2020 compared to 2019 (in %)

Country	Size
Lithuania	0.9
Luxembourg	1.3
Poland	2.7
Sweden	2.8
Finland	2.9
Estonia	2.9
Denmark	3.3
Latvia	3.6
Netherlands	3.8
Germany	4.9
Hungary	5.1
Slovenia	5.5
Czech Republic	5.6
Malta	5.8
Belgium	6.3
Austria	**6.6**
Portugal	7.6
France	8.1
Croatia	8.4
Italy	8.9
Spain	11

Source Österreichs Wirtschaftsleistung im 4. Quartal 2020 (2021)

4.12 Austrian Debates About Compulsory Vaccination

Chancellor Kurz said several times in the spring and summer of 2021, literally or in spirit, that "the pandemic is over for those who have been vaccinated". However, this was clearly incorrect for several reasons. For example, even fully vaccinated people can fall ill with COVID-19: according to Austrian data from the second half of September 2021, 16.7% of COVID patients in hospital intensive care units were doubly vaccinated. However, deaths among vaccinated people are rare (about 1.7% of all cases). No serious source doubts that the unvaccinated have a significantly higher risk of severe, life-threatening courses of the disease. However, politicians, the media and the public not only in Austria have often failed to take into account that vaccinated persons can also pass on the virus to unvaccinated and non-immune persons.

As of December 3, 2021, 71.8% of Austrians had received at least one vaccination dose, 67.5% a second vaccination and 23.3% a booster (compared to 71.4%, 68.8% and 10.8% in the entire EU) (Bevölkerungsanteil mit COVID-19-Impfung, 2021). The virologist Dorothee von Laer from the Medical University of Innsbruck (Tyrol) said that the virus is only under control in an entire country when the proportion of immune individuals reaches at least 80% (Winter & Zwins, 2021). But how can this be achieved when the essence of a pandemic are also, and precisely, its cross-border effects? The World Health Organisation, or WHO, has repeatedly emphasised that a global pandemic cannot be "overcome" in an individual country: As long as the virus meets unvaccinated societies, it will mutate again and again—and at worst destroy all progress in vaccination.—But even this approach was not uncontroversial among experts, who objected, among other things, that selective pressure to mutate the virus would arise precisely when it was confronted with a largely vaccinated population. In any case, such largely "unvaccinated societies" are mainly to be found in the Third World; and should most of the countries there be completely sealed off from the "North" in order to possibly impede the spread of ever new mutations of the virus? This is probably neither logistically and technically possible nor politically desirable or feasible.

From the beginning of 2021, the entire government vaccination policy in Austria was based on a single assumption or assertion, which was very aggressively communicated to society by the government and all nationally significant electronic and print media: "The pandemic is a pandemic of the unvaccinated". This sounds, at first glance, very convincing. The possibility that it could at least be simplified hardly occurred in the public discourse in Austria. But in autumn 2021, a study called "Increases in COVID-19 are unrelated to levels of vaccination across 68 countries and 2947 counties in the United States" by S.V. Subramanian and A. Kumar appeared. Immediately, however, debates began about the interpretation of their results. In any case, Subramanian and Kumar did not reject vaccination; but the population should respectfully be encouraged to do it. They argue that vaccination significantly reduces the risk of hospitalisation and mortality and is an important part of any anti-COVID-19 strategy.

Given its very complex circumstances, the pandemic also posed great challenges to both the social sciences and law, including theories of the state. For instance, what *exactly* does "state effectiveness" mean in the context of the topic of this article? Can this really be the ability of a state to put into practice a policy that may be based on highly simplified (or, in extreme cases, even inaccurate) premises? Or more precisely: Is it *really* so simple that the more people a democratic constitutional state vaccinates and the more restrictions it imposes on its population (several of which were overturned by the Austrian Constitutional Court in 2020 and 2021), the more "effective" it can be considered to be? Viable answers to these questions will (at best) be obtained in a few years after the pandemic has subsided.

The Austrian Federal Government, including Chancellors Kurz and Alexander Schallenberg (both from the People's Party) and Health Minister Wolfgang Mueckstein (Greens), repeatedly explicitly ruled out a new lockdown and compulsory vaccination in the summer and well into the autumn of 2021. But on November 22, 2021, the fourth nationwide lockdown began, and about two weeks later, the first draft of a bill on the introduction of compulsory vaccination became known to the public. It provided for administrative fines of up to €3,600 in case of refusal to vaccinate (for comparison: the median net annual income of an Austrian employee is €22,100, according to the latest available figures).

4.13 "State Failure"!?

Not only in the German-speaking countries, many commentators not only in the tabloid press but also in respectable journalism were very quick to use terms such as "state failure", "system failure", "debacle" etc. during and in view of the pandemic. However, this was mostly a buzzword (or even a swear word) and not a category of political science. In Austria, otherwise level-headed commentators sometimes thought they had to take a similar line. Thus, it was said that the country had shown a "state multi-organ failure" in the face of COVID-19 and had lost control of many events during the lockdowns (Schellhorn, 2020). And Hans Rauscher (2021), one of Austria's best-known journalists, said: The "institutions are already crumbling anyway".

Only rarely—e.g. by the director of the Vienna State Opera, whose core expertise is certainly not in the fields of medicine, virology, disease control, economy, political science and/or constitutional law—the argument was put forward that those who would speak of "state failure" with regard to Austria in the COVID 19 context had "never experienced a 'failed state'" (Hilpold, 2021). This sounds plausible only at first glance, because at the second it should be clear that the term "state failure" in Austria or throughout the EU must refer to a different basic understanding of the state, its tasks and functional efficiency than would be the case, for example, in parts of Africa and the Middle East or in Afghanistan.

The institutions of the state and the public infrastructure have not been in danger in Europe and North America because of the pandemic, and this is not likely to be the case in the foreseeable future. This also applies to Austria: the supply of energy, food and most medicines; public transport; the security agencies (which also had to deal with an Islamist-motivated terrorist attack on November 2, 2020 in downtown Vienna); telecommunications; the media, etc. were by and large functioning. Many educational institutions switched to distance learning, which, after initial difficulties, worked out in principle from the spring of 2020 onwards. The political order is also safe: The authoritarian potential in society—i.e. those who reject democracy, want a "strong man" at the top, etc.—has not increased significantly as a result of the pandemic: it fluctuates between 10 and 15% of the population, as it has for many years (Böhmer, 2021).

At the same time, it was impossible to ignore the fact that there were numerous incidents during the pandemic in Austria that are clearly "unworthy" of a modern industrial and constitutional state. For example, in November 2021, the PCR testing system was at times very unreliable: countless results were reported to the tested persons very late or were lost altogether. Sometimes there was conflicting data on basic facts such as how many patients with COVID-19 were actually in the hospitals—and how many of them were in intensive care units. At the beginning of December 2021, a report temporarily caused a stir, according to which it was not even evident how many PCR tests had been done; infection and death figures were not comprehensible, etc. (Brisantes Papier, 2021): How, then, urgent decisions are to be made in politics, health care and administration if not even just that is clear?

The judiciary also sometimes made decisions that various citizens (including some with law degrees on their own) could not comprehend. For example, in November 2021, the Vienna Regional Court for Civil Matters dismissed lawsuits filed because of the above-mentioned incidents in Ischgl, arguing that individuals had "no right to be protected from contagion by the state". The Austrian state could therefore "neither be blamed for culpable nor unlawful conduct" (Zivilrechtsklagen in Causa Ischgl, 2021). And Heinz Mayer, one of Austria's best-known experts on constitutional law, initially (in December 2020) spoke out against compulsory vaccination (even though he considered it legal) because terms like "compulsion" and "duty" would drive many citizens into the camp of opponents of vaccination. A few months later, however, he demanded not only compulsory vaccination but also (literally) "compulsory isolation" of the unvaccinated. This did not in any way trigger significant criticism in the media (where Mayer has been a sought-after interview partner for many years), the judiciary or politics (Beig, 2021).

4.14 Summary, Conclusions and Outlook for the Future

As can be easily seen from the statistics cited, the performance of the Austrian state in the COVID-19 crisis is mediocre at best when compared within the EU. And it was obvious that the "effectiveness" of the three Austrian lockdowns (between mid-March 2020 and February 2021) was steadily decreasing in the sense that people's willingness to comply with the requirements (and in particular to stay at home) was noticeably decreasing. Kurt Kotrschal, a well-known behavioural scientist in Austria, commented: Austrians "don't like to abide by rules ... Somehow it's snazzy for the Austrian to commit gentle violations of the law. It's not any different in the Corona crisis" (Metzger, 2021).

The discourse in the media, politics and academia in Western Europe and North America, which was related to the state in the face of COVID-19, showed even more contradictions. Thus, in the face of alleged "state failure" in Europe, some—especially left-wing—politicians, economists, scholars, etc. called for the nationalization of vaccine production facilities (Widmann & Stefan, 2021). And how are the diagnoses of a "return" of the state compatible with its alleged "failure"? Is the state "failing" or "returning"? Or is it "failing" in its "return"?

In addition, there is a fundamental analytical problem: what do "strength" and "weakness" of the state actually mean—what content is attached to these terms? "Strength" can be understood to mean military capabilities and centralism of the state system as well as the effectiveness of the administration, social and other security of the population, and so on. In the discourse in the German-speaking countries, including Austria, the—albeit well-founded—opinion that the state is not only not strengthened by the pandemic but *weakened* as a result is rarely expressed—"simply because it is running out of money. When the virus crisis—hopefully—ends at some point, it will in all likelihood be replaced by a budget crisis" (Bollmann, 2020). And it is immediately obvious that without a functioning private sector, an effective public health system cannot be adequately financed. In any case, almost since the beginning of the fight against the pandemic in many EU countries, including Austria, radical parties and groups have tried to instrumentalise the crisis in their own interests.

There is no doubt that COVID-19 is exacerbating the problems in those countries, especially in the "global South", whose bureaucratic apparatus and infrastructure have never been particularly effective anyway. Richard N. Haass, President of the Council on Foreign Relations (United States), even expected an increase in the number of failed states in the wake of the coronavirus crisis (Haass, 2020). Of course, this can only be confirmed or falsified in the long run. But the pandemic has also revealed numerous deficits in state bureaucracy, administration and infrastructure in the EU (including Austria) and North America. Admittedly, this stress test offers the opportunity to learn lessons and remedy weak points. It remains to be seen whether this will actually happen to the necessary extent after the pandemic.

The year 2020 has drastically changed the public perception of what is possible in politics, also and especially in Western and Central Europe—and, of course, in Austria. In politics, the media and the public sphere of all EU members sometimes emotional debates are taking place about state orders against COVID-19, demanded by ones in order to protect public health but vehemently rejected by others as "restrictions on freedom". Much less public attention, however, has been paid to the fact that massive mistakes were made not only since the outbreak of the pandemic in Europe but long before: The EU as well as its member states have allowed many indispensable goods for coping with pandemics, such as medicines, masks, medical technology, etc. to be produced in the EU itself either not at all or to a clearly insufficient extent. Therefore, in many cases, one had to rely on the very China where the pandemic had started and which—as practically all figures available at the beginning of 2021 show—is the main economic and (geo)political winner of the crisis. EU policy is still clearly insufficiently sensitised to the fact that it has made itself dependent in an important area on an authoritarian regime in Beijing that primarily uses its foreign economic policy to create and increase the dependencies of other countries, to pursue geopolitical ambitions in general and, concretely, to turn fantasies of world domination into reality.

References

Bachner, M. (2021, February 21). Schuldenfrei nach 3 Jahren: Neues Insolvenzrecht kommt. *Kurier*, 9.

Bauer, G. (2020). Parteien in der Krise. *Profil, 51*, 29–30.

Beig, S. (2021, November 20). Verfassungsrechtler Heinz Mayer fordert "Zwangs-Isolierung" für Ungeimpfte. *Exxpress*. https://exxpress.at/verfassungsrechtler-heinz-mayer-fordert-zwangs-isolierung-fuer-impfverweigerer/

Bevölkerungsanteil mit COVID-19-Impfung nach ausgewählten Ländern weltweit. (2021, December 3). *Statista*. https://de.statista.com/statistik/daten/studie/1203308/umfrage/impfstoff abdeckung-der-bevoelkerung-gegen-das-coronavirus-nach-laendern/

BIP sank im IV. Quartal 2020 um 4,3%. (2021, January 29). *WIFO*. https://www.wifo.ac.at/news/bip_sank_im_iv_quartal_2020_um_43

Böhmer, C. (2021, January 6). Haben Erinnerung an Pandemien verdrängt [interview with Oliver Rathkolb]. *Kurier*, 6.

Brisantes Papier: Österreichs Corona-Zahlen völlig falsch. (2021, December 6). *Heute*. https://www.heute.at/s/brisantes-papier-oesterreichs-corona-zahlen-voellig-falsch-100177614

Bollmann, R. (2020, December 27). Wie Corona den Staat schwächt. *Frankfurter Allgemeine Zeitung*. https://www.faz.net/aktuell/wirtschaft/konjunktur/schulden-hoch-wie-nie-cor ona-schwaecht-den-staat-17118925.html

Borunda, A. (2020, February 19). Natural gas is a much 'dirtier' energy source than we thought. *National Geographic*. https://www.nationalgeographic.com/science/article/super-pot ent-methane-in-atmosphere-oil-gas-drilling-ice-cores

Coronakrise hat Wirtschaft weiter fest im Griff. (2021, February 23). *BVZ.at*. https://www.bvz.at/in-ausland/513-000-ohne-job-coronakrise-hat-wirtschaft-weiter-fest-im-griff-oesterreich-arbeit slosigkeit-arbeitsmarkt-arbeitsmarktdaten-oesterreich-250573462

Covid: EU's von der Leyen admits vaccine rollout shortcomings. (2021, February 10). *BBC News*. https://www.bbc.com/news/world-europe-56009251

Erstmals seit Jahrzehnten keine Grippewelle in Österreich. (2021, January 29). *Austria Presse Agentur*. https://science.apa.at/power-search/8337606152805984291

FPÖ setzt in Nationalrats-Debatten klare Akzente. (2020, October 14). *FPÖ*. https://www.fpoe.at/artikel/fpoe-setzt-in-nationalrats-debatten-klare-akzente/

Geets, S., & Treichler, R. (2020). Das große Murren. *Profil, 50*, 44–47.

GHS Index—Global Health Security Index. Building Collective Action and Accountability. (2019, October). *Nuclear Threat Initiative, Johns Hopkins Center for Health Security, and The Economist Intelligence Unit*. https://www.ghsindex.org/wp-content/uploads/2020/04/2019-Global-Health-Security-Index.pdf

Haass, R. N. (2020). More failed states. *Foreign Policy, 236*, 13.

Hilpold, S. (2021, November 27/28). Mir ist das zu aufgeregt [Interview with Bogdan Roščić]. *Der Standard*, 31.

4 The Austrian State and the COVID-19 Crisis … 73

Hofbauer, H., & Kraft, S. (Eds.). (2020). *Lockdown 2020. Wie ein Virus dazu verwendet wird, die Gesellschaft zu verändern*. Promedia.

IHS: Lockdown könnte pro Woche 1 bis 1,5 Milliarden Euro kosten. (2020, November 16). *Kurier*. https://kurier.at/wirtschaft/kocher-lockdown-koennte-pro-woche-1-bis-15-mrd-euro-kos ten/401099214

Kleedorfer, R. (2021, January 6). Private Investoren sollen Firmen retten. *Kurier*, 10.

Knapp 533.000 Menschen suchen derzeit Arbeit. (2021, January 12). *ORF*. https://orf.at/#/stories/ 3196986/

Kosten: Wer wird das bezahlen? (2021, January 6). *Kronen Zeitung*, 3.

Krastev, I. (2020). *Ist heute schon morgen? Wie die Pandemie Europa verändert*. Ullstein.

Krise lässt Budgetloch auf 22,5 Milliarden wachsen. (2021, January 31). *ORF*. https://orf.at/stories/ 3199633/

Krupa, M. (2020, December 30). Das Machtbündnis. *Die Zeit* (Austrian edition), 1.

Lampl, A. (2020). Künftig stärker durchgreifen [interview with Johannes Hahn]. *Trend, 51–52*, 48–52.

Langzeitarbeitslose: Rekord. (2021, January 6). *Kronen Zeitung*, 19.

Lauterbach, J. (2020, November 29). Der Angriff des Staates auf das Private [Interview mit Stefan Aust]. *Welt am Sonntag*. https://www.welt.de/regionales/hamburg/article221195938/Ste fan-Aust-Nun-wird-in-die-familiaeren-Einheiten-buergerlicher-Bereiche-eingegriffen.html

Metzger, I. (2021, February 7). Ein Land des "passiven Widerstandes" [interview with Kurt Kotrschal]. *Kurier*, 22.

Nehammer: Rechtsextreme "treibende Kräfte" der Corona-Leugner. (2021, January 5). *Die Presse*. https://www.diepresse.com/5919149/nehammer-rechtsextreme-treibende-krafte-der-cor ona-leugner

Niblett, R. (2020). The end of globalization as we know it. *Foreign Policy, 236*, 10.

Nowak, R., & Hofer, G. (2021, January 3). Debatte über Skilifte ist total scheinheilig [interview with Harald Mahrer]. *Die Presse am Sonntag*, 20.

Österreichs Wirtschaftsleistung im 4. Quartal 2020 um 5,7% gesunken, Rückgang von 6,6% für 2020. Korrigierte Pressemitteilung: 12.461-052/21. (2021, March 3). *Statistik Austria*. https:// www.statistik.at/web_de/presse/125514.html

Parlament segnet CoV-Aufbaufonds in Milliardenhöhe ab. (2021, February 10). *ORF*. https://orf. at/stories/3200868/

Pressekonferenz mit Herbert Kickl: "Initiativen gegen die schwarz-grüne Corona-Diktatur". (2020, December 12). *YouTube*. https://www.youtube.com/watch?v=ruz-fjCcOa0

Rauscher, H. (2021, January 25). Pandemie-Zeiten: Zeichen und Wunder. *Der Standard*. https:// www.derstandard.at/story/2000123605351/pandemie-zeiten-zeichen-und-wunder

Rosner, S. (2020, December 19/20). Wie der Massentest scheiterte. *Wiener Zeitung*, 4–5.

Rosner, S. (2021, February 27/28). Wie Corona die Todessstatistik prägte. *Wiener Zeitung*, 4.

Salomon, M., & Bachner, M. (2021, February 7). Für die Moral der Menschen ist es ein richtiger Schritt [interview with Gernot Blümel]. *Kurier*, 6–7.

Sauer, B. (2004/2011). Staat. In G. Göhler, M. Iser, & I. Kerner (Eds.), *Politische Theorie. 25 umkämpfte Begriffe zur Einführung* (2nd ed., pp. 339–355). VS Verlag für Sozialwissenschaften.

Schellhorn, F. (2016, January 14). Wie viel Staat darf's denn sein? *Die Zeit*, 10.

Schellhorn, F. (2020). Staatliches Multiorganversagen. *Profil, 49*, 34.

Schnauder, A. (2021, Februar 17). Ist der Tourismus wirklich der Hauptgrund für Österreichs Absturz? *Der Standard*, 6.

Schnauder, A., & Laufer, N. (2021, February 2). Österreich erleidet stärksten Wirtschaftseinbruch in der EU. *Der Standard*. https://www.derstandard.at/story/2000123812237/oesterreich-erleidet-staerksten-wirtschaftseinbruch-in-der-eu

Schuster, J. (2020, March 22). Wer wird uns helfen? Der Nationalstaat. *Die Welt*. https://www.welt. de/debatte/kommentare/article206726355/Corona-Nicht-die-EU-hilft-den-Buergern-sondern-Vater-Staat.html

Schweiger, R. (2020). Das 100-Milliarden-Euro-Ding. *Profil, 48*, 26–30.

Sempelmann, P. (2020). Arbeit, nicht um jeden Preis. *Trend, 51–52*, 100–103.

Sieben Prozent der Toten 2020 durch CoV. (2021, February 26). *ORF*. https://oesterreich.orf.at/sto ries/3092331/

Sommavilla, F. (2020, May 2/3). Impfpass an der Grenze. *Der Standard*, 10.

Sozialausgaben. (2020, November 24). *Statistik Austria*. https://www.statistik.at/web_de/sta tistiken/menschen_und_gesellschaft/soziales/sozialschutz_nach_eu_konzept/sozialausgaben/ index.html

Sozialausgaben. (2021, January 20). *Statistik Austria*. Austria https://www.statistik.at/web_de/sta tistiken/menschen_und_gesellschaft/soziales/sozialschutz_nach_eu_konzept/sozialausgaben/ index.html#:~:text=Der%20Gro%C3%9Fteil%20der%20Ausgaben%20f%C3%BCr,%25% 20und%202010%3A%2043%25).

Sozialausgaben in % des BIP. (2020, November). *Wirtschaftskammer Österreich*. http://wko.at/sta tistik/eu/europa-sozialausgaben.pdf

Special European Council, 17–21 July 2020. (2020). *European Council*. https://www.consilium.eur opa.eu/en/meetings/european-council/2020/07/17-21/#

Sperandio, S.-C. (2019). Sicherheitsrisiko Pandemie. In Republik Österreich, Bundesminister für Landesverteidigung (Eds.), *Sicher. Und morgen? Sicherheitspolitische Jahresvorschau 2020* (pp. 219–223).

Staatliche Hilfszahlungen. (2021, January 10). *Kurier*, 4.

Studie: Versammlungsverbot und Schulschließung wirksamste Corona-Maßnahmen. (2020, December 18). *Der Standard*. https://www.derstandard.at/story/2000122618940/corona-versam mlungsverbot-laut-studie-das-wirksamste-mittel

Subramanian, S. V., & Kumar, A. (2021). Increases in COVID-19 are unrelated to levels of vaccination across 68 countries and 2947 counties in the United States. *European Journal of Epidemiology*. https://link.springer.com/article/10.1007/s10654-021-00808-7

Third quarter of 2020. Government debt up to 97.3% of GDP in euro area. Up to 89.8% of GDP in EU. Eurostat Newsrelease, Euroindicators, 13/2021. (2021, January 21). *Eurostat*. https://ec.europa.eu/eurostat/documents/portlet_file_entry/2995521/2-21012021-AP-EN.pdf/ a3748b22-e96e-7f62-ba05-11c7192e32f3#:~:text=At%20the%20end%20of%20the%20third% 20quarter%20of%202020%2C%20debt,3.1%25%20of%20EU%20government%20debt.

Tracking Covid-19's global spread. (2021, February 22). *CNN*. https://edition.cnn.com/interactive/ 2020/health/coronavirus-maps-and-cases/

Übersicht über den Arbeitsmarkt April 2020. (2020, May). *AMS*. https://www.ams.at/content/ dam/download/arbeitsmarktdaten/%C3%B6sterreich/berichte-auswertungen/001_uebersicht_a ktuell_0420.pdf

Ultsch, C. (2021, January 3). Warum impft Österreich so langsam? *Die Presse am Sonntag*, 1.

Verletzte, Festnahmen und Politstreit. (2021, January 31). *ORF*. https://orf.at/stories/3199689/

Walt, S. M. (2020). A world less open, prosperous, and free. *Foreign Policy, 236*, 10.

Widmann, A., Stefan, L., & Schnauder, A. (2021). Ist Impfstoff herstellen Staatsaufgabe? *Der Standard*, 7.

Winter, J., & Zwins, K. (2021, October 1). Corona-Experten zu Kanzler Kurz: "Pandemie ist für keinen vorbei". *Profil*. https://www.profil.at/faktiv/corona-experten-zu-kanzler-kurz-pandemie-ist-fuer-keinen-vorbei/401754486

Winterer, M. (2020, January 30/31). Vom Büro in die Gosse. *Wiener Zeitung*, 17–18.

Zahrer, L. (2021, February 28). 120.000 Menschen durch Lockerungen aus Kurzarbeit oder Arbeitslosigkeit. *Der Standard*. https://www.derstandard.at/jetzt/livebericht/2000124533264/red content/1000221114

Zivilrechtsklagen in Causa Ischgl wurden abgewiesen. (2021, December 1). *Der Standard*. https://www.derstandard.at/story/2000131583733/zivilrechtsklagen-in-causa-ischgl-wur den-abgewiesen

Martin Malek Born in 1965 in Stockerau (Austria), 1991 Dr. in Political Science (Vienna State University). Since 1997 (civilian) researcher at the Institute for Peace Support and Conflict Management, then at the Institute for Strategy and Security Policy, both of the National Defense Academy (Vienna). Several internships in research institutes and think tanks in Germany, Russia, Ukraine and the U.S. Areas of interest and expertise: State failing theories, theories of separatism, theories of ethnic conflicts, security and military policy in the Commonwealth of Independent States (especially Russia, Ukraine, South Caucasus), post-Soviet language policy, military-industrial complex and arms trade of the post-Soviet republics, relations NATO – CIS and EU – CIS, Eurasian energy policy etc. Author/editor of several books and some 300 articles, published in a dozen countries.

Chapter 5
The Changing Dimensions of India's Foreign Relations During COVID-19

Debasish Nandy and Alik Naha

Abstract This chapter intends to critically analyze India's changing dimensions of foreign policy during COVID-19. India's strategy to counter China in association with Australia, the USA, Japan, and other democratic countries of the world has been highlighted in this chapter. India's policy of 'self-reliant' and financial challenges has been sequentially discussed in this chapter. The chapter will further delineate the relations between the domestic factors and external factors in the formulation of the new orientation-based foreign policy of India. COVID-19, it has been discovered, has taught India a valuable lesson. Due to the pandemic, India's foreign policy focus and equations have been steadily altering. India has attempted to improve its acceptability in the post-COVID world with a variety of generous and humanitarian initiatives, as a step toward realizing its global ambitions. The focus is on realizing the idea of Vasudhaiva Kutumbakam.

Keywords COVID-19 · Vaccine diplomacy · Financial · Vande Bharat · Self-reliant

5.1 Introduction

The pandemic COVID-19 has brought about a new global order. Due to coronavirus the entire global economy and international trade, services, and diplomatic relations have been rapidly changing. COVID-19 originated from Wuhan of China (November 2019) and rapidly spread across the globe. Indian economy and foreign policy were badly affected due to COVID-19 and India's relational equations with other countries have been rapidly changed. The future direction of the Indian economy and Indian foreign policy is struck for further development of global order. The global economy has been falling-down from December 2019 to July 2020. The global economic shutdown has raised concerns in the Ministry of Finance. The Government of India on

---

D. Nandy (✉)
Head of the Department, Political Science, Kazi Nazrul University, Asansol, India

A. Naha
Department of Political Science, Vidyasagar College, Kolkata, India

© The Author(s), under exclusive license to Springer Nature Singapore Pte Ltd. 2022
S. Roy and D. Nandy (eds.), *Understanding Post-COVID-19 Social and Cultural Realities*, https://doi.org/10.1007/978-981-19-0809-5_5

24th March 2020 had announced a nationwide lockdown that brought the second most populous country in the world to a standstill. Restricting the spread of the virus was a major challenge for a nation with notable regional and socio-economic incongruities. In such circumstances, much to the surprise of many, India has emerged as a doyen in the global fight against the pandemic through its humanitarian assistance and global diplomatic initiatives, like the *Vande Bharat Mission, Mission Sagar*, and *Vaccine Maitri*. Since its inception as an independent nation, India has been actively involved in assisting countries' victims of civil wars and natural calamities. In the last few decades, the volume of such assistance has increased enormously through development partnerships and entente. Central to India's humanitarian assistance and diplomatic efforts is the principle of "*Vasudhaiva Kutumbakam*" which means the world is one family. The essence of this principle is also reflected in the Indian Prime Minister's efforts to connect, and assure to help the leaders of the nations that were badly affected by the spread of the virus. Under its COVID diplomacy, India facilitated not only the rehabilitation of its stranded citizens but also a large number of foreign nationals (Mohan, 2020). It also extended medical assistance and rapid response teams along with providing food and other items of livelihood and survival to the worst affected nations. Indian foreign policy orientations and equations have been changed due to COVID-19. The pandemic COVID-19 and its consequences led Indian foreign policy-makers to tune foreign policy in a new direction. Vaccine diplomacy and humanitarian assistance as a tool of soft power diplomacy can contribute to India's aspiration of emerging as a great power. In this context, the chapter intends to explore the following ***research questions***—(1) Why India is actively implementing vaccine diplomacy? (2) How India can benefit through vaccine diplomacy in the post-COVID global order?

The present study has been conducted using ***content analysis and observation methods***. We have primarily resorted to examining secondary data sources such as books, book chapters, journals, reports, and other relevant sources conducive to this study. These sources of information have enabled us to work on the key areas detailed in the paper.

5.2   The Context

The Indian approach of global outreach is consistent with Prime Minister Modi's vision of evolving India's role as a responsible Great Power. India's use of Covid diplomacy as a tool of soft power allows it to reconstruct its strained relationship with the neighbors and also to engage closely with nations that are geopolitically important beyond the South Asian region. It also helped to build a positive image for India across the globe. Soon after assuming office in 2014, PM Modi has infused renewed energy in India's foreign policy deliberations. His greater emphasis on the use of soft power is an effort to uplift India's leadership role in a multilateral world. India has already proved its leadership capabilities through its efforts under new initiatives like the International Solar Alliance (2015) and the Coalition on

Disaster Resilient Infrastructure (2019). In this sense, its effort towards containing the spread of the Coronavirus is no different. In all the multilateral summits that were virtually held last year, Prime Minister Modi has stressed the need to redefine the idea of globalization based on the principles of humanity, equality, and fairness. In an op-ed titled *Reimagining Diplomacy in the Post-COVID World: An Indian Perspective*, India's foreign minister Jaishankar observed, "*The general sense is one of trade, finance, services, communication, technology, and mobility... What COVID, however, brought out was the deeper indivisibility of our existence. Real globalization is more about pandemics, climate change, and terrorism*" (Krishnankutty, 2021).

In the South Asian region, India has stressed the need to utilize the SAARC framework for containing the spread of the virus. Under the leadership of PM Modi, a virtual meet of SAARC leaders was held on 15th May 2020. India proposed the creation of a SAARC COVID-19 emergency fund and made a voluntary contribution of US\$ 10 million (*The Hindu*, 2020). Apart from this, since the spread of the virus in the sub-continent and subsequent lockdowns imposed by the South Asian nations, India continued to provide food and medical assistance in the form of PPEs, masks, and ventilators to nations like Nepal, Bhutan, the Maldives, etc. India's stress on multilateral collaboration was to minimize the evolving adverse health and economic impact. Moving beyond the region, India has extended support to Latin America, Caribbean Island nations, Africa, and countries of the Indian Ocean Region. On 10th May 2020, India launched Mission Sagar to send relief assistance to countries in the Indian Ocean Region like Seychelles, Mauritius, Madagascar, Comoros, etc. India has also launched the largest repatriation initiative named "Vande Bharat" to bring back Indians like students studying abroad, people who have lost their jobs during the pandemic, pregnant women, elderly people, etc. It also provided an opportunity for the NRIs to return to the countries where they are employed. Along with Vande Bharat, India has also deployed its Naval ships under Mission Sagar to extend medical relief and humanitarian assistance to its maritime neighbors.

Regarded as the 'Pharmacy of the World', India provided hydroxychloroquine tablets (HQC) on request from the US and Brazil. It also provided 1.54 billion paracetamol tablets to 133 nations (Roche, 2020). In May 2020, India also announced the creation of an INR 1 billion medical assistance fund in the form of testing kits, drugs, and other medical assistance to assist 90 severely affected countries (Gupta, 2020). With the formal approval of the Covishield vaccine by the Indian Drug regulatory authority DGA, India undertook the diplomatic initiative (Vaccine Maitri) to provide vaccines, prioritizing the neighboring countries and, subsequently, to nations across the globe. This Indian vaccine diplomacy is seen by many as an effort to improve the global profile against an aggressive China. As Sreeram Chaulia of the Jindal School of International Affairs observed, "*It's about image and soft power. India wants to be recognized as a global leader. India would like to make a point that in this area, unlike in some others where China usually overshadows India in terms of military and economic might, in this field, in pharmaceuticals, in affordable health care, India has a comparative edge and advantage over China*" (Pasricha, 2021). The Vaccine Maitri initiative has also shut the growing voices of vaccine nationalism or vaccine hoarding i.e., a disparity in the equitable access to vaccines between the advanced and developing countries. Under this initiative, vaccines have been shipped to nations like Bhutan, the Maldives, Bangladesh, Myanmar, Mauritius, Seychelles, Brazil, Morocco, etc. These Indian efforts have been recognized and appreciated by WHO, UN, the US, France, Brazil, and leaders of other countries.

Therefore, India has assumed the role of the leader in the global fight against the pandemic. When other established global powers have struggled to cope with the pandemic, through its efforts and initiatives, India has emerged as a *"responsible and reliable international power"* (Chaudhury, 2020). This essence is also reflected in the speech by the Indian Prime Minister at the 75th anniversary of the UNGA. In the speech, while questioning the effective role of the UN in the global fight against the pandemic, the Prime Minister highlighted India's proactive role in the global fight against the pandemic and assured the world community of India's vaccine production and delivery capability. He remarked, *"As the largest vaccine producing country in the world, I want to give one more assurance to the global community today. India's vaccine production and delivery capacity will be used to help all humanity in fighting this crisis...... India will also help all the countries in enhancing their cold chain and storage capacities for the delivery of Vaccines"* (MEA, 2020). Given this context, the chapter analyses how the pandemic has impacted India's relationship with the US, China, and other regions like Africa, the Middle East, South East Asia, etc.; the evolving socio-economic crises due to the pandemic that have adversely affected the major economies of the world; and, the initiatives implemented by New Delhi to provide humanitarian and medical assistance to its people, neighbors, and countries around the globe. Finally, the chapter focuses on the emerging role of India in the post-COVID world order.

5.3 Impact of COVID-19 on India-US Relations

The pandemic COVID-19 has brought a new equation in Indo-US diplomatic relations. Regarding the supply of hydroxychloroquine to the USA, two questions have been raised—(1) whether India was threatened by the USA to supply the hydroxychloroquine or not? and (2) was it a part of humanitarian diplomacy? However, in the wake of the pandemic COVID-19 diplomatic tug of war between New Delhi and Washington was shown on the one hand and friendly accommodations on the other. To combat COVID-19, hydroxychloroquine and paracetamol are indispensable. The USA came to know about India's large production of hydroxychloroquine. Looking at India's national health security, New Delhi decides to restrict hydroxychloroquine for a time being. The US President Donal Trump has warned India if it stops exporting, then the USA will retaliate against it. India has partially lifted a ban on the exports of a malaria drug following the U.S warning. After receiving the medicine as a substitute by the USA, India was appreciated by Trump. The crazy leadership of Donald Trump was very much uncertain.

The growing synergy between India and the US is very much related to Washington's gradual ascending relational curve with Beijing. The trade war between the world's number one economy and the second-largest economy began in 2017 regarding the imposition of extra tariffs on some goods of China by the US and vice-versa. This war has been intensified with the spread of COVID-19. The US President has been continuously blaming the Chinese government for its irresponsible role in spreading coronavirus. Mr. Trump also strongly argued and propagated that as the virus has originated from China, so, China should be isolated from the global economic system. India's decision to boycott Chinese goods and policies of self-reliance have collectively helped the USA to choose India as a rational choice. Trump has taken this opportunity to corner China. Amid COVID-19, India took over as chair of the World Health Organization's Executive Board, its decision-making panel. Union Health Minister Harsh Vardhan has been elected as the chairman of the WHO Executive Board on May 22, 2020. The US took a key role in cornering the pro-Chinese lobby in WHO. The role of WHO to control COVID-19 is very dissatisfactory and the US President has expressed his discontent over the issue. The increase in the importance of India in WHO is not only a game of the USA but also a step towards the Chinese hegemonic role in South Asia and to make a counter-balance.

The U.S President Donald Trump wanted to reform the G-7 - the advanced economies in the world, to make it a G-10 or G-11 to include India, Australia, South Korea, and Russia. Calling the existing formation 'outdated', Trump revealed the idea of an expanded group after announcing he was subscribing to the G-7 summit he had planned to host at Camp David in June. The announcement of Trump makes two narratives. On 2nd June 2020, US President Donald Trump has formally invited PM Modi to attend the G-7 summit to be held in September 2020. There is diplomacy behind his desire to expand the size and scope of the grouping of major world economic powers. There is a sense of disquiet about Trump's invitation to India and three other nations, especially at a time when he is seeking to isolate Beijing with a raft of measures including withdrawing the special status to Hong Kong. Trump has been also aggressively trying to stop Chinese economic dominance and global supply chains. The tension between the US and China is escalating over the coronavirus pandemic and the ongoing trade war between Washington and Beijing fuelled Washington-New Delhi relations. However, China has rejected all US allegations of a cover-up regarding the COVID-19 outbreak. Firstly, India's advancement in science and technology, economic growth, defense strength, and growing acceptability in world politics gives India an advantage to be considered as a member of reformulated G-7 shortly. And, secondly, to make more strengthen the alliance of the pro-US countries Donald Trump thought about it.

5.4 Impact of COVID-19 on Sino-Indian Relations

The scenario of global economic and strategic order has undergone a massive change due to pandemic COVID-19. The responsibility of China in combating the COVID-19, and sharing information about the effects it raised several questions before the global community. An Anti-China stance has been taken by India along with other countries. The Indian government has been encouraging to abandon the Chinese goods and services. India's dependency on China has been gradually declining not only for COVID-19 but also for Chinese sudden attacks on Indian territory on 16th June 2020 at the Galwan range of Ladakh. The country-wide anti-Chinese waves have been strongly raised that led to the Central government taking the bold decision to ban 59 Chinese apps. On 29th June 2020, the Ministry of Electronics and IT, Government of India has banned 59 mobile apps which are prejudicial to the sovereignty and integrity of India, defense of India, the security of a state, and public order. The Indian Cyber Crime Coordination Centre, Ministry of Home Affairs has also sent an exhaustive recommendation for blocking these malicious apps This ministry has also received many representations raising concerns from citizens regarding the security of data and risk to privacy relating to the operation of certain apps.

Being one of the leading trade partners of India, China's share in India's total export and import are 9% and 18% respectively in 2019–2020. China's share in India's export to the world shows a declining trend from 2010 to 2016 and then, has evidenced a reversal. On the contrary, India's share in total China's exports reveals an increasing trend with a blip in 2016. One recent IMF figure reveals that India has a trade deficit of $60 billion after the US, which has a deficit of $300 billion with China in 2019–2020. It is the primary reason that India has not signed the RCEP treaty. However, India decided to cut up its dependency on Chinese goods and emphasized self-reliance.

India was the first non-communist country in Asia that recognized the PRC and established diplomatic relations avoiding the immense pressure of the USA and other Western powers. The year 2020 is the year of the 70th anniversary of India-China diplomatic relations. But moving forward, China's role in the pandemic is likely to harm the Sino-Indian relationship. China is not transparent regarding the share of actual information to the global community, that is why China has been considering a suspicious country. The Chinese government tried to manipulate the chief executive of the WHO to produce an ambiguous report on the Chinese situation due to COVID-19. The Director-General of WHO Mr. Tedros Adhanom Ghebreyesus has wrongly passed China for its transparency. He advocated the role of the PRC in controlling the COVID-19 and mentioned that China can be a role model for COVID-19. The negative and suspicious role of China has presented a debate in Indian society regarding the reliability of China. Undoubtedly, it can be said China is controlling the global supply chain of goods and services. India has cut up trading with China. It showed a significant impact on India's economy. China is an important supplier of drugs and medicine in India. Nevertheless, due to the sopping of the supply of indispensable medicine, the Indian medical sector has to suffer a lot. India has cut up air connectivity with several affected countries.

5.5 Vande Bharat Mission

The Government of India has taken a very active role in the evacuation of Indian citizens from abroad. The responsibility of the government has been praised by a section of people, but the opposition parties are very critical about this policy because of demanding a high rate of air tickets from the passengers. However, the Government of India can expect credit. Passengers traveling to or through the USA, UK, or Singapore, where foreign nationals are being permitted to travel or transit, are required to show a visa with at least six-month validity. The Indira Gandhi International Airport has been operating chartered flights to and from 28 destinations globally, which were not connected to the city earlier. Indians and foreigners flew out on these first-time direct routes like Auckland, Christchurch, Wellington, and Brisbane in Australia, Dublin in Ireland, Lubumbashi in Congo, and Minsk in Belarus. However, other private airlines also started their charter flights operation from Delhi to various destinations of the globe.

5.6 Mission Samudra Setu

The Indian Navy launched operation Samudra Setu in May 2020 to bring back Indian citizens stranded overseas during the Pandemic. A total of 3992 Indians were brought back by the Indian Navy from Iran, the Maldives, and Sri Lanka through its frigates Jalashwa Airavat, Shardul, and Magar. The operation lasted for 55 days. Also, the Navy's IL-38 and Dornier aircraft were used to ferry doctors and medical assistance to the neighboring countries to tackle the pandemic. Under the operation, 580 tons of food and medical aid were provided to Maldives, Mauritius, Madagascar, Comoros Islands, and Seychelles in 49 days (Indian Navy, 2020).

5.7 Mission Sagar

The countries of the Indian Ocean Region (IOR) are badly affected by the outbreak of the pandemic. The economy of most of the countries of the IOR is significantly dependent on tourism which witnessed a tremendous decline during the period of the pandemic. Countries like the Maldives, Comoros, Madagascar, and Seychelles are already facing the heat. In such a situation the Indian initiative of Mission Sagar was like a boon in disguise. For India, the region of the Indian Ocean is strategically vital for three reasons—firstly, the issue of India's maritime security. India is a strong advocate of freedom of navigation and open and free Indo-Pacific. Therefore, a cordial relationship with the countries in the IOR region will provide it a strategic upper hand 'to counterbalance assertive China' (Naha, 2020) in the region. India has already partnered with Japan, Australia, ASEAN, France, and the US to promote an alternative to the Chinese BRI in the region. Secondly, is the issue of trade and Sea Lines of Communication (SLOCs). Almost '*half of the world's container ships, one-third of the world's bulk cargo traffic, and two-thirds of the world's oil shipments* pass through the Indian Ocean (Singh, 2020). The IOR also has major chokepoints and straits through which huge volume trade takes place and is equally strategically important. The SLOCs of the Indian Ocean is crucial for regional commercial trade. And, Finally, to promote its role as a net security provider in the region. In this respect, India has already undertaken efforts to address crises emanating from non-conventional threats of piracy, natural calamities, and terrorism. Also, to tackle the rising sea levels due to climate change, India is collaborating with like-minded countries for 'sustainable and ocean development' (Naha, 2020).

Given the nature of increasing Chinese hegemony and military assertiveness in the IOR, and also recognizing the geo-strategic and geo-economic significance of the IOR, the Indian Prime Minister in 2015 advocated the doctrine of Security and Growth for All in the Region or SAGAR. The sole objective of the doctrine was to induct the maritime neighbors into India's maritime aspirations and to establish itself as the primary dependable partner to provide humanitarian assistance and maritime security. Keeping in line with this doctrine, India extended support to the countries of the IOR following the global outbreak of COVID-19. It launched Mission Sagar on 10th May 2020 to provide medical assistance and humanitarian aid to countries like the Maldives, Mauritius, Seychelles, Comoros, etc. Indian naval ship, INS Kesari was deployed to send medicine, food, and other essential livelihood commodities to these countries. Seychelles and Mauritius were initially provided live-saving HCQs by India through the initiative.

The second phase of Sagar or Mission Sagar-II was launched on 6th November 2020. INS Ariavat was deployed to extend covid relief materials and assistance to countries like Sudan, South Sudan, Djibouti, and Eritrea (Siddiqui, 2020). This initiative by India helps to legitimize its role as the first responder in the region and also highlights the importance accorded by India to its maritime neighbors to further strengthen the bond.

5.8 Financial Crisis

The entire globe got affected by COVID-19 that resulted in acute financial crises. More than 210 nations are affected in varying degrees (Ghosh, 2020). The slow growth of the Indian economy has been more crisis-prone due to COVID-19. The Government of India has to spend a lot of money in the public health sector due to COVID-19. The government has to spend money on improving health facilities, providing medicines, food, and other associated services. After the withdrawal of the lockdown, the central government has taken some measures for reviving the economy but it remains facing a serious challenge (Nag, 2020). The Central government has announced a lockdown in the entire country from March 22nd, 2020. On 6th April 2020, the Union cabinet had approved an ordinance to cut salaries of the Prime

Minister, all ministers, and siting M. P.s by 30% for one year in the wake of the COVID-19 crisis and also decided to suspend the Local Area Development Scheme for two year. The Central government has given directions to the private sector to continue salary payments to their employees. But, Thousands of people have lost their jobs after COVID-19. It would be continued for a few years as per the analysis of economists.

The COVID-19 pandemic has had an immediate and negative impact on foreign direct investment (FDI) in 2020. The outlook remains dire, with further deterioration projected in 2021 (UNCTAD, 2020). Pandemic COVID-19 had posed a negative impact on the Banking system. Due to long-time lockdown, the domestic and international business and trading were suspended and the transport system was also stopped which made a negative impact on the Banking system. From March 2020 to July 2020, the Reserve Bank of India has reduced the rate of interest. Many people have lost their jobs. The remittance has been almost stopped due to COVID-19. The foreign currency reserve was also reduced due to COVID-19. India is suffering from acute financial hardship and the descending curve of economic development has posed a low economic profile before the global economic order. Regional trade volume has been affected due to COVID-19. The land borders and airlines services are closed, except for emergency services, which resulted in a negative impact on India's regional trade. Except for Pakistan, India is the key supplier of the South Asian states. Due to COVID-19, India's overseas business got a setback in early 2020. Over 20% of export orders have been canceled due to pandemic COVID-19 that resulted in a major amount of funds being locked up, owing to non-payment of dues by large buyers in the USA, Europe, and West Asia, prompting them to seek a bailout from the government. Engineering Export Promotion Council of India has expected the effect of Covid-19 will not be ended soon and exporters can lose up to 80% of their orders. Gems and Jewellery Export Promotion Council has warned of an additional $ 2.7-billion impact in 2019–2020. Similar things happened in the carpet export sector.

5.8.1 Interruptions of Supply Chain and Medical Equipment and Medicines

The supply chain of Indian medicine is extensively dependent upon imports. Most of the medical equipment and medicines of India are imported from China. Due to COVID-19, and the Chinese irresponsible and inhuman role in the wake of COVID-19, Indian's dependency on China for medicinal supply has been interrupted. The positive aspect of the pandemic is that India has concluded agreements with several countries to get the COVID vaccine once it is successfully approved.

5.9 India's Role in SAARC

In COVID-19, India has to face problems in dealing with her South Asian neighbors during the pandemic of COVID-19. China provokes the South Asian countries to continue anti-Indian activities. Pakistan has been continuously using the militants in the Kashmir valley. However, the COVID-19 might reshape India's neighborhood policy with new equations. Nepal has made its new map where some Indian territory has been incorporated. China is asserting its power in bordering areas. In June 2020, India has planned to purchase more modern military equipment from other countries which might affect the Indian crisis-prone economy. However, to normalize the relational continuity cordially India has tried to assist the South Asian neighbors not only through individual effort but also through SAARC. As a responsible member, India initiated raising funds for SAARC countries in cooperation with other members. India's initiatives can be considered as a generous role as the biggest member state of SAARC or initiative for enhancing acceptability in the South Asian region.

India is the second-highest populated country in the world and has been highly affected by a coronavirus that crossed 11,794,407 by the end of March 2021. However, India has initiated to ensure treatment for the citizens of SAARC countries through raising funds by the SAARC countries. When India started to evacuate its citizens from various citizens of India then citizens of other SAARC member countries were also evacuated by Indian national air carriers. India also supplied medical equipment and essential medicines to the SAARC countries like Maldives, Sri Lanka, Bangladesh, Afghanistan, and Bhutan. India initiated a virtual meeting with SAARC countries in March 2020 to raise emergency funds for COVID-19. Except for Pakistan, all countries have contributed as per their capacity. India was the highest contributor and India's paid amount was 10 million USD. As part of India's foreign policy "Neighborhood First" policy (mainly focusing on South Asia), India has extended its generous policy to the SAARC countries by supplying medical instruments.

Coronavirus is a serious threat to the South Asian public health system. There is no doubt India pledged $10 million toward a COVID-19 emergency fund and said it was putting together a rapid response team of doctors and specialists for the South Asian Association for Regional Cooperation (SAARC) nations as part of an initiative led by Prime Minister Modi. Modi made the announcements during a video conference with SAARC leaders that he had proposed amid rising cases of the disease in the region. On March 15, 2020, the leaders of SAARC member nations connected via video conference to formulate a strategy to tackle the outbreak of the novel coronavirus (COVID-19) in the region. Other economically challenged SAARC members contributed as per their capacity. India has contributed the maximum amount. Pakistan has started narrow politics without contributing a single amount. The leaders of South Asia have immediately agreed to participate in the discussion. Leaders of the SAARC states who took part in the video conference. The Maldivian President Ibrahim Mohamed Solih, Sri Lankan President Gotabaya Rajapaksa, Bhutanese premier Lotay Tshering, Bangladeshi Prime Minister Sheikh Hasina, Nepalese Prime Minister K P Sharma

Oli, and Afghan President Ashraf Ghani. Meanwhile, a special assistant to Prime Minister Imran Khan, Dr. Zafar Mirza represented Pakistan.

India's Prime Minister Narendra Modi floated the idea of a COVID-19 Emergency Fund for SAARC member nations. While stating that voluntary contributions will allow this fund to help countries affected in South Asia to tide over economic losses, PM Modi pledged USD 10 million to the fund. Foreign secretaries of SAARC member nations have been asked to take this initiative forward. While addressing SAARC leaders, PM Modi told his contemporaries that a rapid response team of doctors and specialists has been kept on standby and will be at the disposal of India's neighbors if and when required. The Indian Prime Minister also offered online training capsules for the emergency response staff in SAARC member nations. Prime Minister Narendra Modi also offered the expertise of the Indian Council of Medical Research (ICMR) to set up a research platform for diagnostic and therapeutic interventions for disease (Nandy, 2020).

5.10 India's Vaccine Diplomacy in South Asia

India is the largest producer of vaccines. It meets 60% of the global demand for vaccines. India has been supplying medicines and generic drugs to different parts of the globe. About 100 countries have requested India to supply hydroxychloroquine. India supplied it to the USA, Israel, Brazil, and other countries. By May 2020, India had spent US$16 million on pharmaceuticals, test kits, and other medical equipment in 90 countries (Pant & Tirkey, 2021). New Delhi already gifted 49 lakh doses of COVID-19 vaccines to the neighbors, even to Brazil and Morocco. To implement its vaccine diplomacy India has given the caption of 'grant assistance' to neighbors (Business Line, 2021).

India has played 'vaccine diplomacy' with Bangladesh by promising the supply of 'COVID Vaccine' to Bangladesh on a priority basis. Amidst the corona pandemic crisis, Indian Foreign Secretary Harsh Vardhan Shringla has paid a surprise visit to Dhaka on 18th August 2020. During his visit to Dhaka, Mr. Shringla has said, "for India, Bangladesh is always a priority country" (The Times of India, 2020). He also promised that once the COVID Vaccine is available, then India will immediately supply it to Bangladesh. This visit was very significant because this was his first visit to the neighboring during the pandemic that gave a signal to understand the importance of Bangladesh to India. He met with key policymakers in Bangladesh. Indian High Commissioner in Dhaka Riva Ganguly Das was also present in all meetings. India's relations with other South Asian neighbors have been very problematic in recent times. So, it was a very timely initiative to normalize the diplomatic engagement with Bangladesh from the Indian end. Finally, India started to supply vaccines to Bangladesh in January 2021.

India has been the key supplier of COVID vaccines to the neighborhood. India is exercising its vaccine diplomacy in the manner of humanitarian actions to the neighbors. India is supplying vaccines to Nepal, Bangladesh, Sri Lanka, Myanmar, and other countries (Krishnan, 2021). Despite having some relational complexities, India is playing an admirable role in combating coronavirus. It is very challenging for New Delhi to maintain a balance between domestic demands and commitment to help other countries. India also shipped COVID-19 vaccines to Bhutan, Maldives, Mauritius, Seychelles, and other countries (Giri, 2021). The role of China is very negative in this regard.

5.11 COVID-19 and India's Response to South-East Asia

India has extended its cooperation towards selected South-East Asian countries to combat COVID-19. The Indian government has talked to Vietnam, Singapore, and Indonesia about healthcare and economic challenges caused by coronavirus. India has also agreed to supply HCQ tablets to Malaysia and received a donation of COVID-19 testing kits. The Indian embassy in Manila has supplied masks, sanitizers, and medicines to Philippine government officials, university students, and regular citizens. The Indian healthcare industry already has made a significant contribution to ASEAN. The health industry of India has occupied several segments of India-Cambodia bilateral trade. and India's Export–Import (EXIM) Bank has prioritized funding for Indian healthcare operators to expand operations in the country. The EXIM-led healthcare initiatives have been considered for Myanmar in the post-COVID-19 period. India has been supplying vaccines to Southeast Asian countries. Some vaccines were supplied free of cost, and the rest of the vaccines were supplied at minimum cost. Through supplying vaccines India has tried to exercise diplomacy. India has used the so-called "Quad" group in exercising vaccine diplomacy. A quad is a strategic group of four countries, such as India, Australia, the USA, and Japan to counter Chinese supremacy in the Pacific region. India is the world's largest vaccine manufacturer country. India will be supported by the USA, Australia, and Japan in producing large-scale vaccines. The Quad aims to discard the Chinese hegemonic presence in the Southeast Asian region and other parts of the globe.

5.12 India and Middle-East in Response to COVID-19

The pandemic spread rapidly across the country, the government exploited diplomatic opportunities to demonstrate leadership both within South Asia and globally (Taneja & Singh, 2021). In the wake of the pandemic COVID-19, India has provided medical assistance to Middle-eastern countries for strengthening its cooperation in the post-CAA period through 'extended neighborhood policy'. In the 2018–2019 FY, Saudi Arabia and the UAE were India's fourth and the third-largest trading partners respectively. Both these Gulf countries are aspiring to increase their trade volume and investments with India. India has established its friendly relations with Oman, Israel, Jordon, Kuwait, Qatar, and other countries for extending its exports and securing

5 The Changing Dimensions of India's … 89

energy security. India is not only providing medical equipment and medicines to the Middle-eastern countries to deal with COVID-19 but also providing advice. The UAE, Jordon, Saudi Arabia, Jordon, and other strategic partners of the Arab world are also in close consultation with India on the COVID-19 pandemic. India's director-general of civil aviation (DGCA) had considered bringing Indian laborers and other professionals from the Middle-eastern countries.

5.13 India's 'Vaccine *Maitri*' Initiative

As the 'pharmacy of the world', India manufactures around sixty percent of the total global vaccines (Sajjanhar, 2021). In this regard, its efforts toward vaccine diplomacy become crucial, more so, when the President of WHO has expressed dissatisfaction over vaccine nationalism by the developed countries, while depriving the developing and underdeveloped states. India's 'vaccine *maitri*' initiative is, therefore, a humanitarian effort of providing vaccines as a 'gift' to the neighbors as well as the developing nations of the world in containing the spread of the virus. This initiative is in symphony with India's policy of "Neighborhood First".

Under this Vaccine diplomacy, Bhutan and the Maldives were the first recipients of the India-made Covishield vaccine produced by the Serum Institute of India (SII). On 20th January 2021, both these nations received 1.5 lakh and 1 lakh doses of vaccines respectively. On 21st January, Bangladesh and Nepal received their first batch of vaccine aid from India. Together they received 30 lakh doses of the vaccine. On January 22nd, Myanmar, Seychelles, and Mauritius received their first doses of vaccine from India. Sri Lanka, too, received 5 lakh doses by January 27th. Apart from facilitating the vaccines, the medical staff from these neighboring states were also provided training by India to carry out the vaccination program. India's prompt response to Bangladesh's need for the vaccine was hailed by its health minister. For Nepal too, India sent the first consignment of vaccines within one week of request by the Nepali foreign Minister. From a regional geopolitical perspective, this holds much significance given the current discourse of increasing Chinese economic and political influence over both these nations. The vaccine diplomacy has provided India with the opportunity to increase and strengthen its regional as well as global outreach. India-made vaccines reached Canada. The Serum Institute of India (Pune) will send 1.5 million more doses of the Covishield vaccine as per commitment.

Beyond the South Asian region, India provided doses of vaccines to Brazil and Morocco, 20 lakh doses each. The Brazilian President Bolsonaro equated India's gesture with lord Hanuman bringing 'Sanjeevani Booti'. Doses of Vaccines were also provided to the Island nations of the Caribbean like Antigua & Barbuda, Guyana, Jamaica, Nicaragua, and the region of CARICOM. A total of 10 million vaccine doses has been sent to African nations like South Africa, Egypt, Rwanda, Ghana, the Democratic Republic of Congo, Senegal, and Cote d' Ivoire. An additional 1 million doses were provided to the UN health workers under the COVID-19 Vaccines Global Access (COVAX) facility (Dhar, 2021). Middle Eastern nations like Bahrain, UAE, and Kuwait were also supplied with doses of vaccine. Following the request by the Dominican Prime Minister Skerrit, India airlifted doses of vaccines to help the Republic in its fight against the pandemic. In the East, countries like Mongolia and the Philippines have been provided with the doses. This has effectively established India's leadership role in fighting the pandemic. This initiative is in continuity with the Prime Minister's assurance at the 75th UNGA speech that emphasized on availability of vaccines for the welfare of all humanity.

This Indian effort has received widespread accolade and praise. World bodies like the UN, WHO, and leaders of various nations and MNCs have congratulated India for providing vaccines to nations that were once feared of being deprived of getting the vaccine. The Africa, Caribbean, and Pacific groups (ACP) and the CARICOM have made heaps of praise for India at the WTO (Sen, 2021). The South and Central Asia Bureau of the US State Department termed India as a "True Friend" for helping the world community by supplying vaccines (PTI, 2021). Nepali Prime Minister K.P. Oli thanked India for its friendly gesture. The foreign minister of Bhutan also expressed his gratefulness for India's unconditional support in Bhutan's fight against COVID-19. The Prime Minister of Bangladesh also thanked the Indian Government for this initiative. Yaroslav Trofimov and Bellman wrote in the Wall Street Journal that through Covid diplomacy India has established itself as a "Vaccine Superpower" (IANS, 2021). Therefore, India has effectively utilized its soft power diplomacy as a development partner to support these developing nations.

Amidst the fear of vaccine nationalism, India's 'vaccine maitri' has been a standout initiative. According to a report by Duke University's Global Health Institute, developed countries like Canada, the US, Australia, Chile, the UK, and some other member states of the European Union have emerged as the biggest 'vaccine nationalists' (Marcus, 2021). They have stocked piled doses nearly six to ten times of their population. In contrast, India has shared doses of vaccines with other nations while simultaneously meeting its own domestic needs. As of 12th February 2021, a total of 229.7 lakh doses (64.7 lakh doses as grant and 165 lakh doses on a commercial basis) has been supplied to various nations across the globe. This suggests that during a medical emergency, vaccines must be treated as humanitarian goods and not as a commodity of profit.

The vaccine diplomacy of India has also taken China by surprise. In South Asia, where China has assumed a greater aggressive role, this Indian initiative could contribute to even out the playing field (Dhar, 2021). As of March 2021, China could supply vaccines to only 28 countries while in the same period India has extended 5.84 crore doses of vaccine to nearly 70 countries (The Wire, 2021). China's ruling Communist Party mouthpiece the Global Times has begun to spread lies about the efficacy of the Indian-made vaccines even when many countries have rejected to approve the Chinese-made vaccines over the quality issue (Sajjanhar, 2021). Also, to China's disliking the QUAD (India, Australia, Japan, and the US) has undertaken the Quad vaccine initiative emphasizing *"Indian manufacturing paired with the US technology, Japanese and American funding as well as Australian logistics capabilities*" (Financial Express, 2021). The Quad vaccine initiative aims to deliver doses of vaccine to the ASEAN nations and the nations of the Indo-Pacific by the end of 2022.

5.14 India's Vaccine Diplomacy in Africa

The Continent of Africa has also been severely affected by the pandemic. But due to a vigorous response launched immediately after the outbreak of the virus by some of the African nations, the continent has done comparatively better in containing the spread of the virus in comparison to some other parts of the world (Coronavirus in Africa tracker, 2021). With the African nations, India shares friendly relations. Even during the pandemic, India was diplomatically committed to the region. Cooperation in the health sector has been one of the key aspects of India-Africa ties. There lies an underlying harmony between the health policies of India and African nations. Over time India has been the major source of low-cost generic drugs and vaccines for the African nations to combat TB, malaria, HIV, and other such diseases. Pharmacy giant Cipla (India) has provided anti-retroviral drugs at cheap costs for the treatment of Aids. Likewise, another pharmaceutical giant Ranbaxy Laboratories is also very active in Africa (James et al., 2015). Therefore, the initiative of 'vaccine maitri' provides a renewed scope of cooperation in the healthcare sector between India and Africa.

As of March 27th, 2021, Africa has a total confirmed case of 4.03 million with 3.07 million active cases. Countries like South Africa, Nigeria, Morocco, Libya, Kenya, Ethiopia, Ghana, Egypt, and Algeria are most affected (Coronavirus in Africa tracker, 2021). India has been continuously engaged with the region and has shared crucial information from time to time with the African region on handling the pandemic (UNI, 2020). Since the outbreak of the virus, India has stood up to its reputation as the 'pharmacy of the world' by availing HCQs, Paracetamols, PPEs, Testing kits, and masks to 90 countries (including 25 African nations) around the world. It has also provided health care training through e-ITEC courses on COVID management and protocol to several of the African nations (Beri, 2021).

Among most of the African nations, there is also the fear of 'vaccine nationalism'. Rwandan President Kagame pointing towards vaccine nationalism by the US and Europe observed that [it] "*could undermine decades of progress in human development while investing in vaccination for all would benefit international trade shortly*" (Rwanda's president Paul Kagame warns on delayed vaccination in Africa, 2021). The South African President has also raised his voice against the 'hoarding' of vaccines by the developed nations, and the consequent suffering by the developing states (President Cyril Ramaphosa bemoans the rise of nationalism, 2021). India, too, has raised its voice against vaccine nationalism and demanded global collaboration for equal access to vaccines (PTI, 2020). In these circumstances, the Indian 'vaccine friendship initiative provides much-needed relief for these poor and developing African nations. Under the initiative, India has provided 10 million doses of Covishield vaccine to several African nations like South Africa, Egypt, Rwanda, Ghana, the Democratic Republic of Congo, Senegal, and Cote d' Ivoire. Seychelles was the first African nation to receive 50,000 doses of these Made-in-India vaccines as a gift.

This Indian initiative has been much appreciated by the African nations. The foreign minister of Seychelles observed, "[this] gesture cements the ties of solidarity, friendship, and cooperation which exists between our two countries." (Seychelles: India gifts Seychelles with Covishield vaccines, 2021). Similar feelings were expressed by leaders of Algeria, Botswana, Egypt, Ethiopia, Ghana, Kenya, Mali, Mauritius, Morocco, Mozambique, Nigeria, Rwanda, Senegal, Sierra Leone, Somalia, South Africa, the Democratic Republic of Congo, and Uganda. This Indian initiative will contribute to Africa's fight against the pandemic and will further cement the India-Africa relations.

5.15 Effects on Tourism/Service Sector and Global Connectivity

Tourism makes important contributions to development in both developed and developing countries. The sector has been severely affected by the crisis, given the severity of the restrictions on movement, border closures, and other restrictions imposed on travel in response to the pandemic. The significant projected economic impact of the crisis arising from the decline in tourism is because of the strong backward linkages of the sector in destination countries, including with accommodation, catering, and beverage-related services and transport. Such indirect services employ millions of people worldwide, who have lost their livelihoods during the pandemic. Of increasing concern to policymakers is the impact of the decline in tourism on cultural heritage and creative industries. Because of the crisis, museums have had to close, traditional festivals have been postponed and the activities of workers who sell traditional crafts and souvenirs have been brought to a standstill.

The coronavirus pandemic has badly impacted India's tourism sector. Around 4–5 crore people may lose their jobs. The total loss can be reached around Rs 1.58 lakh crore in 2020–2021. India earned $27 billion from foreign tourists in 2017 which is approximately Rs1,75,000 crores. In the same year, the foreign exchange earnings went up by 20.2%. The Indian tourism sector has been contributing 6.88% to the country's total GDP. The World Travel and Tourism Council COVID-19 will make a negative impact on the global travel and tourism Sector. The entire tourism industry is interlinked with foreign exchange, airlines, online booking systems, travel agents, hotels, resorts, transport systems, and so on. All related fields have been highly affected which might be a difficult task for India for recovery. Medical tourism, religion-based tourism, cultural tourism, heritage, and other service sectors have fallen into a severe crisis.

5.16 Post-COVID-19 Global Order and Role of India

As the Indian economy is closely linked with the global economy that is why the slowdown of global economic impact largely affects the Indian economy. Economic liberalization has given priority to the private sectors, and MNCs. During the COVID-19, it has been noticed that the role of MNCs and the private business houses are very less regarding social responsibility and maintaining economic stability. Now, states of the globe are thinking about de-globalization. The role of the state is very much visible which can be called 'state role back in'. Some scholars are arguing that like other countries, a paradigm shift can happen in India's foreign policy. India has performed its humanitarian responsibility towards 123 states of the globe to combat coronavirus. Where the Chinese role has been criticized during the COVID-19, the Indian responsibility to the global community has been highly praised. The post-COVID global order can be established without China to avoid Chinese economic hegemony. The Western democratic countries have been united to discard China from the global economic order. The USA has taken the key role and India might be a key factor in balancing the post-COVID global order. Indian humanitarian role in supplying hydroxychloroquine (HCQ) and paracetamol tablets initially to 123 countries and subsequent sending of millions of Covishield vaccine doses as gifts has been regarded as a very responsible job. After the commencement of India's supply of vaccines to different countries, The Prime Minister of India felt proud. He said in the Indian parliament in January 2021, "*It's a matter of pride for every Indian and an occasion to move forward*" (*The Hindustan Times*, 2021).

The 15th round of the G20 summit held virtually in November 2020 demonstrates the extraordinary challenge posed by the pandemic COVID-19 and the emerging changing nature of the post-pandemic world order. Given these circumstances, and the leadership role assumed by India during this pandemic, the world is looking towards India as a "*compelling, credible, and trustworthy major power*" (Bhattacharya, 2021) in the changing world order. The existence of strong political leadership, the pursuance of the multi-faceted policy both at home and globally during COVID-19, and a recovering economy have given it a position to provide stability to the disordered global order. India's deep-rooted commitment to multilateralism, global rules, and the ability to collaborate with the international community on issues like climate change, technology development, and leadership in medical diplomacy has put it to the center stage of reshaping the tormented world order.

As the virus continues to grapple the world, established Great Powers like the US is still a major victim of the pandemic coupled with the issue of domestic racial fights and presidential transition. The European Union is suffering from an economic slowdown and an increase in the number of COVID-19 cases. China, on the other hand, as the source of the virus, is being grasped with fear of global isolation. The UN has also failed to provide leadership and has become marginalized. In such a geopolitical conundrum, the stage is all set for India to bridge the strategic gap by exhausting its hard-earned reputation as a responsible power as well as utilizing its strategic and economic resources. In the post-COVID world order, the centrality of India's role can be well expressed by Prime Minister Modi's statement: *"Like today, the world is facing a huge challenge in the form of CoronaVirus. Financial institutions have also considered it a big challenge for the financial world. Today, we all have to face this challenge together. We have to be victorious with the power of our resolution of 'Collaborate to Create"* (Saran, 2020).

India's development and large-scale production of vaccines and its pursuance of vaccine diplomacy when the developed nations are accused of vaccine hoarding have made it a messiah for the developing states. Justifying its name as the 'pharmacy of the world', India has provided Covishield vaccines to nearly 70 countries of the world. Leaders of 60 nations have also visited the production unit of the indigenously produced Covaxin vaccine. These leaders have expressed confidence in India's leadership role in vaccine diplomacy and in eradicating the virus. Also, in this period of crisis, India continues to be a leading voice for climate and environmental protection. The pursuance of 'Atmanirbhar Bharat' and 'Vocal for Local', as enunciated by Prime Minister Modi, is expected to further strengthen India's position as a dependable factor in the China-minus global economy and supply chain in the post-COVID new world paradigm.

But as India struggles to tackle the second wave of this deadly virus, opposition voices began to question the need for India's vaccine diplomacy. The second wave hit the second-most populous country in February and has since then created havoc across its length and breadth. There has been a sharp increase in the number of cases due to the mutation of the virus. As of 6th May 2021, the number of active cases stood at 3.64 million while 1.96% of people have been fully vaccinated (Covid Tracker, 2021). This situation has challenged India's health care machinery. There have been reports of shortage or unavailability of hospital beds, vaccines, oxygen cylinders, and other vital medicines like Remdesivir. The Supreme Court and the High Courts of Kolkata, Delhi, and Madras have criticized the government for its mishandling of the situation. The demand for vaccine stocks is growing every day across various states. The situation demands urgent help from the world community. India required reciprocity from the world whose medical needs have been urgently fulfilled by India through its vaccine diplomacy drive.

This grim situation in India has been a catalyst fuelling the already tense US-China relations. This can have ramifications for the post-covid regional balance of power. With the US initially declining India's call for help by allowing the export of raw materials required by the Indian companies for the production of vaccines, China exploited the opportunity to criticize the strong relationship between the two democratic partners as artificial. The CCP backed Global Times in a series of editorials blasted the US for not providing humanitarian assistance to India, thereby stressing closer Sino-Indian ties. The editorial noted, *"This pandemic shows that the West's getting closer to India is more in a geopolitical sense. There is actually a gap of people's livelihoods and public interests between them. Their closeness to each other is fragile and superficial"* (The Global Times, 2021). In another article, the Global Times noted, *"In the past few days as India is battling the deadly surge of COVID-19 infections and deaths, it has clearly felt how "unreliable" its close partner, the US, is. If there had not been pressure from China and other countries, the US may not offer any substantial assistance to India, not even a verbal promise*" (Wenwen, 2021). While the Chinese political leadership has shown their intent to support India in overcoming the crisis, India's reaction towards Chinese efforts has been rather cautious. Even New Delhi has been hesitant to participate in the meeting called by Chinese Foreign Minister Wang Yi on forging South Asian cooperation for handling the COVID crisis. But despite this sharp criticism over the US initial inaction, the suspension of the Chinese state-run Sichuan Airlines carrying oxygen concentrators for 15 days is a mark of Chinese hypocrisy and propaganda. Facing domestic criticism for its sloppy response to the prevailing crisis, the Biden administration has allowed the export of raw materials and vital medical equipment to India on 25th April 2021. The breakthrough happened after the National Security Advisors of both countries had a telephonic conversation. The US President tweeted, *"Just as India sent assistance to the United States as our hospitals were strained early in the pandemic, we are determined to help India in its time of need"* (Chaudhary & Czuczka, 2021). This late US response towards its global strategic partner has put to question the effectiveness of the QUAD partnership in the Indo-Pacific. There have been growing Indian voices calling for strategic autonomy rather than allying with the US. The US assured India of providing 7 lakhs of rapid testing kits and 60 million doses of the AstraZeneca vaccine. India has received 545 oxygen concentrators and more than 2 lakh vials of Remdesivir from the US. However, this delay in response has again put to debate the issue of vaccine nationalism by the rich countries. The US is reported to have stockpiled vaccines over what its total population would require after receiving the prescribed two doses.

Apart from the US and China, several other countries around the world have rushed to support India by providing oxygen cylinders, oxygen concentrators, and other medical supplies. France was the earliest to come to India's rescue. French President Macron stated, *"Solidarity is at the heart of our nation. It is at the center of friendship between our countries. We will win together"* (The Times of India, 2021). French solidarity mission consisted of oxygen generators, liquid oxygen containers, ventilators, etc. Russia too came forward to support its old friend, India. Following President Putin's telephonic conversation with Modi, India received 22 tonnes of equipment, including 20 oxygen production units, 75 ventilators, 150 medical monitors, and 200,000 packs of medicine (Laskar, 2021). The first consignment of 1.5 Lakhs doses of Russian-made 'Sputnik V' vaccines reached India on May 1st. The decision to set up the 2 + 2 dialogue of foreign and defense ministers between India and Russia will further boost this close partnership. This can have ramifications for the post-covid global and regional power play. Japan, India's undoubtedly closest partner has also expressed concern over the growing crisis in India. In a statement, the Japanese Foreign Ministry observed, *"Japan stands with India, our friend and partner, in her efforts to fight against Covid-19 pandemic through this additional emergency assistance. Japan will continue to extend further support promptly in order to contain the Covid-19 situation"* (*The Hindustan Times*, 2021. Japan has provided 300 oxygen concentrators and 300 ventilators as assistance. Australia has also provided India with oxygen, ventilators, and personal protective equipment. Several Australian Cricketers and Australian Cricket Media have donated money to the PM-Cares fund. The United Kingdom has supported India by providing 160 ventilators, 495 oxygen concentrators, 5 lakhs anti-viral face coverings, and 450 oxygen cylinders. Also, countries like Germany, Pakistan, Poland, the UAE, Canada, Romania, Mauritius, Singapore, Thailand, Uzbekistan, Belgium, etc. have extended their support to India by providing essential medical equipment. In late April 2021, the Indian Navy launched *"Operation Samudra Setu-II"* to bring oxygen-filled cryogenic containers to meet growing domestic demand. INS Kolkata and INS Talwar were sent to Bahrain as the first deployment under the operation. INS Talwar is bringing 40MT of liquid oxygen to Mumbai. INS Kolkata will dock at the port of Doha (Qatar) and then at Kuwait to bring essential medical supplies along with liquid oxygen. In the Eastern sector, INS Airavat is sailing to Singapore and INS Jalashwa to Bangkok for the same purpose. The Indian Navy in its tweet commented, *"India Navy launches Operation Samudra Setu-II to augment ongoing national mission Oxygen Express. Mission deployed warships will undertake shipment of liquid Oxygen filled cryogenic containers & associated medical equipment in support of nation's fight against Covid-19"* (Bhalla, 2021).

The prevailing crisis in India over the shortage of essential medicines and vaccines has once again intensified the debate over the global north–south divide. When the developing countries of Asia, Africa, and Latin America are struggling to vaccinate all their citizens, the rich countries of the West are closer to achieving herd immunization and have been accused of stockpiling excess vaccines than required. This widening of the gap between the haves and have-nots has fuelled the possibility of a shifting geopolitical arrangement (Pratt & Levin, 2021). Though the US allowed exporting of essential raw materials for vaccine production in India, on a broader scale these have-nots are more exposed to global coercion and enchantment. The West has been primarily concerned with addressing the vaccination needs of its people. They have been largely unaccommodating of the global demand. For instance, the EU has distributed millions of doses of vaccines to its member states. Canada, which is not a vaccine producer by itself ranks behind the US and the UK in terms of total vaccination. This reflects the inequitable distribution between the global north and the global south. Even the COVAX initiative of WHO has fallen short in ensuring fair distribution. This vacuum in global cooperation has given opportunities to countries like Russia and China to pursue vaccine diplomacy and anti-west geopolitical reconfiguration. For instance, China's criticism of the initial US reluctance to help India and an attempt to provoke anti-US sentiment consolidates this argument. China is also accused of bribing and pressuring countries like Paraguay and Brazil for strategic and economic concessions against vaccine shipments. Russia, too, has provided its homemade Sputnik V vaccines to the Central Asian and East European nations in an attempt to bring them under its influence. In this respect, the vaccine diplomacy pursued by India, to achieve its global geopolitical and geostrategic aspirations can be a game-changer provided India successfully overcomes the deadly second wave and move closer towards herd immunization at the earliest.

5.17 Policy Recommendations

1. India's medical diplomacy has been bolstered as a result of the pandemic. India has made attempts to reach out to everyone in need, from hydroxychloroquine treatments to Covid-19 vaccines, and upholding its age-old concept in 'Vasudhaiva Kutumbakam'. When there was a rising fear of 'vaccine nationalism,' New Delhi provided a considerable volume of vaccine dosages to the neighbors and other countries in need. India's initiative has also been praised by neighboring countries. It's Mission Sagar to provide Covid-19-related assistance to the island states of the Maldives, Mauritius, Madagascar, Comoros, and Seychelles in an attempt to outsmart China. In this evolving post-Covid world, India should further its soft power diplomacy to calibrate its relationship with its neighbors to secure regional strategic goals and negate the influence of China in the region.
2. Engaging with the QUAD may help India achieve two geo-strategic goals: opposing China's aggressive stance on the border with India's aggressiveness in the marine domain, and emerging as a net security provider in the region. The Quad Vaccine Partnership has set the goal of producing 1 billion vaccine doses by the end of 2022. India, as the leading manufacturer of pharmaceuticals, has the potential to make a substantial contribution to the program.
3. Now that India has become the second country to vaccinate more than 100 crore people with at least a single dose of vaccine in record time, it must re-launch its vaccine diplomacy to assist countries in the region and around the world that are struggling to obtain sufficient vaccine dosages. There is also the opportunity to contribute through the UN COVAX program. With its mass production capability, India must reclaim its title as the 'World Pharmacy'.
4. With the markets showing indications of recovery, India has a unique opportunity to re-emphasize its 'Atmahnirbhar Bharat' program. This would encourage MSMEs and new start-ups to enter the market after suffering severe economic implications as a result of the pandemic. A new trade strategy would allow them to expand their reach beyond national borders, boost the competitiveness of Indian brands, and position India as a worldwide leader.

5.18 Conclusion

Pandemic COVID-19, has given a comprehensive lesson to India. Indian foreign policy orientation and equations have been gradually changing due to COVID-19. Despite facing a financial crisis, India has been trying to resurrect its economy. The setback of relations between India and China amid COVID-19 on the issue of the border compelled India to formulate the 'policy of self-reliant'. After the border standoff on 15th June 2020, India has decided to boycott Chinese goods. At the same time, India and global democratic forces have been united to suppress China. India's long-awaited goal to be a global power can be fulfilled through the formulation of an anti-Chinese global lobby. During COVID-19, through various generous and humanitarian measures, India has tried to enhance its acceptability in the post-COVID world. That may give India extra mileage in fulfilling its goal. From South Asia, Southeast Asia, and the Indian Ocean Region, India has been supplying vaccines and medical equipment. Despite the existing domestic challenges emanating out of the pandemic, India has decided to help countries like the United States, a few European, African, and Latin American countries by providing medicines and sending medical professionals (Nandy, 2020).

India has been propagating the ancient Sanskrit dictum *Vasudhaiva Kutumbakam,* meaning "the world is one family." For a highly populated country like India, it would be a very difficult task to overcome the financial crisis caused by COVID-19. The present interdependent pattern of the global order might be changed in the post-COVID-19 period. India has already decided to opt for self-reliance. The Prime Minister has thus begun to advocate 'vocal for local'. The over-dependence on foreign goods and services has taught India a great lesson. The COVID-19 might be beneficial for India in implementing the project of 'Make in India'.

The second wave of the pandemic has wreaked havoc on India, with cases reaching over 4 lacs per day and deaths numbering in the thousands. India, on the other hand, has been able to successfully vaccinate more than 100 crore people because of a well-coordinated immunization policy that began early this year. This historic event has also supported the stock market, which is showing signs of a quick rebound. India, which had to halt sharing of vaccines to other countries due to mounting domestic pressure in the face of a vaccination shortage, has resumed the process of vaccine sharing under the COVAX program. There has been a change of administration in the United States, the re-Talibanization of Afghanistan, increasing significance of QUAD, formation of a new security alliance between the US, Australia, and Britain, and rising tensions between China and the United States over trade and free navigation during this time. Also, when countries around the world progressively open up and return to business as usual, it will be interesting to see how global power politics unfold in the following days, and how this may affect or benefit New Delhi.

References

Beri, R. (2021). *India's Vaccine Maitri with Africa.* New Delhi: Manohar Parrikar Institute for Defence Studies and Analyses.

Bhalla, A. (2021, April 30). Indian Navy launches operation Samudra Setu-II to bring medical oxygen from abroad. *India Today.* Retrieved May 5, 2021, from https://www.indiatoday.in/cor onavirus-outbreak/story/indian-navy-launches-operation-samudra-setu-ii-to-bring-medical-oxy gen-from-abroad-1797073-2021-05-02

Bhattacharya, D. (2021). *India at the centre stage in the G20: Strategic role in post COVID-19 world order.* Observer Research Foundation.

Chaudhary, A., & Czuczka, T. (2021, April 26). On Slow US Response To India's Covid Crisis, China's Strategic Digs. *NDTV.* Retrieved April 30, 2021, from https://www.ndtv.com/world-news/superficial-closeness-chinas-digs-over-us-response-to-india-crisis-2422329

Chaudhury, D. R. (2020, April 10). Covid diplomacy establishes India as a reliable and responsible global power. *The Economic Times.* Retrieved March 21, 2021, from https://economictimes.ind

iatimes.com/news/politics-and-nation/covid-diplomacy-establishes-india-as-a-reliable-and-res
ponsible-global-power/articleshow/75080356.cms?from=mdr

(2021). *Coronavirus in Africa tracker.* BBC. Retrieved March 24, 2021, from https://www.bbc.co.
uk/news/resources/idt-4a11d568-2716-41cf-a15e-7d15079548bc

(2021). *Covid Tracker.* The Times of India. Retrieved May 7, 2021, from https://timesofindia.indiat
imes.com/coronavirus

Dhar, B. (2021). *India's vaccine diplomacy for the global good.* East Asia Forum. Retrieved March
21, 2021, from https://www.eastasiaforum.org/2021/02/08/indias-vaccine-diplomacy-for-the-glo
bal-good/

Financial Express. (2021). *India treading on vaccine diplomacy! 58 million doses to 71 countries
bolsters Quad vaccine initiative.* Retrieved March 25, 2021, from https://www.financialexpress.
com/lifestyle/health/india-treading-on-vaccine-diplomacy-58-million-doses-to-71-countries-bol
sters-quad-vaccine-initiative/2212288/

Ghosh, N. (2020). The Indian Imperatives in the Post-COVID World. In P. De, &
S. Gupta, *COVID-19 Challenges for the Indian Economy: Trade and Foreign Policy
Effects.* (p. 25). New Delhi: India Habitat Centre. Retrieved March 19, 2021, from
file:///C:/Users/XYZ/Desktop/Covid19_Report.pdf,

Giri, A. (2021, January 26). How India is using vaccine diplomacy to recalibarate its neighbourhood
first policy. *The Kathmandu Post.* Retrieved March 19, 2021, from https://kathmandupost.com/
national/2021/01/26/how-india-is-using-vaccine-diplomacy-to-recalibrate-its-neighbourhood-
first-policy

Gupta, S. (2020, May 11). India draws up Rs 1 billion Covid-19 medical assistance plan, targets
90 countries. *Hindustan Times.* Retrieved March 26, 2021, from https://www.hindustantimes.
com/india-news/india-amps-up-covid-19-medical-assistance-plan-targets-to-reach-90-countr
ies/story-0X1H8z1Zqi9piw6n4FDu8J.html

IANS. (2021). *India's vaccine diplomacy garners praise from global media.* India Tv. Retrieved
March 26, 2021, from https://www.indiatvnews.com/news/india/global-media-praise-india-vac
cine-diplomacy-covishield-covaxin-latest-news-684704

India Gifts 49 Lakhs Doses to Neighbours. (2021, January 22). *Business Line.* Retrieved March 25,
2021

Indian Navy. (2020). *Indian Navy Completes "Operation Samudra Setu".* Retrieved April
2, 2021, from https://www.indiannavy.nic.in/content/indian-navy-completes-%E2%80%9Coper
ation-samudra-setu%E2%80%9D

James, T., Shaw, P., Chatterjee, P., & Bhatia, D. (2015). *India Africa Partnership in Health Care:
Accomplishments and Prospects.* New Delhi: Research and Information Systems for Developing
Countries (RIS).

Krishanan, A. (2021, January 19). Explaining India's Vaccine Diplomacy in the neighbourhood
and beyond. *The Hindu.* Retrieved March 23, 2021, from https://www.thehindu.com/podcast/
explaining-indias-vaccine-diplomacy-in-the-neighbourhood-and-beyond-the-hindu-infocuspo
dcast/article33611425.ece

Krishnankutty, P. (2021, February 11). India has set an example in global diplomacy with Covid, climate change, says Jaishankar. *The Print.* Retrieved March 26,
2021, from https://theprint.in/diplomacy/india-has-set-an-example-in-global-diplomacy-with-
covid-climate-change-says-jaishankar/603477/

Laskar, R. H. (2021, April 29). Covid-19 second wave: Russia extends support to India. *The
Hindustan Times.* Retrieved April 30, 2021, from https://www.hindustantimes.com/india-news/
covid19-second-wave-russia-extends-support-to-india-101619637043753.html

Marcus, M. B. (2021). *Ensuring Everyone in the World Gets a COVID Vaccine.* Duke University's
Global Health Institute. Retrieved March 25, 2021, from https://www.eastasiaforum.org/2021/
02/08/indias-vaccine-diplomacy-for-the-global-good/

MEA. (2020). *English translation of Prime Minister's address at 75th United Nations General
Assembly.* Ministry of External Affairs, GoI. Retrieved March 26, 2021, from https://www.

mea.gov.in/Speeches-Statements.htm?dtl/33064/English_translation_of_Prime_Ministers_address_at_75th_United_Nations_General_Assembly

Mohan, G. (2020). *Vande Bharat Mission: India launches massive repatriation drive for Indian nationals*. India Today. Retrieved March 26, 2021, from https://www.indiatoday.in/india/story/vande-bharat-mission-india-launches-massive-repatriation-drive-for-indian-nationals-1675040-2020-05-06

Nag, B. (2020). Post-COVID-19 Global Econmic Order and China Scenario Building for India's 2050 Strategy. In P. De, & S. Gupta, *COVID-19 Challenges for the Indian Economy: Trade and Foreign Policy Effects* (p. 25). New Delhi: India Habitat Centre. Retrieved March 19, 2021, from file:///C:/Users/XYZ/Desktop/Covid19_Report.pdf

Naha, A. (2020). India & the Indo-Pacific: An appraisal. In N. H. Lashkar (Ed.), *International Relations: Emerging Issues* (pp. 69–77). Authors Press.

Nandy, D. (2020). *Revisiting India's Post-Cold War Foreign Policy: Since 1991 to Present Day*. Avenel Press.

Neighbour's pride. (2021, January 21). *The Indian Express*. Retrieved March 24, 2021, from https://indianexpress.com/article/opinion/editorials/coronavirus-vaccine-bangladesh-nepal-myanmar-south-asia-7155004/

New world order emerging post-Covid, India can be a leader: PM Modi. (2021, February 10). *The Hindustan Times*. Retrieved March 24, 2021, from https://www.hindustantimes.com/india-news/the-way-india-handled-and-helped-itself-and-the-world-during-covid-19-was-a-turn-101612952912722.html

Pant, H., & Tirkey, A. (2021). India's Vaccine Diplomacy. *Observer Research Foundation*. Retrieved March 20, 2021, from https://www.orfonline.org/research/indias-vaccine-diplomacy/

Pasricha, A. (2021, January 24). COVID-19 global reality check, from China, South Africa to Cuba. *Voice of America*. Retrieved March 26, 2021, from https://www.voanews.com/covid-19-pandemic/india-launches-neighborly-vaccine-diplomacy

Pratt, S. F., & Levin, J. (2021). Vaccines Will Shape the New Geopolitical Order. *Foreign Policy*. Retrieved May 1, 2021, from https://foreignpolicy.com/2021/04/29/vaccine-geopolitics-diplomacy-israel-russia-china/

(2021). *President Cyril Ramaphosa bemoans rise of nationalism*. eNCA.

PTI. (2020). *India co-sponsors resolution calling for equitable access to COVID-19 vaccines*. The Hindu.

PTI. (2021, January 23). 'India a true friend,' says US; lauds move to gift COVID-19 vaccine to several countries. *Business Today*. Retrieved March 26, 2021, from https://www.India a true friend,' says US; lauds move to gift COVID-19 vaccine to several countriesbusinesstoday.in/current/economy-politics/india-a-true-friend-says-us-lauds-move-to-gift-covid-19-vaccine-to-several-countries/story/428847.html

Roche, E. (2020, May 11). Despite challenges, India provided medical assistance to 133 countries: Shringla. *Mint*. Retrieved March 26, 2021, from https://www.livemint.com/news/india/despite-challenges-india-provided-medical-assistance-to-133-countries-shringla-11589209146018.html

(2021). *Rwanda's president Paul Kagame warns on delayed vaccination in Africa*. Africa News.

Sajjanhar, A. (2021). *India's 'Vaccine Maitri' Initiative*. Manohar Parrikar Institute for Defence Studies and Analyses. Retrieved March 25, 2021, from https://idsa.in/idsacomments/indias-vaccine-maitri-initiative-asajjanhar-290121

Saran, S. (2020, March 25). A revival of multilateralism, steered by India. *The Hindu*. Retrieved March 27, 2021, from https://www.thehindu.com/opinion/lead/a-revival-of-multilateralism-steered-by-india/article31093421.ece

Sen, A. (2021, March 21). India's 'Vaccine Maitri' initiative earns praise at WTO. *Bussiness Line*. Retrieved March 26, 2021, from https://www.thehindubusinessline.com/news/national/indias-vaccine-maitri-initiative-earns-praise-at-wto/article33979754.ece

(2021). *Seychelles: India gifts Seychelles with COVISHIELD vaccines*. Africa News.

Siddiqui, H. (2020, November 8). Mission Sagar II – India extends a helping hand to IOR countries; After Sudan, Eritrea receives food aid. *Financial Express*. Retrieved March 26, 2021, from https://www.financialexpress.com/defence/mission-sagar-ii-india-extends-a-helping-hand-to-ior-countries-after-sudan-eritrea-receives-food-aid/2123677/

Singh, N. (2020). Mission Sagar: Key to the Indian Ocean. *ORF Young Voices.* Retrieved March 24, 2021, from https://www.orfonline.org/expert-speak/mission-sagar-key-to-the-indian-ocean/

Taneja, P., & Singh, B. (2021). India's Domestic and Foreign Policy responses to COVID-19. *The round Table, 110*(1), 46–61. https://doi.org/10.1080/00358533.2021.1875685

The Global Times. (2021, April 24). Lack of international cooperation glaring in India's epidemic ballooning: Global Times editorial. Retrieved April 30, 2021, from https://www.globaltimes.cn/page/202104/1221945.shtml

The Hindu. (2020). *Coronavirus | Prime Minister Modi calls for COVID-19 Emergency Fund for SAARC.* Retrieved March 26, 2021, from https://www.thehindu.com/news/national/coronavirus-pm-modi-participates-in-saarc-videoconference-to-formulate-joint-strategy-to-combat-covid-19/article31074653.ece

The Hindustan Times. (2021, April 30). Japan to send oxygen concentrators, ventilators for India's Covid-19 response. Retrieved May 1, 2021, from https://www.hindustantimes.com/india-news/japan-to-send-oxygen-concentrators-ventilators-for-india-s-covid-19-response-101619758247166.html

The Times of India. (2021, April 29). 'Together we will win': France President Macron's message to .. Retrieved April 30, 2021, from https://timesofindia.indiatimes.com/india/covid-19-crisis-will-provide-all-assistance-to-india-french-president-emmanuel-macron-says/articleshow/82275673.cms

The Wire. (2021). *India Has Exported 5.84 Crore Doses of COVID-19 Vaccines To 70 Countries: Data.* Retrieved March 24, 2021, from https://science.thewire.in/health/india-has-exported-5-84-crore-doses-of-covid-19-vaccines-to-70-countries-data/

UNCTAD. (2020). *Impact of the COVID-19 Pandemic on Trade and Development: Transitioning to a New Normal.* Geneva. Retrieved March 20, 2021, from https://unctad.org/system/files/official-document/osg2020d1_en.pdf

UNI. (2020, April 17). PM Modi speaks to South African and Egyptian Presidents on COVID-19. *United News of India.* Retrieved from http://www.uniindia.com/pm-modi-speaks-to-south-african-and-egyptian-presidents-on-covid-19/india/news/1958949.html

Wenwen, W. (2021, April 27). US selfishness hits partnership with India, but China blamed. *The Global Times.* Retrieved April 30, 2021, from https://www.globaltimes.cn/page/202104/1222271.shtml

Debasish Nandy PhD is an Associate Professor and Head in the Department of Political Science, Kazi Nazrul University, Asansol, West Bengal, India. Dr. Nandy is the Coordinator of the Centre for Studies of South and South-East Asian Societies at the same University. He is a visiting faculty member in te Department of Foreign Area Studies at Tajik National University, Republic of Tajikistan.

Alik Naha is a Faculty Member in the Department of Political Science, Vidyasagar College, Kolkata, India.

Chapter 6
Pandemic and the Administrative Rationality: Understanding the Administrative Response to the Pandemic

Arindam Roy

Abstract The outbreak of the Corona Virus Disease 2019 or COVID 19 pandemic has literally dashed our enlightened scientific rationality. It has claimed more than six million lives around the globe. The struggling humanity has adopted a series of strict legal-administrative protocols like lockdown, quarantine, isolation, to contain the spread of the virus. However, the strict adherence to the above-mentioned protocols has brought several collateral damages like the disruption of normal socio-economic activities; suspension of political and civic engagements of the people. The situation gets further complicated as endless suggestions and opinions have been offered by several experts. The scientific community, till today, is grappling with the possible antidote of the virus in the form of vaccines. Several research laboratories across the globe have been actively engaged in devising full-proof vaccines of which, some have already started manufacturing commercially. Despite the tall claims of these companies, the efficacy of these vaccines is still not very clear. Moreover, the modality of administering these vaccines is another difficult issue, involving delicate distributive management that requires something more than mere scientific rationality. Further, given the nature of neoliberal governance, where delivery of services is a collective venture of all the stakeholders like state, civil society, market, and community, administrative rationality is perhaps the most important means. Drawing on the existing literature, the paper intends to explore the administrative responses to the pandemic of COVID-19 through the lens of administrative rationality. Finally, the paper with an optimistic note concludes that the administrative rationality of the bureaucracy has the potential to devise a bailout programme for all the stakeholders concerned.

Keywords Epidemic · Neoliberal governance · State · Civil society

---

A. Roy (✉)
Department of Political Science, University of Burdwan, Burdwan, West Bengal, India

© The Author(s), under exclusive license to Springer Nature Singapore Pte Ltd. 2022
S. Roy and D. Nandy (eds.), *Understanding Post-COVID-19 Social and Cultural Realities*, https://doi.org/10.1007/978-981-19-0809-5_6

6.1 Introduction

There is no denying that the entire humanity has been passing through an epidemiological disaster. From its outbreak in December 2019 to its present state of havoc, the novel coronavirus has claimed above six million people across the globe[1] (WHO Coronavirus Disease (COVID-19) Dashboard, n.d.) Apart from the primary implications of the pandemic like physical casualties, there are several other secondary implications of the pandemic that have gone well beyond the physical casualties to include economic disaster, social dislocation, psychological disorder, and polity disorder. For example, the economic impact of the virus is far more devastative in nature. In fact, it has surpassed the extent of the damage done by the global financial (liquidity) crisis of 2008. The pandemic has affected all sectors of the economy. From agriculture to industry almost all the sectors of the global economy have registered negative growth rates. For example, farmers have been suffering from broken supply chains, poor demand, dipping output prices, lack of market outlets, and so on. Similarly, the industrial sector has also suffered a serious setback. From hospitality, travel, and tour, aviation, real estate, to retail almost all the sectors of industry have sustained massive losses. However, an economic crisis of such magnitude fails to generate much-coveted multilateralism. In fact, a typical protectionist geo-economic strategy of putting the nationalist agenda above everything else has marked the post-Covid economic reconstruction on the part of the rich countries (Gregosz et al., 2020). For example, economic revival package like 'America First' or '*Atma Nirbhar Bharat*' may be mentioned. Consequently, multilateral organizations which could have provided immense help to the developing countries in fighting the economic shock have lost their relevance. In fact, the compulsion of doing business in the interconnected world has facilitated the pandemic to get global via growing air connectivity and free flow of labour from one part of the globe to another. Similarly, the pandemic has left an enduring socio-psychological imprint for the generations to come.

The prolonged period of social distancing and lockdown following the pandemic has led to social isolation and a drastic change in inter-human relations. Moreover, a constant fear of being exposed to the contagion in addition to irregular social contact leads to typical post-traumatic stress disorders like anxiety, depression, and distress. A state of uncertainty has obscured our conscience and existence. With no possible breather, either in the form of epidemiological breakthrough or in the way of pharmacological safeguard insight at the beginning, the struggling humanity has settled down for the legal- administrative protocols to resist the pandemic. Consequently, law and order administration took the centre stage in the fight against the pandemic bypassing any credible health measure. A Series of administrative measures have been imposed upon the people to contain the spread of the virus but to no effect. These authoritarian measures have brought severe collateral damages like the disruption of normal socio-economic and political activities, violation of civic and personal liberties of

---

[1] The actual numbers are 852,758 on 2nd August 2020.

the people, and so on. Hence, the pandemic has provided a sweeping administrative authority in the hands of the government to address the exigency situation that emerged out of it. It has not only disrupted public health but also dislocated democratic and governance processes worldwide. For example, some governments on the pretext of the pandemic have expanded their executive powers by restricting individual rights, delaying the electoral process, and disrupting the basic governance functioning. Further, the pandemic has also unsettled the ideal relationship between national and local governments in the federal setup (Frances et al., 2020; Yung Yung Chang, 2020).

Interestingly, bureaucratic rationality propelled all these decisions on an exigency basis became truncated. Except for the medical communities, especially the doctors, no other stakeholders were consulted in the administrative process. In fact, fighting the pandemic through the protocols like physical distancing, lockdown, quarantine, isolation, maintaining social and personal hygiene, public awareness, sensitization, etc., also demanded proper planning and responsive execution. But bureaucratic rationality viewed the pandemic mainly through the lens of law and order, which could be restored with appropriate arrangements like placing roadblocks, checkpoints, declaring night curfew, activating mobile squads to ward off defiant pedestrians, or motorists, etc. The state applied the new invasive digital surveillance mechanism in the wake of a pandemic by restoring the ethics of the old surveillance state which has intruded upon the private/personal space of the people and has grossly violated the fundamental human rights on the pretext of containing the spread of the virus. Moreover, in a hurry of arresting the further aggravation of the COVID-19 virus, all the regular health services were suspended for an indefinite period in the public hospitals (Porecha, 2020).

The role of the people, the primary stakeholders, especially the affected section of them, in the ongoing war against the pathogen, was not taken into consideration. In fact, in these arrangements, what was found missing, was proper planning and coordination among the multiple stakeholders. This caused endless misery of the stranded home-bound laborers (reverse- migration) in different parts of the country due to sudden lockdown. It is often called 'reverse migration' as people/workers are heading back home, which is opposite to migration where laborers leave their homes in search of a job in the city. The pandemic -induced hardship was not confined to the misery of the home-bound laborers alone. In fact, utter mismanagement of the public distribution system compelled the people to depend upon mercy and charity despite having surplus food reserves in the state granaries. These raised public service debates over the last few months.

The situation got further worsened as several experts via electronic and print media gave their seemingly endless and often contradictory opinions, suggestions, and advice. Under these circumstances, a serious existential question is begging our attention as to what should be the people's response to the present situation. In our country, there has been a parallel tradition of civic activism and civic engagement in delivering goods and services vis-a-vis the structuralist perspective of the statist administration. In fact, there have been some sporadic attempts at the community level to address the pandemic. But at the beginning of the crisis, the state had adopted an overbearing role, leaving no room for civic action. In fact, drawing on the colonial templates, the government had resorted to several measures to contain the pandemic which put serious roadblocks for civil society activism. Hence, given the nature of the epidemic, it would be too ambitious to think in terms of a non-structured way of handling the situation as the so-called third sector or non-governmental sector in India has no significant presence. Under the circumstance, the pandemic of COVID 19 compels us to repose our faith on the good old 'administrative rationality' to cope with this 'new normal'. The 'New Normal' depicts a state of economy, society, and polity following a crisis which differs markedly from the situation that was prevailing before the problem. In other words, the new normal signifies the adaptation of humankind to the unprecedented situation by bringing about several new modalities. The term has been in vogue following the financial crisis of 2007–2008, the aftermath of the 2008–2012 global recession, and the COVID-19 pandemic (Buheji, M., & Ahmed, D.A.A. in Business Management and Strategy, 2020).

The need for administrative solutions does not cease with the Covid 19 situation alone. In fact, its importance increases manifold in the management of the post-Covid situation. Since the handling of the pandemic requires a fine balancing between research and its application, specialized know-how alone is not enough. Hence, identifying the cause of the pandemic or devising an antidote alone cannot bail out humanity from the scourge of the virus. For, returning to the pre-pandemic stage involves the most important issue of distribution of the antidotes in addition to a host of logistic issues. Thus, the complexity of the post-COVID-19 situation demands holistic generalist intervention based on the virtue of administrative rationality. The scientific community across the globe has launched a massive drive to know the nature of the virus, its probable behavioural pattern including its pace of mutation, aggravation, and its life cycle so that a credible antidote in the form of vaccine can be devised. Eventually, at the end of 2020, there are more than 200 vaccines are in the making worldwide and governments are busy dealing with the modalities to distribute those vaccines. Dodd et al. (2020). Even amid the jubilation of the discovery of vaccines, worrisome news of mutation of a new more lethal variant of SARS-CoV-2 was reported in the UK. As per the various scientific modeling exercises, the new variant unlike its earlier version is 70% more transmissible. This new variant was first reported in September 2020 in the UK when it was just one of the four diagnosed cases. But by mid-December the new variant has reached almost two-thirds of the new cases in London, leading to strict tier-4 lockdown across the country. (). Recently, an alarmingly new and potentially more fatal COVID-19 strain is spotted in South Africa which is claimed to have neutralized the immune system developed by the vaccines. Researchers claimed that the mutations on the specific part of the virus's outer spike protein would enable it to escape antibodies. In fact, the mutation they studied in South Africa (i.e. E484K) has demonstrated that there has been a frightening transformation in the shape of the spike protein, used by the virus to latch onto cells in the body. Such scientific revelations undoubtedly put the efficacy of vaccines into question as to the recent trend of mutation of the virus, spotted in South Africa, has the potential to make the recently developed vaccines redundant.

6.1.1 Methodology

The paper tries to make sense of the problem of the so-called bureaucratic handling of the pandemic of the Covid 19 and calls for an immediate infusion of administrative rationality in administrative deliberations. The paper is premised on a working hypothesis that bureaucratic organization with administrative rationality turns out to be the most reliable means of provisioning public goods and services. Drawing on the recent experiences of Covid management in India, the paper has demonstrated how administrators have resorted to administrative rationality in delivering public services. For testing the above working hypothesis, the paper has conducted an ethnographic study in purposively chosen two districts of West Bengal-one reported with the highest percentage of Covid positive cases and another with lowest cases. Further, two sets of respondents have been identified for the study viz. the administrators for getting the administrator's/ deliverer's perspective; and from the common citizens to know the beneficiary's perspective. A sample of a total of 300 citizens, 150 each from each district (with 75 each from two blocks) have been chosen for the ethnographic survey. However, garnering information from the administrators, especially on the management of day-to-day affairs is a daunting task as bureaucrats hardly share information. Hence, as a technique of data collection, the paper has primarily opted for qualitative methods especially ethnomethodological techniques like in-depth interviews, focused group interviews, and narrative analysis to grasp the administrator's rationale of administrative deliberations.

6.2 Theoretical Framework

As a theoretical framework, the paper has subscribed to the ideal-type construction of bureaucracy by Max Weber, bounded rationality by Herbert Simon, disjointed incrementalism by Lindblom, and pathological theory of bureaucracy by Parkinson and Peter. Whereas Weber, made strong advocacy for ideal-type construction of bureaucracy to streamline administrative deliberation (Albrow, 1970); Herbert Simon has questioned the notion of absolute rationality and emphasized the improvising capacity of the administrator to draw a line in the perennial search for absolute rationality (Simon, 1957). Lindblom has advised his administrator to master the art of muddling through (Lindblom, 1959, 1979). Parkinson C. Northcote (1957) and Peter (Peter and Hull 1969) have made pathological profiling of bureaucracy and explained how bureaucracy gets bulkier and inefficient.

Besides that, the article intends to explore the concept of administrative rationality and identifies the significant shortcomings of administrative rationality. It concludes with an argument in favour of administrative rationality to cope with the 'new normal' with an analytical discussion.

6.3 In Search of Administrative Rationality

The present section fields in the concept of 'administrative rationality' to overcome the current pandemic situation, especially in addressing the collateral damages of the pandemic on society, polity, and economy. Administrative rationality springs out and presupposes the existence of an administrative state. Since the endorsement of it by Dwight Waldo in his famous book of the same title in 1948, the administrative state had secured a permanent berth in the development discourse until the New Right philosophy dethroned it. Before we move on to spell out the concept of administrative rationality, as we set out in the beginning, a caveat seems to be in order so that administration rationality should not be treated as an unmixed blessing for humanity. At the outset, a few unsettling questions merit our attention: what do we mean by administrative rationality in the first place? Whether administrative rationality is self-sufficient? Do they comprise other types of rationalities like economic or political rationalities? Shall we go for homogenous administrative rationality or shall we go for multiple rationalities? These are but a few conceptual puzzles that may interrogate the efficacy of administrative rationality in fighting the pandemic. In the course of the discussion, the paper tries to address the above conceptual puzzles. However, responding to these puzzles demands a brief discussion on the concept of administrative rationality in the first place.

6.4 Administrative Rationality: The Conceptual Explorations

Administrative rationality is a capacious term that includes among others instrumental rationality, technical rationality, formal/legal rationality (Stout, 2013) in addition to patrimonial values and the 'art of judgment' (Vickers, 1965). In common parlance, administrative rationality is often getting blurred with bureaucratic rationality and subjects to public opprobrium and bureau-bashing. But in reality, it is too wider a concept to be confined within the oppressive idea of bureaucratic rationality. Unlike bureaucratic rationality, administrative rationality does not spring automatically. It is a product of continuous engagement with administrative deliberations. Hence, for the sake of conceptual clarity, the concept of administrative rationality needs to be differentiated from some of the associated concepts. However, before we move on to untangle the idea of administrative rationality a clear definition of the vexing issue of rationality warrants some space here as endless debates have been spawning around the very meaning of 'rationality'. Moreover, the idea of rationality has taken several theoretical forms such as rhetorical, historical, normative, political, and social, leading to conceptual confusion (Curtis Ventriss, 2003). Nicolaidis in one of his path-breaking research on administrative decision making has demonstrated that the nature of rationality in the traditional model was primarily based on the following propositions: economic man, the 'one best way' of scientific management and industrial engineering; and the ideal type of bureaucracy postulated by Max Weber (Pfiffner, 1960). To him, the classical concept of rationality is striving for a universal logic, which is independent of time, space, and principle. However, the administrative decision-making is not linear, but more circular in nature. To him, administrative rationality is a constellation of numerous individual decisions based on three important elements viz. muddling through, eliminating uncertainty, and clothing with reason. Moreover, the concept of rationality becomes more complicated as it comes in different combinations. For instance, technical rationality is often wrongly equated with administration rationality.

Technical rationality undeniably constitutes the core of administrative rationality, but it is not equal to administrative rationality. From the administrative point of view, technical rationality tends to repudiate all the values and reposes its commitment to facts. However, conceptually speaking, it is a philosophical idea associated with the Frankfurt school and to be more specific with Herbert Marcuse (Marcuse, 1964). He had introduced the concept in 1941 in a journal of philosophy and developed it in his famous book entitled 'One Dimensional State' in 1964. According to Marcuse, technological innovations and progress have the potential to liberate a human being from the bondage of labour and erstwhile rationalities of humankind. The formal/legal rationality, on the other hand, has a legal/constitutional sanction to exercise authority. Max Weber had dealt with it in a very comprehensive manner in discussing the nature of ideal type bureaucracy. The formal/legal rationality in the form of legal/constitutional sanction may ensure much-needed legitimacy in administrative deliberations, but it alone cannot guarantee the holistic assurance of administrative rationality. Administrative rationality is also confused with instrumental rationality. In common perception, instrumental rationality is understood as a kind of rationality that is specially constructed to suit a particular objective. It is an indispensable part of practical rationality. Max Weber had distinguished between instrumental rationality and value rationality. Geoffrey Vickers has highlighted the importance of making a judgment in the overall process of decision-making. To him, appreciation, which is an inherently human activity, lies at the heart of human judgment (Vickers, 1965). Vickers has identified three distinct components of appreciative judgment: first, is the *making of reality judgment*, which is based on detail reality check; secondly, the *making of value judgment,* which is based on the assessment of underlying value bases; and thirdly, the making of instrumental judgment. Moreover, administrative rationality also includes the deontological commitments of the administrator. However, deontological commitment does not necessarily mean dry and arid mechanical compliance to technical rationality, embedded either in the administrative rule book or in the Constitution. Though the concept of deontological commitment has a long philosophical root, in common perception, it signifies duty bounded-ness, which is not interrupted by any other considerations. More importantly, deontological commitment has a dangerous potential of falling into a bureaucratic or administrative evil if it is not properly checked by contextuality.

There are several unwritten contextual considerations and conventions are embedded in the organizational culture that is equally significant in the making of administrative rationality. Despite their reservations, none of the administrative thinkers has denied the importance of administrative rationality in administrative management. There is a continuity of thought on administrative rationality, which can be traced back to the ideas of Max Weber, Lindblom, and Herbert Simon. Though not expressed inconclusive terms except Max Weber, both Herbert Simon and Lindblom reposed their faith in the improvisations of administrators, which is nothing but administrative rationality. For example, Herbert Simon leaves his administrator to decide what would be the rational decision in a given context in his famous concept of 'bounded rationality. To him, the rationality criterion of a decision is not predetermined. In fact, it is dependent upon his judgment based on his point of satisfaction or what Simon called 'satisfying' (Simon, 1957). Similarly, Lindblom has reposed his faith in administrators' capability of muddling through in his famous thesis of disjointed incrementalism. Administrative decision-making, according to the bargaining approach, demands a lot of persuasion and flexibility on the part of the administrators. Charles E. Lindblom, a Yale economist and a profound scholar of public policy has introduced this approach of (administrative) decision making in his seminal essay 'The Science of Muddling through' in 1959. In the said essay, Lindblom has interrogated the systematic and rational nature of planning and decision making. To him, administrative decisions are not always the product of solid reasoning and rationality. In fact, in a real-life situation, administrative decision-making demands much more discretion on the part of the administrators to arrive at any conclusive decision. Hence, it would be a gross over expectation to think that an administrator stationed at the ground level to go by all the possible value choices available at that given point of time, weigh the potentials of those options and finally settle down for a particular option as a decision. These types of rational approach or what is generally known as a rational comprehensive approach, views Lindblom, is inadequate for three reasons: intellectual, behavioural, and political. Intellectually, going through all the possible alternatives to arrive at a specific option as a decision is seldom possible as it is beyond the capabilities of a common man. Behaviourally, also the rational comprehensive approach is inadequate as the approach fails to explain why people behave the way they do in a practical situation. Similarly, from the political point of view, absolute rational decision-making is not feasible as the planning and policy-making cannot be disassociated from the overarching political structure of the society. Moreover, arriving at the value consensus, which is supposed to be the core of rational decision making is not always possible in a pluralistic democracy.

Hence, to salvage his administrator from the practical policy -dilemma, Lindblom has brought a new approach of decision making, entitled 'disjointed incrementalism'. For him the concept of disjointed incrementalism may be summed up in the following points: first, decision making is essentially incremental in nature as administrative decisions are reached through small and adjusted steps, not in a single go as it is wrongly perceived in some theoretical constructions. Secondly, it is thought to be incomprehensible as the administrator cannot consider all options into account. Thirdly, the comparison which constitutes the heart of the branching technique of decision-making is not an end in itself. Decisions are 'made and remade seamlessly through small chains of comparisons between narrow choices'. Fourthly, decision-making in practice 'suffices rather than maximizes' from among the options available. Fifthly, decision-making is based on a pluralist notion of the public sector, where competing interest groups struggle over policy issues. Hence, decision-making is the political art of compromise, dependent upon negotiating skills of the administrator. Caught among the contesting demands mooted by several interest groups for greater control over the policymaking process, the administrator has to navigate very cautiously to arrive at any decision finally.

The next important issue regarding administrative rationality that deserves some space here is the nature of administrative rationality. It should be noted that administrative rationality is not an autonomous construction. It is constructed by several other types of rationalities like economic rationality, political rationality, socio-cultural context, and so on. Hence, to consider administrative rationality as a lucid and homogeneous construction would be an oversimplification of reality. Administrative rationality though often presented as a homogenous construction, in actuality, however, it is composed of multiple nationalities. Hence, administrative rationality is not a magic wand that can bail out humanity from a catastrophe like COVID 19. In fact, it has several shortcomings and maybe degenerate into administrative evils, if it is not counterbalanced by flexibility and contextuality. In the following section, an attempt will be made to highlight the dangerous potentials of administrative rationality that need to be excluded in practice.

6.5 Blues of Administrative Rationality-A Devil's Advocacy

This section engages into a devil's advocacy of sort, which has identified the major objections regarding administration, especially the typical dehumanizing tendency of the bureaucratic rationality to distinguish it from the administrative rationality. To begin the section, it should be noted that unlike in common parlance, where bureaucratic rationality is getting blurred with administrative rationality, the present paper has deliberately distinguished it from administrative rationality, which is qualitatively different from the former. Hence, the dehumanizing tag is more appropriate for bureaucratic rationality. Even the most important protagonist of bureaucratic rationality, Max Weber, did not deny the dehumanizing effect of it. Weber had anticipated the birth of an administrative man, who would reduce administration to a typical dehumanizing organization dotted with submissive individuals, without any critical faculty of comprehension. To him 'administrative man', is not a normal social being, rather a queer fusion of half-man and a half-machine committed to the technical rationality of organization. He had voiced his concern about bureaucratization in the following words: 'It is horrible to think that the world could one day be filled with those little cogs, little men clinging to their jobs and striving towards ones - a state of affairs which is to be seen once more as … playing an increasing part in the spirit of our present administrative system … world should know no men but these: it is in such an evolution that we are already caught up, and the great question is therefore not how we can promote and hasten it but what can we oppose to this machinery to keep a portion of mankind free from parceling-out of the soul, from this supreme mastery of the bureaucratic way of life' (Turner et al., 1998). Herbert Simon was equally apprehensive of the dehumanizing element of bureaucratic rationality. Hence, he had scaled down the eternal search for absolute administrative rationality and wanted his administrators to abide by the limits of rationality in his famous conception of bounded rationality. In fact, there is an alarming possibility lies embedded in the technocratic rationality of bureaucracy. In this context, a fascinating joint publication, entitled *Unmasking Administrative Evil* in 2004 by Guy B. Adams and Danny L. Balfour deserved some space here. They have demonstrated that such evils are neither benign nor unintentional nor accidental. The text had brought forth the shortcomings of technocratic rationality codified in bureaucratic rationality as they appear on many occasions. Those acts of applying bureaucratic, technical rationality are deadly lethal. But the puzzle lies in the fact that it is presented in an out and out rational-legal and formal organizational framework. Hence, administrative evil should not be belittled as a mere act of a 'crazy leader, personal failings, lax controls or racist ideologies' (Adams and Balfour 2004).

No act of a leader can be that lethal until and unless there is a bureaucratic backup in terms of efficiency and professional commitment. The horrific extermination campaign during the Nazi rule in Germany and the holocaust bear a very vivid imprint of administrative evil. Interestingly, this kind of administrative evil is often indistinguishable from any other normal administrative malpractices. Moreover, serious theoretical discussion on it is rather non-existent in administrative theory. However, a solid theoretical foundation of administrative evil was provided by Hannah Arendt in her celebrated publication *The Origin of Totalitarianism*, way back in the 1950s. In exploring the intricacies of totalitarianism, Arendt has demonstrated how bureaucracy becomes instrumental in rationalizing the application of terror or what she termed as the 'logicality of terror'. In *The Human Conditions* Arendt had mentioned the instrumentality of bureaucracy in the following words: 'As we know from the most social form of government, that is, from bureaucracy …the rule of nobody is not necessarily no-rule; it may indeed, under certain circumstances, even turn out to be one of its cruelest and most tyrannical versions' (Arendt, 1958). The distinguishing characteristics of administrative evil may be summarised as follows: first, the hallmark of this evil is the deontological commitment towards one's professional responsibilities. Secondly, a corollary of the earlier point it's the inversion or abdication of any moral overtone. Here moral standpoint is discounted to suit the objective of the organization.

The act of malice is administratively 'sanitized' and accepted as rational and proper in terms of efficiency. In other words, the technical-rational approach to public services is valorized to the extreme. The grisly example of official communication between the German Rail Authority and the Gestapo under the rule of the Third Reich was a case in point, where the Gestapo sought concession from the German Railway Authority for transporting groups (group rates) and children to their death. Thirdly, deceptive simplicity is another important feature of administrative evil. If we draw on the example of the Gestapo, discussed in the last point, we will find the impression of deceptive simplicity. The gruesome act of eliminating Jews was presented in such a nonchalant and matter-of-fact manner, that it appears on the surface as a mere routine task of administration. Hence, a lethal potential of relegating into administrative evil is embedded in the useful and innocuous concept of bureaucratic rationality, and utmost care should be taken to temper it with flexibility, commitment, contextuality. The concept of administrative rationality has the strength of overcoming the inadequacy of bureaucratic rationality. In the context of the 'new normal', the concept of administrative rationality is perhaps the only wherewithal we have at our disposal.

6.6 Making Sense of the Administrative Perplexity in the Postcolonial Societies

The pandemic of COVID 19 has exposed the severe administrative fault line of the postcolonial states. Administration in these societies has been subject to severe criticism. Since the reportage of the first COVID positive case in India to its present state of devastation, the administration appears to be in a state of disarray. Indeed, the administrative perplexity is the manifestation of administrative confusion in every executive deliberation in the post-COVID times. Interestingly, critiques of different ideological orientations have come together in criticizing the organizational responses to the pandemic. The allegations are ranging from inefficiency, lack of commitment, to lack of professionalism. However, it would be completely misleading to accuse the administration alone as the administrative realities in most of the postcolonial countries are caught among the several alternatives or trade-offs which have acted as impediments to administrative efficiency and effectiveness. In the following section, an attempt will be made to spell out the said trade-offs.

The **first** and perhaps the most intractable alternatives that the administration has to grapple with is the ***trade-off between life and livelihood***. The unprecedented pace of the aggravation of the microorganism of COVID 19 demanded equally exceptional measures like coercive compliance of the Covid protocol. However, implementation of those coercive policies is not an easy task as the success of the said policies is directly proportional to the loss of livelihood. Hence, the pandemic -hit administration finds itself in a tight spot as the risk of life is equally poised between the virus and poverty (or pathogen and starvation). Sandwiched between the two inflexible options, the administration has to tread very cautiously so that there will be a proper balance between life and livelihood. Recent pandemic has demonstrated that the trade-off between life and livelihood has curtailed administrative efficiency to a great extent. The lockdown as a significant step to contain the spread of the Coronavirus is a case in point. The exponential rise of Corona positive cases in India in the recent past demanded immediate suspension of all the social and economic activities through the imposition of complete lockdown. Such measures might have solid scientific reasoning, but the application of these measures for an indefinite period would involve economic repercussions, especially livelihood issues. Hence, caught between the two complicated options, administrators have to strike a proper balance to fight the 'new normal'.

Ensuring livelihood security has been a serious preoccupation for the administration in India since independence. The general administration has been roped in the task of guaranteeing livelihood security to undo the sorry legacy of underdevelopment under colonial governance. The arrangement continued until the onset of globalization. Globalization, with its associated string of conditionality, has brought a body blow for livelihood security as the neoliberals are discarding the positive interventionist role of the state. Consequently, the administration finds itself in a difficult position to deliver services with limited capacities. Hence, the apparent untidiness of the administrative deliberations during a present pandemic can be attributed to the said macroeconomic compulsions as well.

6.6.1 Secondly, the Trade-off between Transparency and Public Order

There is little doubt that transparency constitutes the heart of good governance. It compels the government to behave the way it should behave. But if we approach the issue of transparency from the administrative perspective, the concern for public order cannot be entirely ignored as it often restricts the free flow of information. Further, transparency cannot be unrestrained in nature. This is more so if we consider the relative importance of the issue of transparency in the era of post-truth.

Further, it should be noted that the live streaming of events in the name of transparency is also dangerous for social order. Hence, being the repository of law and order in society, the administration cannot afford to ignore the fallout of the 'overexposure to information for greater social cohesion. An example of the recent pandemic of COVID 19 is a case in point. There is a lot of hue and cry about the suppressing of actual data of patients and death. It was argued that the administration in a bid to cover up their inefficiency in handling the pandemic had suppressed the real picture and such an act of suppression is no less a criminal offense. But viewing from the administrative perspective, the apprehension of public hysteria due to overexposure to unadulterated dissemination of information cannot be overlooked. The administration prefers to exercise restraint in the dissemination of information as such restraint has nothing to do with the quality of administrative deliberations.

6.6.2 Thirdly, the Trade-off between Welfarism and Pareto Optimality

The exchange between welfare versus Pareto optimality boils down to the most unsettling problem for the administration under neoliberal governance. Pareto's optimality, the essence of market transaction, is explained as 'the economic situation when the circumstances of one individual cannot be made better without making the situation worse for another individual'. Pareto's optimality takes place when the resources are optimally utilized. It was theorized by the Italian economist and engineer Vilfredo Pareto. Administrations across the globe have been wrestling with this dilemma. On the one hand, the ground realities of most of the postcolonial societies demand welfare intervention or welfare measures in the social sector. Still, the neoliberal conditionalities based on Pareto optimality of the market, on the other hand, preclude any welfare measure on the part of the administration as such providentialism might distort market dynamism. Administration perplexity in the wake of the recent pandemic is indicative of this trade-off. Caught between the contesting priorities of social optima and Pareto optima, the administration fails to deliver the services it is expected to deliver.

6.6.3 Fourthly, the Trade-off between Permanency and Adhocracy

The administration is also caught in the contesting priorities between permanency and adhocracy. Permanency, which was the hallmark of traditional bureaucratic administration has gone past the phase of so-called 'sheltered bureaucracy', where bureaucracy enjoyed benign support of the state and entered into a phase of adhocracy, indicative of the post-bureaucratic administration, marked by 'temporary work system', *contractualization*, casualization and outsourcing. Consequently, administrative deliberations have been replaced by a partnership, popularly christened as Public–Private- Partnership. Hence, the shift from permanency to adhocracy has incapacitated the bureaucratic administration to the extent of a mere facilitator of public services. Consequently, administrative response to any situation is rather helpless and feeble.

6.6.4 Fifthly, a Trade-off between Continuity and Discontinuity

Finally, the administration is also trapped in a trade-off between continuity versus discontinuity, which has also bounded administrative efficiency to a great extent. Whereas, on the one hand, right to the spirit of neoliberalism, the administration clings to the present and refuses to learn anything from the past. Still, then on the other hand, as an intrinsic behavioural feature, the administration cannot forget its continuity with the past. The post-pandemic administrative response bears the mark of the said trade-off, where administration as a part of the neoliberal scheme of things refused to learn any lesson from the past events like the bubonic plague of the Bombay province in 1897, but approached the present pandemic by drawing on the legal administrative templates of colonial administration like Epidemic Disease Act of 1897 and maintained continuity.

Hence, administrative indecision or failure vis-à-vis the unprecedented pandemic has to be understood in light of the above trade-offs. Most importantly, there is adequate intersectionality among the trade-offs mentioned above. The administrative bewilderment in the face of the pandemic of COVID 19 is indicative of the fact that administration, especially that of postcolonial state finds itself in the tangle of multiple trade-offs. The above discussion on the administrative disorientation notwithstanding, it is quite evident that as of now there is hardly any radical alternative to administrative handling of the situation. Hence, reposing on the administrative acumen or what this paper calls 'administrative rationality' is perhaps the only rational choice that humanity has at its disposal. The section that follows spells out the essence of administrative rationality.

6.7 Administrative Rationality and the 'New Normal'

With no immediate escape route to normalcy in sight, the pandemic -hit humanity has been forced to enamour the 'new normal' lifestyle. The 'new normal' lifestyle, as it unfolds in the wake of the pandemic of COVID 19, appears to have accepted the fact that our life is not going to back on track at least for now. That our activities remained suspended, and our confinement seems to be unending. All the normal civic activities have been arrested. The typical political activities like organizing rallies, campaigning, and elections have been postponed. The escalating number of COVID-positive patients further intensified the restrictions. Hence, for the new normal, mere bureaucracy armed with technocratic rationality is not sufficient, even if it enjoys requisite legal/formal sanctions. It runs the risk of dehumanizing tendency in administrative deliberations. History is replete with examples where typical bureaucratic interventions of containing exigency often deteriorated into dehumanized tendencies. For example, armed with the combined power of technocratic rationality and legal/formal authority, colonial administration during the epidemic of Spanish influenza or Bubonic plague had devastated the living conditions of the native people. From Weber to Simon, all the scholars have warned us not to become a victim of the 'iron cage of rationality. However, as it appears now that our policymakers seem to have learned very little from history. In fact, drawing on the same legal/formal templates of the colonial government, the present administration (both at the center and as well as in the states) appears to have repeated the same error of entrusting bureaucratic rationality to address the pandemic. For example, to keep a tab on the rising graph of infection, the present government has resorted to a digital surveillance mechanism. Consequently, the citizens have been robbed of their rights to movement, rights to assemble, rights to livelihood, and so on. On the contrary, giving priority to the improvising capacity of the administrators, administrative rationality enables bureaucrats/administrators to fight the situation unfolding in the era of the new normal. It equips administrators with a rationality that can steer humanity out of the pandemic. Hence, administrators being the frontline warriors are supposed to customize their decisions following the local level needs and priorities, keeping a broad policy outline in mind.

The centrality of the concept (administrative rationality) in administrative deliberations can be better understood if we draw on the experiences of Covid management in a postcolonial society like India. This section has cherry-picked a few revealing narratives of the administrators and general citizens, originated in course of the ethnographic study conducted in two districts of West Bengal-one reported to have the highest percentage of Covid positive cases and another with the lowest cases.

6.7.1 Administrator's Perspective

In course of the interaction with the administrators, three prominent issues have emerged viz the life versus livelihood, transparency versus public order, Pareto optimality versus social optima, which compelled them to go beyond the narrow, positivist approach of bureaucracy. In delivering public goods and services if anything that causes a serious dilemma for the administration it is the trade-off between life and livelihood issues. Several narratives, generated in course of the interview had indicated that administrators had well surpassed the legal-formal templates to fight the Covid exigency. One Mr. Srivastav (the name has been changed to maintain the administrative anonymity), a middle-aged state cadre sub-divisional officer, encapsulates this perennial duality between life versus livelihood in the following words: *'We are literally in a fix. The pandemic has pushed us to a point of no return!!! The severity of the spread of the virus forced us to implement the strict legal-administrative protocol. But we are well aware of the hardship caused by lockdown, quarantine, and the suspension of the public transport system. Hence, in real-life situations, I instruct both general and police officials working under my supervision to handle the situation with empathy and give reasonable concessions to the marginal section of the society especially those working in the informal sector".* A similar kind of response was echoed by a police officer, Mr. Jafar, aged 32, working in the industrial belt of North 24 Parganas (one of the worst affected districts of West Bengal), where the said officer applied his judgment and empathy to strike a balance between the intractable duality between life and livelihood. He said:

> No doubt, we come down heavily on casual offenders and transgressors who were breaching the Covid protocol but remained soft on those who earned their living on daily basis. Hence, we had to customize the Covid protocol a bit to ensure the living of the marginal section of the society

Similarly, another important issue like transparency vis-à-vis public order was surfaced in course of the discussion. The administrators, both general and law and order, have expressed the dilemma of maintaining a fine balance between transparency and public order in the Covid management. One government official, working in tandem with the Ministry of Health and Family Welfare in the Covid corridor, has explained the dilemma in the following words: *"we were literally sandwiched between government agencies, media, and political parties to disclose every detail of the Covid data on the one hand, and our concern for public order on the other hand. My long experience tells me that disclosing government concern in the media would create public hysteria, let alone disclosing data relating to Covid"*. In an almost similar vein, one administrative officer added *"we should exercise a lot of restraint in disseminating information. There should be a reasonable difference between information and speculation. And those who are familiar with administrative temperament knew it pretty well that it would be disastrous to share all classified information in the name of transparency. Being at the heart of the Covid corridor we have to improvise the possible repercussion of the sharing of information as well. Hence, we meticulously pass on information to the Ministry of Health and Family Welfare, the Govt. of India, but do not allow media to focus on area-specific news as that would stigmatize affected areas"*.

Another issue that has surfaced over and over again in the official narratives is the trade-off between Pareto optimality and social optima. Though known as the perennial dilemma of the postcolonial governance, the pandemic hit administration has opted for social optima to bail out the beleaguered humanity from the scourge of the Covid 19, as evident from the following narratives: One block-level administrator has mentioned how he was compelled to repose his faith on public institutions instead of the market. "Covid situation has finally busted the myth of market efficiency."

6.7.2 Citizen's Perspective

The several ways of customizing legal-formal approaches to bureaucracy to deliver public services during the pandemic of Covid 19 have been validated by the citizen respondents. A cross-section of people during the focused group interviews had confirmed that the administrators have tried different approaches, sometimes evening going beyond the legal-rational framework to bail out humanity during the Covid pandemic. Among the revealing narratives, emerged out of focused group interviews, a few deserved some space here. One Sulema Bibi, a 48 old domestic help, narrated her experiences during the lockdown: *"We had a miserable condition as my husband was confined home due to sudden lockdown. And most of the families where I had worked as domestic help refused to take my help in the fear of infection. But we will remain indebted to BDO sahaab for personally taking care of foods and other utilities and giving special concession card to my husband to go for work"*.

The above narratives have amply showcased how the administration could handle a challenging task like Covid management by transforming mere professional bureaucratic values into qualitatively more humane administration by applying administrative rationality.

6.8 Concluding Observations

In the foregoing analysis, an attempt has been made to demonstrate that we have been suffering from a typical 'poverty of epistemology'. The pandemic has caught us on the wrong foot. No one knows what is in store for us. The entire human race has been at the disposal of the so-called 'tyranny of survivalism'. In this context proposing 'administrative rationality' as trusted wherewithal is somewhat naïve. For example, administration alone, no matter how rational it might be, cannot provide any solution to the emergent crisis. In fact, it is the scientific community, especially the medical scientists who can offer scientific solutions. Administrators at best only can operationalize the solution provided by the specialists. However, there was no reliable alternative to the government that could bail out humanity from the scourge of COVID 19. Under neoliberal governance through the non-governmental sector is posited as the smart alternative to state/government in the management of public affairs, in reality, its performance is anything but inspiring. Moreover, the development of the non-governmental sector is not uniform across the globe. It grows contextually depending upon differential political cultures. Hence, the fight against the pandemic differs from country to country. If we compare the experiences between the United States and India the above statement can be validated. For example, unlike India, civil society and non-governmental sectors in the US have contributed immensely to the fight against the Coronavirus. The American society is known for its intrinsic value of civic voluntarism and embedded tradition of spontaneity. The civil society or the so-called third sector, which could have complemented, if not compensated the bureaucratic handling of the pandemic, is relatively non-existent in India. Thanks to the legacy of colonial rule in India for more than two hundred odd years, the alternative tradition of civic activism, which has had a long tradition in India, was never allowed to flourish. A healthy colonial state had deliberately throttled any spark of voluntarism and civic activism in fear of nativist backlash. The post-Independent India, especially its administration, had carried forward the legacy of colonial governance. Consequently, the legacy of mistrust and suspicion towards civic alternatives had dominated India's official narrative of civic activism. The official handling of the pandemic by India is indicative of the relative weaknesses of the non-governmental sector, which is deliberately reduced its role to a mere auxiliary part of the government. Hence, administrative rationality is of utmost necessity. The importance of administrative rationality is also felt in the post-Covid situation which is utterly volatile in nature.

For instance, by the end of the last year when a word of reassurance comes from the scientific communities that they are very close to putting a brake on the pandemic by developing vaccines, the need for administrative rationality has become multiplied. From the initial stage of the haplessness of not having any pharmacological shield available before us to beat the pathogenic pandemonium to devising an antidote in the form of vaccines is indeed a glorious journey. It has substantially recovered our very pride of scientific rationality, which was put to test by the pandemic. However, due to relentless efforts by scientists in several research institutes across the globe, we are finally having full-proof vaccines. But possessing vaccines is no end to the ordeal. For example, the economic impact of the pandemic is said to be worse than the liquidity crisis of 2008. Hence, rebuilding the economy in the post-Covid requires a lot of administrative skills. Therefore, administrative rationality in the present context is perhaps the only way out that we have at our disposal. Moreover, the modality of administering these vaccines is another difficult issue, involving delicate distributive management. Further, given the nature of neoliberal governance, delivery of services is considered to be a collective venture involving all the stakeholders, including the state, civil society, market, and community. Hence, armed with administrative rationality, it is only the bureaucracy/administration that could devise a dependable bailout programme for us by roping in all the stakeholders concerned.

References

Adams, G. B., & Balfour, D. L. (2004). *Unmasking administrative evil*. M.E. Sharpe.

Arendt, H. (1958). *The human condition*. The University of Chicago Press.

Buheji, M., & Ahmed, D.A.A. in Business Management and Strategy. (2020, May). Planning for 'the new normal'—Foresight and management of the possibilities of socio-economic spillover due to COVID 10 Pandemic. *Business Management and Strategy, 11*(1), 160–169.

Dodd, R. H., Pickles, K., Nickle, B., Cvejic, E., Ayre, J., Batcup, C., et al. (n.d.). What is Pareto's efficiency? Definition of Pareto's Efficiency, Pareto's efficiency meaning. Retrieved from https:// economictimes.indiatimes.com/definition/paretos-efficiency

Dodd, R. H., Pickles, K., Nickle, B., Cvejic, E., Ayre, J., Batcup, C., Bonner, C., Copp, T., Cornell, S., Dakin, T., Isautier, J., & McCaffery, K. J. (2020, December 15). Concerns and motivations about Covid 19 vaccination. *Lancet Infectious Diseases, 21*(2), 161–163.

Francesz, Z. B., Brechenmacher, S., & Carothers, T. (2020, April 6). *How will the Coronavirus reshape democracy and governance globally*. Carnegie Endowment for International Peace, Commentary.

Gregosz, D., Koster, T., Morwinsky, O., & Schebesta, M. (2020). *Corona virus infects the global economy: The economic impact of an unforeseeable pandemic*. Source: http://www.jstor.org/sta ble/resrep25284/. Accessed on 15 January 2021.

Marcuse, H. (1964). *One-dimensional man: Studies in the ideology of advanced industrial society*. Beacon Press.

New normal. (2020, 25th August). Retrieved from https://en.wikipedia.org/wiki/New_normal

Parkinson, C. N. (1957). *Parkinson's law, and other studies in administration*. The Riverside Press.

Peter, L. J., & Hull, R. (1969). *The Peter principle*. Buccaneer Books.

Pfiffner, J. M. (1960). *Administrative rationality*. Public Administration Review, Source: http:// www.jstor.org/stable/973965. Accessed on 22 December 2020

Porecha, A. V. (2020, 27th July). *Covid's 'other victims': Delaying treatment is injurious to health*. Retrieved from http://www.thehindubusinessline.com/news/national/covids-other-vic tims-delaying-treatment-is-injurious-to-health/article32206173.ece

Simon, H. A. (1957). *Administrative behaviour: A study of decision-making processes in administrative organisation*. Macmillan.

Stout, M. (2013). *Logics of legitimacy: Three traditions of public administration praxis*. CRC Press.

Ventriss, C. (2003). Rethinking rationality. *Administrative Theory & Praxis*, source: http://www. Jstor.org/stable/25610596. Accessed on 22 December 2020

Vickers, G. (1965). *The art of judgment: A study of policymaking*. Chapman & Hall.

WHO Coronavirus Disease (COVID-19) Dashboard. (n.d.). Retrieved from http://covid19.who.int/.

Yung Yung Chang. (2020). The post pandemic world: between constitutionalized and authoritarian orders—China's narrative—Power play in the pandemic era. *Journal of Chinese Political Science, 26*, 27.

Arindam Roy is an Associate Professor in the Department of Political Science at the University of Burdwan, West Bengal, India.

Chapter 7
Negotiating Access to Maternal Health Services During COVID-19 Pandemic in Kilifi County, Kenya: Rapid Qualitative Study

Stephen Okumu Ombere

Abstract Globally, women do a lot of unpaid work even before the onset of the COVID-19 pandemic. COVID-19 has delivered a blow to existing gender systems that could recalibrate gender roles, positively affecting population health. Initial research suggests that the crisis and its consequent shutdown responses have resulted in an intense increase in this burden. There is a dearth of information on expectant mothers' negotiation mechanisms to access maternal health services during COVID-19 in Kenya. This rapid qualitative study draws data from purposefully selected 12 mothers who were either pregnant or had newborn babies during the COVID-19 pandemic in Kilifi county. Data were analyzed thematically and presented in a textual description, with at least five ideal typologies of emic alternatives to negotiating access to maternal health care. This chapter describes experiences of of women with their husbands' presence or absence and how this impacted access to maternal health services. In this study, the household economic situation, in particular, emerged as a crucial gendered factor associated with negotiation for access to maternal health care. For the migrant husbands, most women used a range of other options to ensure that they fed or get money to sustain their families. Therefore, most households had minimax strategies to buffer risk in accessing maternal health services during COVID-19. The findings show that gender norms sustain a hierarchy of power that reinforces a systemic inequality that undermines women's rights and restricts them from accessing maternal health services during pandemics.

Keywords Coronavirus · Covid-19 · Birth · Kilifi county · Maternal health services · Qualitative

7.1 Introduction

Coronavirus Disease-2019 (COVID-19) has delivered a shock to existing gender systems that could recalibrate gender roles, with beneficial effects on population health. While women were already doing most of the world's unpaid care work

---

S. O. Ombere (✉)
Department of Sociology and Anthropology, Maseno University, Kisumu, Kenya

© The Author(s), under exclusive license to Springer Nature Singapore Pte Ltd. 2022
S. Roy and D. Nandy (eds.), *Understanding Post-COVID-19 Social and Cultural Realities*, https://doi.org/10.1007/978-981-19-0809-5_7

before the onset of the COVID-19 pandemic, initial research suggests that the crisis and its consequent shutdown response have resulted in an intense increase in this burden (Power, 2020). Gender is not accurately captured by the traditional male and female dichotomy of sex. Instead, it is a complex social system that structures the life experiences of all human beings (Heise et al., 2019). Moreover, the gender equality and women's empowerment agenda is recognized in the Sustainable Development Goals (SDGs) and by various United Nations (UN) and government commitments before the SDGs. However, mainstream public health and public policy have yet to invest substantially in research and action to tackle gender inequalities in health (George et al., 2019). The health sector's inability to accelerate progress on a range of health outcomes brings a sharp focus on the substantial impact of gender inequalities and restrictive gender norms on health risks and behaviours (Heise et al., 2019).

The differences in how women fare during a pandemic compared to men are largely due to long-existing inequalities and social disparities, which are exacerbated by the pandemic, rather than biology (World Health Organization, 2007). Inequalities created and compounded by outbreaks leave women in a more vulnerable position (Wenham et al., 2020). Policies and public health efforts have not addressed the gendered impacts of disease outbreaks (Smith, 2019). Experience from past outbreaks shows the importance of incorporating a gender analysis into preparedness and response efforts to improve the effectiveness of health interventions and promote gender and health equity goals. During the 2014–2016 west African outbreak of Ebola virus disease, gendered norms meant that women were more likely to be infected by the virus, given their predominant roles as caregivers within families and as front-line health-care workers (Davies & Bennett, 2016). Women were less likely than men to have power in decision making around the outbreak, and their needs were largely unmet (Harman, 2016). Studies indicate that sexual reproductive health, including maternal health services, has been disrupted by the COVID-19 pandemic (Hussein, 2020; Oluoch-Aridi et al., 2020; Ombere, 2021; Wangamati & Sundby, 2020). Studies have also shown that during such pandemics, pregnant women face particular challenges because of their duties in the workforce, as caregivers of children and other family members, and their requirements for regular contact with maternity services and clinical settings where the risk of exposure to infection is higher (Ombere, 2021; Rasmussen et al., 2008, 2020). Pregnancy and childbirth are often regarded as the women's exclusive concerns in patriarchal societies (Kwambai et al., 2013; Mangeni et al., 2012). Therefore, during pandemics, women are often left alone to negotiate access to maternal health services. Research has also shown that gender inequity negatively affect maternal health and maternal health care access and utilization in multiple ways (Tolhurst et al., 2009).

Maternal health remains a challenge in low-resource countries (Machel, 2010). The numbers of women dying every year from maternity-related causes have remained high in such countries despite various efforts to bring them down (Otieno et al., 2020; WHO, 2019). As much as there has been an improvement in access to maternal health services, improved access depends on the availability of health services and community factors that influence individuals' decision-making (Manda-Taylor et al., 2017). Therefore, integrating gender (one of the community factors) into maternal and child health interventions has positively affected intervention outcomes. A review of gender-integrated interventions in reproductive and maternal-child health, for example, found that while the effects of integrating gender into interventions were mixed, overall, the studies suggested that addressing social and structural factors within maternal and child health interventions, such as gender norms and inequalities, is beneficial for effective intervention outcomes (Morgan et al., 2017; Tolhurst et al., 2009).

Kenya introduced free maternity services (FMS) in all public hospitals in 2013 to encourage skilled care deliveries and provide financial risk protection and equitable access to maternal health services (MHS) for poor and vulnerable populations. Since the introduction of FMS, Kenya has made remarkable progress towards reducing mortality rates and improving health services coverage (Kenya National Bureau of Statistics [KNBS] et al., 2015). Despite such successes, considerable inequities in health outcomes and uptake of health services remain low in interior rural areas, disadvantaging the most vulnerable individuals (KNBS et al., 2015). Kenya recorded an increase in facility-based deliveries from 44% in 2008 to 61% in 2015 (KNBS et al., 2015). This increase in skilled care deliveries has been partly attributed to the FMS policy introduced in June 2013 (KNBS et al., 2015; Pyone et al., 2017).

The construction of masculinity in patriarchal societies often limits how men are "allowed" to engage in pregnancy, birth and child-rearing (Farré, 2013). Therefore, just like in other patriarchal communities, in Kilifi County, birth is gender-constructed. A majority of women from such rural areas have low bargaining power and decision-making on issues of their health. However, to date, despite FMS's availability, there is a dearth of information on mechanisms used by expectant mothers to negotiate for access to maternal health services during the COVID-19 pandemic in Kenya. Although a study by Wangamati and Sundby (2020) explored the ramifications of COVID-19 on maternal health in Kenya, their study did not look at how women or pregnant mothers negotiate for maternal health services access. However, their study recommended that there was a need for reflection on the impacts of robust response and future planning for pandemics measures to ensure that vulnerable populations such as pregnant women and mothers are not left behind.

Recent studies in Kenya have shown that COVID-19 mitigation strategies are known to have an indirect negative impact on women's well-being. For example, many hospitals have put restrictions on visits by partners and relatives during admission at the hospitals for delivery (Eunice et al., 2020; Ombere, 2021). This is despite the fact that women are customarily denied companionship during delivery in most hospitals due to privacy concerns (Afulani et al., 2018). The COVID-19 period presents new challenges for women with the lockdowns and curfews, instilling fear and necessitating birth companionship. Lockdowns have also resulted in varied economic consequences such as job loss, food, and housing insecurity, further aggravating health outcomes (Shupler et al., 2020; Zar et al., 2020).

This chapter presents four exemplified case studies of purposefully selected poorest women because they typically represent different categories of husbands and how they either assist or fail to help pregnant mothers and how this affects maternal health care during COVID-19. These women had complications, delivered at home, came to health facility later, or used free maternity (giving birth for free in all public health facilities), which was not 'free'. The categories presented here show how maternal health care utilization is related to individual choice or characteristics. To a large extent, it depends on communities' socio-cultural arrangements and social capital (Shaikh et al., 2008). Typical cases in this chapter are derived from the poorest peasant households. A Russian agricultural economist, Alexander Vasilevitch Chayanov, noted that peasants are always balancing the drudgery of work against the return, and they have few desires beyond food and security (Hunt, 1978). In peasant households, food produced is consumed within the house, and each wife grows food for her children and her husband. Women are also responsible for farms or gardens owned by their husbands where together with their children and other close relatives, they could plant, weed, spray and harvest the farm produce.

7.2 Methods

This chapter is based on author's PhD ethnographic fieldwork on local perceptions of social protection schemes in maternal health in Kenya, conducted between March-July 2016 and February-July 2017 (Ombere, 2018). "Social protection schemes" include free maternity services in all public health facilities and maternal vouchers in selected accredited public and private health facilities. (These vouchers were no longer in supply during my fieldwork). The author conducted a rapid-qualitative study with -up interviews to explore additional gender dynamics in negotiating access for maternal health services during the COVID-19 pandemic in Kilifi County, Kenya.

Data analyzed for this paper is from the follow-up interviews from a previous ethnographic study. This rapid qualitative study explored how women from the Giriama community in Kilifi County negotiate access for maternal health services in a patriarchal societal set-up during the COVID-19 pandemic.

Since March 2020, when the first case of COVID-19 was reported in Kenya, out of 40 mothers I followed during my ethnographic fieldwork in Kilifi County, I managed to reach 20 of them between June 13 and July 24, 2020. Data for this article were derived from the responses of 8 of these mothers who were either pregnant or gave birth during the COVID-19 pandemic. Kenya's maternal mortality rate is still high at 342 per 100,000, while Kilifi County has 289 per 100,000 (Kenya National Bureau of Statistics & ICF International, 2015).

The qualitative data was analyzed through two main approaches: (a) the hermeneutic analysis of the ethnographic data, and (b) content analysis of interview and focus group data (Braun & Clarke, 2013). Transcription was done by the author using computer-aided transcription software (F5 transcription-free). The findings are presented in textual descriptions and illustrated using verbatim quotations. No identifying name tags have been used in reporting the study findings to maintain confidentiality and minimize the potential of identification of study participants. Ethical approval was obtained from Maseno University Ethical Review Committee-reference number MSU/DRPI/MUERC/00206/015.

7.3 Findings

This section unbundles four threads of different typical cases where women negotiate access to maternal health services. The cases are follow-ups from the previous ethnographic research. The cases represent various women's experiences in relation to their husbands' presence or absence and negotiating access to maternal health services during the COVID-19 pandemic. Typical cases are:

– a husband who was away and helping,
– a husband who was around but not helping,
– a husband who was away and not helping
– a husband who was around and helping.

Although among the Giriama community men play a key role in the family as the main decision-makers, sometimes pregnant women are forced to find alternatives to access maternal health care in cases where the husband is away from home but reliable and helping, the husband may be around but not helping, the husband may be away and not helping. In some cases the husband may be around and helping. For instance, like in 'scenarios' presented below.

7.3.1 Scenario 1: Mama Hussein: Reciprocal Arrangement with Neighbours based on Reliable Migrant Husband

I met Mama Hussein in May 2016 during my first phase fieldwork when she came with her newborn baby at Ngoni Health center. At the health center, we agreed to visit her at her home some 15 kms from the health facility. The woman got married at the age of 20, and she did not go to school at all. She is now 40 years old with twelve children (4 girls and eight boys). Before I left the field after the first phase in July 2016, she had eleven children and gave birth to another boy child in June 2017. Apart from the lastborn who was delivered in the hospital, all other children were born at home through a traditional midwife. The husband worked as a caretaker in an Indian home in Malindi town and could come home every weekend or send money and food to the family every end of the month. When the first case of COVID-19 was reported in Kenya, Mama Hussein was pregnant and was in her second trimester. The husband was always in Malindi town hustling to feed the family. During emergencies such as a child's sickness, the husband allowed her to borrow money from the neighbour which he pays later. Our continuous conversations made it clear that Mama Hussein's husband was very reliable during a health crisis and supported her during COVID-19 when she wanted maternal health care access. For instance:

> My husband is away from the village, but I still borrow money from the neighbours to feed the family. Clinics are closed so I go to a private one but it is expensive however, my husband always encourages me to borrow from the neighbours and later he pays back (Interview with Mama Hussein).

7.3.2 Scenario 2: Bahati's Case: Multiple Reproduction Roles and Selling Own Production with Present Non-helping Husband

Bahati, is one of the village elder's wife in Magarini Sub-county. She has eight children and six are in school. One child is disabled. Therefore, Bahati is mainly indoors or goes with him wherever she goes before other children come from school. Most of the time, Bahati's husband, a village elder, was always present at home and depended on the little money he got from attending meetings at the chief's camps or resolving local disputes and conflicts. Therefore, Bahati had to look for casual labour to supplement whatever little her husband could give her to feed the family. Occasionally, her husband helped, but she was the one fending for the family in most cases.

Fieldwork in 2016–2017, documented cases where the husband would leave home in the morning and come back in the evening. When he arrived home, they always disagreed with Bahati over some issues I did not know initially. As I continued visiting this family and spending more time with them, I came to learn from Bahati that she was not happy with her husband's 'I don't care attitude and approach to the family issues.' The quarrels were mainly based on the husband's refusal to assist Bahati in getting regular casual work in the local chief camp. She also quarreled because he rarely supported the family and the little money, he got was mainly spent at what villagers called *mang'weni, a* local palm wine drinking bar. Bahati was not very happy and blamed the local chief for failing to take action against her husband who neglected his duties as the house's head. This had been their lifestyle, and even neighbours branded Bahati's family as quarrelsome. Bahati told me she was not a quarrelsome woman when things are in the right direction, but when she felt all was not okay, and then she had to quarrel.

Bahati mainly relied on *vipande* (casual work- digging and weeding on people's farms) to get money to feed her family. The present but not helping Bahati's husband also demanded his share of food when he arrived home. This provoked Bahati and sometimes resulted in verbal quarrels. During COVID-19 and with several government restrictions, Bahati had difficulty feeding the husband and saving little money to go for routine maternal clinics.

> Steve, the situation has not changed much. The behaviour is still the same. He is just around but drinks alcohol, lazy around in the neighbors' compound and in the long run he quarrels as he expects food to eat. I am heavily pregnant now but still work on people's farms, fetch firewood, look for food to feed my children including him. With the restrictions due to the coronavirus, I tell you it is so hectic for me here saving money for the clinic, feeding my children and the lazy husband anyway what can I do? It is also what society expects a woman like me to do.

This discourse shows what society expects married women to do. Too much pressure is on women's side, for instance, feeding the children and a lazy or a present but not helping husbands. Lazy husbands also expect women to work hard and not demand any help from them. Moreover, this case shows how the present and not helping husbands expect their wives to perform both production and reproduction roles. The excerpt suggests that the additional household chores were meant for the women, and Bahati had to look for ways of feeding the husband and the children.

7.3.3 Scenario 3: Chima: Relying on Traditional Midwife with Husband Not Present and not Helping

I first met Chima during my first fieldwork phase at a local public health center in Kilifi County in 2017. Chima was 38 years old and stayed with her 12 children in a village in the Mavueni market approximately 20 km from Kilifi town. She dropped out of school in upper primary (class five) after her father's death, the breadwinner. At the age of 15 years, she got pregnant and married a wine tapper locally referred to as *Mgema*. Therefore, the husband is mostly away in another village in Jibana sub-county, mainly known for palm wine production in Kilifi County. In 2017, Chima was among my respondents who struggled to access maternal health services due to economic hardships.

Her husband, 53 years old, only came home when there was anything urgent to attend to, such as when close kin passed on or his family member was critically ill. Chima narrated how her husband had abandoned her and their children in this village, and now it was two years since they last met. She attributed her husband's refusal to come home to witchcraft which made him forget about his responsibilities as a family man. However, occasionally when the extended family pressurized him, he remitted some little money home for upkeep, which was never enough. Issues of health care were just a burden to Chima's family, and in some cases, she relied on traditional herbal medicine to treat her children.

She delivered ten children at home assisted by a traditional midwife and traditional birth attendant (TBA) who could compensate in installment and without much pressure. She could pay money in bits and sometimes help the TBA attend to the visitors, wash dishes and clean the house. The wealthy neighbour trusted her and occasionally could send her shopping in the local market, and at least she could get some little money to buy flour for the family. Whenever she borrowed money from this neighbour, she notified her husband to send some money to pay back. Sometimes the husband delays sending cash or fails to respond to her requests and forces Chima to work on the wealthy neighbour's garden, clean the house and wash dishes. During my fieldwork in 2017, she helped get money for the hospital to give birth, but she did not go to the hospital and resorted to a TBA. She argued that the health facility was far and could not afford transport expenses. She was also sure of paying some little money in the health facility because free maternity services were never free. For instance:

> I also delivered at home because I did not have money to go to the hospital to deliver. The health facility was far, and my neighbour gave me the little money I used part of it to compensate TBA and the rest buying my newborn a few items. Thank God our local TBA

helped me, but I compensated her without pressure anyway (In-depth interview with Chima in 2017).

According to her, giving birth at the TBA offered companionship and support. It was also cheap to deliver with a TBA since she accepted any payment form that Chima had. Despite not being supported by Kenya's government, delivering at TBAs was a locally crafted institution that played a key role in increasing the poor women's bargaining power and negotiating access to maternal health services such as delivery.

During a follow-up interview in June 2020, Chima was pregnant, and the husband was away. She mentioned that the situation is the same as the husband was away and offered no support thus, she still relied on TBA for assistance and was sure to give birth at TBA's home. According to her, an absent and not helping husband adds more burden and additional work to the women. Therefore, maternal health care and facility delivery become very difficult. Consequently, many poor women like her who lack support from their husbands end up delivering on TBA care, which was cheaper and easily accessible.

7.3.4 Scenario 4: Halima: Using Own Limited Resources and Help of Present Husband

Halima, a 39 years old mother of twelve children, comes from Ganze sub-county in Kilifi County. The presence of her husband at home brings a sense of security. she said her children could rarely go hungry. Even when she was away, she believed her children were well fed by their father. Just before COVID-19, Halima informed me that she was expecting another child. When the first COVID-19 was reported in Kenya, Halima panicked that she could no longer go for the routine ante-natal clinic in the public health facilities, which were temporarily closed following government directives on COVID-19 measures. However, she could occasionally go to a private health facility because her husband could save a little money for the hospital visit. Halima's case represents a scenario of eased pressure on pregnant women whose husbands are available and helping. The women can easily negotiate access to maternal health services during pandemics to access private health facilities with assistance from their husbands. For instance, during an interview-

> Steve, I am expecting another baby, but there is no public health facility operating again. My husband who is always at home has been supportive and he gives me money to go for antenatal check-ups in the private hospital in the market centre (Interview with Halima, June 2020).

The findings give us a primary conclusion that those women who manage to get broader community support and the support not just of their husbands but their kin and even in a more extensive social network found it easier to meet the maternal health costs and thus were able to go to the health centers with ease. Women with multiple reproduction roles and who sell their own production with present non-helping husbands experienced more pressure and are burdened to negotiate access to health-care and take care of family needs. To ease the pressure of husbands who were away and not helping, such women relied on traditional midwives to access maternal services. Such arrangements were cheaper for poor women as they could pay the traditional midwive in kind by working on their farms or paying in instalments. Therefore, it might be better to be honest regarding the costs for the delivery and to see this as not just a personal family-based duty but also one of a larger community. Rotating credit associations or locally defined insurance schemes helped some women in this endeavor. Women who were integrated into self-help groups were better prepared to cover all the costs than those who were not. Therefore, community-based measures might also discuss how people want to include even their poorer members in the network of local security systems for easy access to maternal health services in the future.

7.4 Discussion

Globally, men's involvement in maternal health programs has been associated with positive reproductive health outcomes, such as an increase in contraceptives. Moreover, male involvement in maternal health care utilization is essential to maternal health, especially in patriarchal societies (Chattopadhyay & Govil, 2020). Findings from this study show how the differences in how women fare during a pandemic compared to men are primarily due to long-existing inequalities and social disparities, which are exacerbated by the pandemic rather than biology (Simba & Ngcobo, 2020).

Findings show how apart from patriarchal dominance, women's weak bargaining power and position in the household also determined the utilization of maternal health services in Kenya. In most households among the Giriama of Kilifi County, women have restricted roles, for instance, caring for family and children, cleaning, and cooking. The women whose husbands are away from home are often unable to access antenatal health services for various reasons, including transport problems, family restrictions, and lack of control over the household's finances. Therefore, in this study, household economic situation, in particular, emerged as an important gendered factor associated with alternatives to financing and accessing maternal health care. For the migrant husbands, most women used a range of other options to ensure that they feed or get money to sustain their families. Therefore, most households had minimax strategies (diversification of choices made or a means of having a wide range of access to resources, which can minimize the risk of being without resources) to buffer risk in production (Michael, 1988). Still, not all of them can cope with changing conditions.

My analysis is built on intersectional feminist and Neo-Marxist theories in response to this call. Intersectional feminist postulates that the bargaining power and hierarchy exhibited in health systems make some people more likely to benefit, support, and advance. In contrast, others are more likely to be marginalized or disempowered (Davis, 2008). Neo-Marxist theory shows how exploitation of women takes place in the household. Meillassoux and Edholm (1981) used the neo-Marxist notion of exploitation in smallholder contexts to explain that women are the exploited group, especially in patriarchal societies. Men control property, resources and most agricultural products realized from the land through the workforce of their spouses and children (Meillassoux & Edholm, 1981). Women are also responsible for reproducing labor in other types of production (contract farming, casual labourers or working in informal sectors). This depicts a clear picture of poor women in the Giriama community who are exploited and has to devise mechanisms for negotiating access to maternal health services.

Consequently, the study findings show how gender norms sustain a hierarchy of power that reinforces a systemic inequality that undermines women and girls' rights and restricts them. In the Giriama community, just like in other male-dominated African societies, the so-called good women are expected to care for and prioritize family members' needs at the expense of their own health. Without alternatives to negotiate for assistance during pandemics, gender norms influence what are considered to be women's or men's domains, a practice that excludes men from engaging with maternal and child health-care in many settings (Greene & Biddlecom, 2000). Gender inequality falls most heavily on women, especially poor women. This is based on the historical legacy of gender injustice. The rigid gender norms undermine the welfare of all people regardless of age, sex, gender, or income setting (Heise et al., 2019). If the response to disease outbreaks such as COVID-19 is to be effective and not reproduce or perpetuate gender and health inequities, it is important that gender norms, roles, and relations that influence women's and men's differential vulnerability to infection, exposure to pathogens, and treatment received, as well as how these may differ among different groups of women and men, are considered and addressed (Wenham et al., 2020).

Studies have shown that husbands can play a crucial role in pregnancy and childbirth in deciding about seeking appropriate health care services especially in patriarchal societies of developing countries (Kwambai et al., 2013; Othman et al., 2011; Wai et al., 2015). However, this rapid qualitative study shows different categories of men and their involvement in maternal health services. From the theoretical rankings in this study, women whose husbands migrate and those whose husbands are present and helping had less pressure and burden to access maternal health services in private health facilities during COVID-19. However, women whose husbands were away and not helping and those that had multiple reproduction roles and selling their labour with present and not helping husband and those women who relied on traditional midwives to assist in maternal health care when the husband was present and not helping, experienced multiple pressure and felt exploited too. A recent study in Kenya shows how women relied on the traditional midwives to access maternal health care during COVID-19 because it was cheaper negotiating with the traditional midwives' payment modalities (Eunice et al., 2020; Ombere, 2021).

Moreover, recent findings by Pant et al. (2020), noted that decreased access and utilization of skilled care maternal health services could have dire consequences for both women and newborns. Pregnant and postpartum women are already at high risk of nutritional deficiency due to decreased nutritious food supply during the lockdown.

On top of that, when they cannot have regular antenatal and postnatal services, they are deprived of the micronutrient supplements they get from the clinics. In addition, without regular check-ups, there are chances of certain danger signs going unidentified, making them vulnerable to pregnancy and childbirth complications.

7.5 Conclusion

This chapter highlights the gendered perspective on negotiating access to maternal health services during the COVID-19 pandemic. It presents typical cases from four households with the theoretical ranking of husbands. Poor mothers whose husbands were present and helping, away and helping, experienced less pressure on negotiating access to maternal health services. Mothers whose husbands were present and not helping, away and not helping experienced a lot of pressure from multiple roles and had difficulties in accessing maternal health services. From the four typical cases, the household economic situation, in particular, is a crucial gendered factor associated with negotiation for accessing maternal health care during the pandemic. The findings suggest that the COVID-19 pandemic outbreak exacerbated the already existing gender inequalities. Therefore, women's health needs to be prioritized as women are more vulnerable and have multiple roles that would otherwise exacerbate access to maternal health services in Kenya. Thus, sexual and reproductive health rights and health care access should not be neglected during the pandemic crisis. Thus, gender-informed responses and strategies addressing the gender inequalities that persist during outbreaks must be the norm. Since this rapid qualitative study was a follow-up from previous fieldwork, some respondents might have exaggerated their response however, the author asked one question repeatedly on different days to ensure that the response was accurate.

7.6 Recommendations

There is a need to ease pressure on women who engage in multiple roles in the family. There is a need to include men in maternal health promotion and education to increase their knowledge and participation in the birth process while recognizing various important considerations. Therefore, further research is needed to explore how the variations in the theoretical ranking of husbands affect male involvement in maternal and child health practices, particularly between rural and urban communities. Moreover, there is also a need for a longitudinal study to explore all aspects of gender inequality during disease outbreaks, preparedness and response of men and women to such outbreaks.

Acknowledgements I am grateful to all women who participated in this study some under difficult circumstances and to Kilifi County Department of Health who granted me permission and access to health facilities to conduct this study. This research received financial support from the Josephine de Karman scholarships (2018), administered by the University of Bern-Switzerland. French Institute for Research in Africa (IFRA) in Kenya also financed fieldwork for the study. I am also indebted to Prof. Tobias Haller, Dr. Sonja Merten, and Prof. Erick Otieno Nyambedha for their comments and guidance during my study and fieldwork.

Funding The research study underlying this chapter was funded by Netherlands Organization for Scientific Research-WOTRO Science for Global Development grant *number W 08.390.006* awarded to Dr. Sonja Merten, Swiss Tropical and Public Health Institute-Switzerland and Prof. Erick Otieno Nyambedha, Maseno University, Department of Sociology and Anthropology-Kenya. A research project on social protection and part of knowledge agenda of INCLUDE, the knowledge platform on Inclusive Development Policies.

References

Afulani, P., Kusi, C., Kirumbi, L., & Walker, D. (2018). *Companionship during facility-based childbirth Results from a mixed-methods study with recently delivered women and providers in Kenya* (pp. 1–28).

Braun, V., & Clarke, V. (2013). *Successful qualitative research: A practical guide for beginners.* Sage.

Chattopadhyay, A., & Govil, D. (2020). Men and maternal health care utilization in India and in selected less-developed states: Evidence from a large-scale survey 2015–16. *Journal of Biosocial Science.* https://doi.org/10.1017/S0021932020000498

Davies, S., & Bennett, B. (2016). A gendered human rights analysis of Ebola and Zika: Locating gender in global health emergencies. *International Affairs, 92*(5), 1041–1060. https://doi.org/10.1016/S0140-6736(14)60497-9

Davis, K. (2008). Intersectionality as buzzword: A sociology of science perspective on what makes a feminist theory successful. *Feminist Theory, 9*(1), 67–85. https://doi.org/10.1177/1464700108086364

Eunice, P., Mary G., N., Rose, M., & Valerie, F. (2020). The impact of covid-19 on midwives' practice in Kenya, Uganda and Tanzania: A reflective account. *Midwifery, January.* https://doi.org/10.1016/j.midw.2020.102775

Farré, L. (2013). *The role of men in the economic and social development of women: Implications for gender equality* (pp. 22–51). https://doi.org/10.1093/wbro/lks010

George, A. S., Amin, A., García, C., & Sen, G. (2019). Gender equality and health: Laying the foundations for change. *The Lancet, 393*(10189), 2369–2371. https://doi.org/10.1016/S0140-6736(19)30987-0

Greene, M., & Biddlecom, A. (2000). Absent and problematic men: Demographic accounts of male reproductive roles. *Population and Development Review, 26*(1), 81–115. https://doi.org/10.1111/j.1728-4457.2000.00081.x

Harman, S. (2016). Ebola, gender and conspicuously invisible women in global health governance. *Third World Quarterly, 37*(3), 524–541. https://doi.org/10.1080/01436597.2015.1108827

Heise, L., Greene, M. E., Opper, N., Stavropoulou, M., Harper, C., Nascimento, M., Zewdie, D., Darmstadt, G. L., Greene, M. E., Hawkes, S., Henry, S., Heymann, J., Klugman, J., Levine, R., Raj, A., & Rao Gupta, G. (2019). Gender inequality and restrictive gender norms: Framing the challenges to health. *The Lancet, 393*(10189), 2440–2454. https://doi.org/10.1016/S0140-6736(19)30652-X

Hunt, D. (1978). Chayanov's model of Peasant household resource allocation and its relevance to Mbere division, Eastern Kenya. *The Journal of Development Studies, 15*(1), 59–86. https://doi.org/10.1080/00220387808421701

Hussein, J. (2020). COVID-19: What implications for sexual and reproductive health and rights globally? *Sexual and Reproductive Health Matters, 28*(1). https://doi.org/10.1080/26410397.2020.1746065

Kenya National Bureau of Statistics. (KNBS). Ministry of Health/Kenya, National AIDS Control Council/Kenya, Kenya Medical Research Institute, & National Council for Population and Development/Kenya. (2015). *Kenya Demographic and Health Survey 2014.*

Kenya National Bureau of Statistics, & ICF International. (2015). *Kenya 2014 demographic and health survey key findings* (Vol. 6). KNBS and ICF International. https://doi.org/10.5261/2013.GEN1.04

Kwambai, T. K., Dellicour, S., Desai, M., Ameh, C. A., Person, B., Achieng, F., Mason, L., Laserson, K. F., & ter Kuile, F. O. (2013). Perspectives of men on antenatal and delivery care service utilisation in rural western Kenya: A qualitative study. *BMC Pregnancy and Childbirth, 13,*. https://doi.org/10.1186/1471-2393-13-134

Machel, G. (2010). Maternal Health: Investing in the lifeline of healthy societies and economies. *Africa Progress Panel, September*, 1–36. http://scholar.google.com/scholar?hl=en&btnG=Search&q=intitle:Maternal+Health+:Investing+in+the+Lifeline+of+Healthy+Societies+&+Economies#0%5Cn

Manda-Taylor, L., Mwale, D., Phiri, T., Walsh, A., Matthews, A., Brugha, R., Mwapasa, V., & Byrne, E. (2017). Changing times? Gender roles and relationships in maternal, newborn and child health in Malawi. *BMC Pregnancy and Childbirth, 17*(1), 1–13. https://doi.org/10.1186/s12884-017-1523-1

Mangeni, J. N., Mwangi, A., Mbugua, S., & Mukthar, V. K. (2012). Male involvement in maternal healthcare as a determinant of utilisation of skilled birth attendants in kenya. *East African Medical Journal, 89*(11), 372–383.

Meillassoux, V., & Edholm, F. (1981). *Maidens, meal and money: Capitalism and the domestic community.* Cambridge University Press.

Michael, L. (1988). The poor and the poorest: Some Interim Findings. In *The sociology and politics of health: A reader* (Issue April). The World Bank. https://doi.org/10.2307/j.ctt1t89jmr.24

Morgan, R., Tetui, M., Kananura, R. M., Ekirapa-Kiracho, E., & George, A. S. (2017). Gender dynamics affecting maternal health and health care access and use in Uganda. *Health Policy and Planning, 32*(December), v13–v21. https://doi.org/10.1093/heapol/czx011

Oluoch-Aridi, J., Chelagat, T., Nyikuri, M. M., Onyango, J., Guzman, D., Makanga, C., Miller-Graff, L., & Dowd, R. (2020). COVID-19 effect on access to Maternal Health Services in Kenya. *Frontiers in Global Women's Health, 1*(November). https://doi.org/10.3389/fgwh.2020.599267

Ombere, S. O. (2018). *Local perceptions of social protection schemes in Maternal Health in Kenya : Ethnographyn i coastal Kenya* (PhD Thesis). http://biblio.unibe.ch/download/eldiss/18ombere_so.pdf

Ombere, S. O. (2021). Access to Maternal Health Services during the COVID-19 pandemic: Experiences of indigent mothers and health care providers in Kilifi County, Kenya. *Frontiers in Sociology, 6*(April), 1–8. https://doi.org/10.3389/fsoc.2021.613042

Othman, K., Dan, K., & Michael, O. (2011). Male involvement in birth preparedness and complication readiness for emergency obstetric referrals in rural Uganda. *Reproductive Health, 8*(1), 1–7. http://ovidsp.ovid.com/ovidweb.cgi?T=JS&PAGE=reference&D=emed10&NEWS=N&AN=2011337341

Otieno, G. A., Owenga, J. A., & Onguru, D. (2020). *Determinants of Maternal Health Care Choices among Women in Lunga Lunga Sub County in Kwale, 5,* 76–85.

Pant, S., Koirala, S., & Subedi, M. (2020). Access to Maternal Health Services during COVID-19. *Europasian Journal of Medical Sciences, 2*(2), 48–52. https://doi.org/10.46405/ejms.v2i2.110

Power, K. (2020). The COVID-19 pandemic has increased the care burden of women and families. *Sustainability: Science, Practice, and Policy, 16*(1), 67–73. https://doi.org/10.1080/15487733.2020.1776561

Pyone, T., Smith, H., & Broek, N. Van Den. (2017). *Implementation of the free maternity services policy and its implications for health system governance in Kenya, 1963*(figure 1), 1–11. https://doi.org/10.1136/bmjgh-2016-000249

Rasmussen, S. A., Jamieson, D. J., & Bresee, J. S. (2008). *Pandemic in Fl Uenza and Pregnant Women, 14*(1), 95–100.

Rasmussen, S. A., Smulian, J. C., Lednicky, J. A., Wen, T. S., & Jamieson, D. J. (2020). Coronavirus Disease 2019 (COVID-19) and pregnancy: What obstetricians need to know. *American Journal of Obstetrics and Gynecology, 222*(5), 415–426. https://doi.org/10.1016/j.ajog.2020.02.017

Shaikh, B. T., Haran, D., & Hatcher, J. (2008). Where do they go, whom do they consult, and why? Health-Seeking behaviors in the northern areas of Pakistan. *Qualitative Health Research, 18*(6), 747–755. https://doi.org/10.1177/1049732308317220

Shupler, M., Mwitari, J., Gohole, A., & De Cuevas, R. A. (2020). *COVID-19 Lockdown in a Kenyan Informal Settlement : Impacts on Household Energy and Food Security.*

Simba, H., & Ngcobo, S. (2020). *Are Pandemics Gender Neutral ? Women' s Health and COVID-19. 1*(October), 1–6. https://doi.org/10.3389/fgwh.2020.570666

Smith, J. (2019). Overcoming the 'tyranny of the urgent': Integrating gender into disease outbreak preparedness and response. *Gender and Development, 27*(2), 355–369. https://doi.org/10.1080/13552074.2019.1615288

Tolhurst, R., Joanna, R., & Sally, T. (2009). Maternal and child health: Global challenges, programs, and policies. *Maternal and Child Health: Global Challenges, Programs, and Policies, 1–582.* https://doi.org/10.1007/b106524

Wai, K. M., Shibanuma, A., Oo, N. N., Fillman, T. J., Saw, Y. M., & Jimba, M. (2015). Are husbands involving in their spouses' utilization of maternal care services?: A cross-sectional study in Yangon, Mya. *Plos ONE, 10*(12), 1–13. https://doi.org/10.1371/journal.pone.0144135

Wangamati, C. K., & Sundby, J. (2020). *The ramifications of COVID-19 on maternal health in Kenya The rami fi cations of COVID-19 on maternal health in Kenya.* https://doi.org/10.1080/26410397.2020.1804716

Wenham, C., Smith, J., & Morgan, R. (2020). COVID-19: The gendered impacts of the outbreak. *The Lancet, 395*(10227), 846–848. https://doi.org/10.1016/S0140-6736(20)30526-2

World Health Organization. (2007). *Addressing sex and gender in Epidemic-Prone infectious diseases.*

World Health Organization (WHO). (2019). *Maternal mortality.* https://www.who.int/news-room/fact-sheets/detail/maternal-mortality

Zar, H. J., Dawa, J., Fischer, G. B., & Castro-, J. A. (2020). Challenges of COVID-19 in children in low- and middle-income countries. *Paediatric Respiratory Reviews.* https://doi.org/10.1016/j.prrv.2020.06.016

Stephen Okumu Ombere is an anthropologist with a lot of research experience in social protection and sexual reproductive health. Stephen is a lecturer in the Department of Sociology and Anthropology Maseno University-Kenya. His general areas of expertise are maternal health, sexual reproductive health, youths, vulnerable and marginalized groups, gender and climate change, and project monitoring and evaluation. Stephen is well-grounded in qualitative research approaches and methods.

Chapter 8
#I Stay Home (If I Can): COVID-19 and Social Inequality in Peru: A View from Auto-Ethnography

Cristian Terry

Abstract The chapter aims to analyze the COVID-19 pandemic from an auto-ethnography carried out in Cusco (Peru). This highlights the social differences and socioeconomic conditions that influence the way of living the pandemic and suffering its effects, which, in the Peruvian case, has more critically affected the most vulnerable populations. Thus, the privileged people can stay at home while the rest must go out to live/survive. The chapter invites us to think about a new social pact, more equitable and fairer, that divorces the pandemic-social inequality marriage, observed in different parts of the planet, particularly in the Americas. This is necessary to avoid future problems of equal or greater magnitude that tend to take their toll on vulnerable populations that often do not have the means to pay, or pay at the risk of their lives.

Keywords COVID-19 pandemic · Social inequality · Auto-ethnography · Peru

> All animals are equal, but some animals are more equal than others
>
> —George Orwell.

On March 16th 2020, Peru began a national quarantine decreed by the Government. The State of Emergency, which should have lasted two weeks, lasted for months. The #YoMeQuedoEnCasa (#IStayHome)—promoted by the Government, the media and even advertising—became *leitmotiv* (until mid-June).[1] The President of the Republic constantly called for #YoMeQuedoEnCasa, implementing certain measures such as the "Yomequedoencasa" bonus, the Government's monetary aid to overcome the difficulties of those most in need (for other bonds, see Trivelli, 2020). Despite good intentions, this aid would not be enough and many Peruvians found the need to leave their homes to work and eat, to survive. In spite of knowing the risk of contagion as Peru was the seventh country of the world with the most official cases and the fifth

---

[1] Then #PrimeroMiSalud (my health first).

C. Terry (✉)
Independent researcher, Lausanne, Switzerland
e-mail: cristain.terry@graduateinstitute.ch

© The Author(s), under exclusive license to Springer Nature Singapore Pte Ltd. 2022   137
S. Roy and D. Nandy (eds.), *Understanding Post-COVID-19 Social and Cultural Realities*, https://doi.org/10.1007/978-981-19-0809-5_8

in deaths per capita (Worldometers, 2020, date 08 August 2020; see also Ahílesva, 2020).

COVID-19 has affected the world in a heterogeneous way, "even within the same country" (Asensio, 2020b, p. 13), both socially and individually. This chapter aims to analyze the phenomenon from an auto-ethnography carried out in the city of Cusco (Peru), which highlights the social differences and socioeconomic conditions that influence the way the pandemic is lived and how people suffer its effects, particularly in the Peruvian case. This country is crossed by strong social inequalities that precede the health crisis (Contreras & Cueto, 2013; Figueroa et al., 1996; Franco, 2007) and that COVID-19 has brought to light and accentuated (Asensio, 2020a; Macher et al., 2020). Through the Peruvian case, this chapter seeks to respond to the following research questions: how has COVID-19 unequally affected people's lives? How have socioeconomic conditions shaped the pandemic effects? How have they impacted on the government measures to stay home to prevent contagions?

The auto-ethnographic accounts will allow us to see a privileged reality that contrasts with that of many Peruvians in situations of poverty, vulnerability and precariousness, and many others who cannot stay at home because they must get "the piece of bread for each day." These stories are based mainly on personal and family experiences. They show how COVID-19 prolongs the country's socioeconomic differences. This point will make it possible to argue that COVID-19 is not a "democratic virus" as some intended (see Abrahão, 2020; Benites Alvarado, 2020; García-Sayan, 2020), but one that is more actively participating in social inequality, particularly in Latin American (Bidegain et al., 2020) and American countries (DeWitte, 2020). This fact makes it possible to understand in a better way that while some may stay at home, many simply cannot do so, they must go out to survive.

For this chapter, I will first present the methodology and the data used. Then I will develop the auto-ethnographic stories selected in this text. As a final reflection, based on the auto-ethnographic elements, I will address the issue of inequality and social injustice, contrasting the diverse realities of a country as unequal as Peru and entering into a dialogue with other works that address the issue.

8.1 Methodology and Data Collection

In this chapter I use auto-ethnography, which has gained an increasingly recognized place in the social sciences (Anderson, 2013; Ellis & Bochner, 2013; Sikes, 2013b), that has been used, for example, to study tourism (Brougère, 2014; Morgan & Pritchard, 2005; Noy, 2008; Terry, 2020a), contemporary dance (Vionnet, 2018) and viruses such as HIV (Dijstelbloem, 2014) or H1N1 (Aylesworth-Spink, 2017). Some scholars have begun to use it to study COVID-19 (Gerbaudo Suárez et al., 2020), faced with the difficulty of being able to perform a face-to-face ethnography in times of pandemic.

Auto-ethnography is "a method that allows ethnographers to use their own experience as a way to generate academic knowledge" (Pink, 2009, p. 64) or "theoretical understanding" (Anderson, 2013, p. 83), being both a method and a type of writing (Ellis & Bochner, 2013; Reed-Danahay, 2013; Sikes, 2013b).[2] It should be emphasized that every ethnography—a classical method in anthropology—is "an unknown auto-ethnography"[3] (Brougère, 2014, p. 152) and whose vindication depends on the author (Ellis & Bochner, 2013, p. 138). There is thus an auto-ethnography/ethnography continuum, which varies from author to author. For this reason, the term "auto-ethnography" must be understood for its dual component, between individual and collective (Stanley, 2013), between history, social structure and biography (Popkewitz, 2013). Beyond criticism of its alleged subjectivity and narcissism (see Atkinson, 1997; Coffey, 1999; Delamont, 2013), a series of works defend this method that allows the understanding of the social world of the author (Lancaster, 2011), inter-subjectivity (Pink, 2009) and through it, the understanding of social phenomena (Essén & Winterstorm Värlander, 2012). Carolyn Ellis and Arthur Bochner (2013) insist on the importance and relevance of auto-ethnography in understanding, from intimacy, phenomena that go beyond the person and are somewhat shared by a collective, as it is the case of the COVID-19 pandemic.

The auto-ethnographic data referred to in this text, were prepared during the pandemic, between March and July 2020 in the city of Cusco (Peru). These fall within the context of the State of Emergency decreed by the Government from 16 March to date, characterized by governmental measures, mainly quarantine (generalized first and targeted from the first of July) and curfew.[4] It is in this context of the health crisis that the #YoMeQuedoEnCasa (#IStayHome) promoted by the Government and replicated by the media must be understood.

The auto-ethnographic data was completed based on other information, mainly provided in the television media. This has allowed me to contrast what has been lived at home, individually and familiarly, with the reports of other Peruvians suffering the effects of the pandemic, for its socioeconomic situation. This makes the difference between #YoMeQuedoEnCasa (I stay home) and #YoNoPuedoQuedarmeEnCasa (I can't stay home), something that made the Government take longer to understand and implement effective measures to address social inequalities between Peruvians.

It should be noted that every story provided here should be regarded as "an orderly and consistent textual construct that cannot be compared to the raw field notes taken during empirical research" (Voirol, 2013, p. 51). Thus, the auto-ethnographic stories

---

[2] For more information on its use, relevance and criticism, see Terry (2019, pp. 86–90), Méndez (2013), and Sikes (2013a).

[3] Any subpoena or concept of a source in Spanish or French provided throughout the article was translated by the author.

[4] "Generalized quarantine" applies to the entire country while "targeted quarantine" applies only to some high-contagion regions. The curfew has been maintained throughout the State of Emergency, with variations in schedules and regions (it starts earlier in those with the highest contagion). Until the end of June, lockdown will be all day on holidays (valid even for regions in targeted quarantine). Lockdown will be progressively vanished (it will be restored for specific days afterward like Halloween festivities).

were elaborated from moments lived in these months of the pandemic; both, the ones spent at home (in an upper middle-class family) and outside while in the street. This textual construction contains some thoughtful passages and references to academic and press works, as well as some supplementary information detailing elements evoked in auto-ethnography.

8.2 Pandemic Auto-ethnography

Since my return from Europe to Cusco on the first of March, I have been at my maternal family's house. Having decreed the State of Emergency in Peru two weeks later, since then I have had to live with the health crisis in Cusco. Fortunately, we live in a spacious building (4 floors) that belongs to my maternal family. My mother, Daría (my sister) and Rio (her son) live on one of the floors, and I live upstairs. The rest of the building is occupied by my grandmother and uncle's family. We also have a large garden where you can breathe fresh air and sunbathe (if it does not rain). Inherited from my grandfather, the land was useful not only to build the family abode (with its ten members), but also to help the family business: an event center which remains closed since the beginning of the State of Emergency, and it's unable to function (large crowd meetings are not allowed).

Tuesday, April 21.

It's supermarket day. I protect myself as it should be done: face mask, lenses and disposable gloves.[5] I also carry alcohol with me to disinfect my hands when necessary. Every two weeks we go shopping. This time I carry a suitcase—which I used to use on trips—to transport as much as I can, delaying the next shopping trip. In the supermarket, I see several people with their bags full, I even see couples, even though it is not authorized.[6] At the cash register, I pay by card a sum of 300 soles (about 85 dollars), which corresponds to approximately one third of the minimum salary in Peru. With the suitcase full and a few extra bags, I'm on my way home. We are "lucky" to have a refrigerator to store the fruits, vegetables and meats I bought. A lot of Peruvians do not have a refrigerator, so they usually go out more often for shopping, being difficult for many to stay at home (Radio Ambulante, 2020).

I arrived home, I take off my shoes (I put on some spare shoes) and leave the clothes to put them in the washing machine. These are COVID-19 prevention measures that we adopt at home. At lunch, Daría tells us about her fears of not being able to carry out any activity related to events and theater in which she usually works. She used to go to her classes with kids. Now she only works with them virtually once a week, reducing her income considerably (twenty-five soles a week, less than 6 dollars).

---

[5] At first the use of gloves was required for banks and markets (Supreme Decree No. 083–2020-PCM). Subsequently, their disuse was recommended (faith of wrong decree) for not being an effective prevention measure, as suggested by the infectologist Peruvian Juan Villena (ATV Noticias Edición Matinal, 05/12/20).

[6] The supermarket warns that "only one person in the family is allowed out from Monday to Saturday (Supreme Decree No. 064–2020-PCM)".

Like other self-employed people, she is suffering from the lack of work, without fixed wages and without state assistance for not being eligible to receive the state benefits. At least, she does not have to pay rent, she lives at home with my already retired mother, who, in part, lives off the family business and especially the rents she receives from our house in Chile. "Imagine the ones who are tenants!" exclaims Daría. One of my cousins, a computer scientist, can work remotely just like me. In my case I advise exchange students on their research work. Compared to my sister, I worry less, because I live off my savings, having worked in Switzerland for the previous seven years. I also do not pay rent and prefer to occupy this time to write some awaiting academic papers. The rest of my family is living off their savings, without being able to reopen the event center (this one will open only on July 7th as a restaurant, though without generating further profits). Interestingly, Talus—one of my cousins—received the "Yomequedoencasa" bonus. He probably earned it because of his declared low income (see Barrantes, 2020).

Lunch is pleasant, despite the health situation we are going through. We usually cook as a family, although sometimes we buy food by delivery, mainly grilled chicken, burger and pizza. It's not common, but during quarantine we've done it a few times.[7] It gives us the feeling of going to the restaurant, which we used to do every weekend, before COVID-19.

In the afternoon, wearing masks and gloves, Santos arrives. He is *a comunero*[8] Q'ero to whom I must give 100 dollars on behalf of Gael, an anthropologist close friend of his. He lives with part of his family and other Q'eros in San Sebastían, a district of the Cusco province.[9] Having once been to his house, this one is much smaller than ours, even more proportionally to the number of people who live there. "I don't know when tourism will resume," he tells me worried. As a guide, he has groups that have already cancelled their trip. He has no income and claims not to have received the "Yomequedodoencasa" bonus. He says he wanted to go back to his community, because "at least there's food, and you live in the countryside. [But] they [villagers] no longer let you in." In fact, many *comuneros*—called "returners" (*retornantes*)—have returned to their villages for lack of income, "labor precariousness and consequent lack of means to survive in cities" (Burneo & Castro, 2020, p. 136), to live in the countryside and with their relatives (Centro Bartolomé de las Casas [CBC], 2020). I say good-bye by handing him the money, some backpacks and flashlights that Gael had left me for Santos. At least in his case, he has contacts with foreigners such as Gael, who help him monetarily and materially to deal with the situation. Other Q'eros work as shamans giving lectures abroad on the Pachamama (mother Earth). But it is not the case for everyone, many Q'eros suffer from precariousness and poverty (Terry, 2019, p. 108) and even the effects of climate change on

---

[7] To be exact, once my mother asked for a "clandestine" delivery grilled chicken, as the activity was not yet admitted by the Government. In May, the delivery will be authorized. On other occasions we went to buy a "take out" directly from the restaurant, the opening restaurants will be authorized in July.

[8] *Comunero*: native inhabitant of rural communities in the Andes.

[9] As other Peruvian regions, the Cusco region is divided into provinces and districts. The province of Cusco (that has the same name of the region) holds seven districts that make up the city of Cusco.

the field and livestock (Cometti, 2015; Cometti et al., 2018). I am "lucky" that I do not have to go through these difficulties and the poverty that often strikes the rural Andes (Franco, 2007; Mayer, 2018; Morlon, 1992; Terry, 2011, 2017).

At night we meet with other cousins via Messenger. With a glass in hand, we try to emulate our past encounters, often in bars or nightclubs. Since quarantine I have increased the use of these platforms (WhatsApp, Skype, Zoom, etc.) with cousins and friends from South America and Europe. Although at home the internet connection is not always optimal, at least we can communicate, work remotely (as in my case) or do virtual classes (the case of Rio).[10] "Having an internet connection is a kind of privilege" (Cuenca, 2020, p. 55), even more so today. Many children of *comuneros* have no internet connection in their communities and find it difficult to follow the government's educational program "Yo Aprendo en Casa" (I learn at home), even if it is also broadcasted on radio or television (see limitations in Reátegui, 2020). Nothing compared to the tiny cable TV problems me and my mother had once or when I broke my smartphone and had no internet access for a moment.

That night we shared our "covidian" experience among cousins, staying at home, except to stock up on food or medicine. Others like Oscar—Paty's boyfriend, my cousin—must work at the bank, one of the sectors that has continued to work. We should have celebrated at their wedding a week ago. But it has been impossible with the COVID-19 pandemic. Other regional events such as the *Inti Raymi* (celebration for solstice) have already been suspended (Terry, 2020b, 2021). I had two conferences in Italy and Spain scheduled for June, both postponed. In fact, in the face of the closure of borders, it will be impossible for me to return to Europe.[11] It's a hard blow for me because I usually travel a lot, for research and tourism.

Friday, July 10.

Watching TV with my mother, Talus tells me "I went early in the morning to Juliaca to meet my girlfriend." I was surprised because it is not possible to take inter-provincial trips. Juliaca province is about 345 km from Cusco city. The Government has not yet authorized these trips. I then learned that his girlfriend had traveled from Arequipa to Juliaca, which surprises me even more, Arequipa being a region where targeted mandatory quarantine was still in force for the high number of contagions.[12] Talus went to Juliaca by driving my uncle's Peugeot, bringing her to Cusco before the curfew at 10 p.m.

The reason for the "transgressive act" is the couple's marriage had initially been scheduled for mid-July in Cusco, and later postponed by the end of September. Their idea is to carry out the formalities in Cusco to have everything prepared, at least for

---

[10] Since March 6th 2020, the Government prohibited face-to-face classes in schools, universities and institutes.

[11] Until July 1st 2020, inter-provincial borders were closed (closure remained in targeted quarantined regions). International borders will open in October (November for flights from and to Europe).

[12] As of July 30th, there are seven regions who follow a targeted quarantine: Ancash, Arequipa, Huánuco, Ica, Junín, Madre de Dios and San Martín. Targeted quarantine also includes children under the age of 14, adults over the age of 65, and those with comorbidities (El Peruano, 2020). In August, other regions including, within which is the province of Cusco and the Convention (both from the Cusco region).

civil marriage. Interestingly, this coincided with a couple's wedding held the next day at my family's event center. Exclusively, my uncle who runs the place agreed to perform such a marriage, a service that was already paid for but had to be postponed because of the pandemic. That Saturday afternoon observing from the garden, I found that while couples like Oscar and Paty decided to postpone their marriage, others would go through it as soon as they can, despite the health crisis and the need for physical distancing, which on that Saturday wedding was not fully respected (see also Terry, 2020d).

Saturday, July 25.

My grandmother (90 years old) is ready to return to Mollepata, her homeland. Being the daughter of a farmer owner (*hacendado*), she grew up on her father's estate before the land reform at the end of the 1960s, gave the land back to the peasants (see Contreras & Cueto, 2013). She now has a country house in Mollepata where she used to go (sometimes alone) to spend a few days to rest and water her plants. In fact, the main motivation of her trip is to water her plants. Faced with the possible quarantine declaration next week, my uncle takes advantage of taking her by car so he can also enjoy a country day with his wife and children.

On her return, on Sunday night, my grandmother cheerfully tells me that she was able to see her sister, who has been living there with her husband for about a month. She gives me details on how they drank wine accompanied by a neighbor. She confesses without greater concern about the necessary physical distancing and in spite of being her (because of her age) a person at risk to COVID-19, a pandemic that is on the rise in the Cusco region (see Terry, 2020c). In fact, I find out from my uncle that a person in Mollepata tested positive, being the first case in Mollepata. It was someone, who just like them, came from the suburbs, bringing the disease unknowingly.

8.3   Final Reflection: Who Stays Home?

This chapter highlights the social differences and socioeconomic conditions that influence the way of living the pandemic and suffering its effects, which, in the Peruvian case as shown through auto-ethnography stories, has more critically affected the most vulnerable populations: the privileged people can stay at home while the rest must go out to live/survive. I could not completely abstract myself from these stories that show some contempt of government norms and the call to stay home. I have also given myself the "luxury" of going outside in the middle of quarantine (not to the supermarket, for shopping or banking), because of the need to breathe fresh air and also out of anthropologist's curiosity to see the world during the pandemic. Thus, I have lived the phenomenon auto-ethnographically in large part, by experiencing the COVID-19 effect not only inside the house, but also outside, in "clandestine" outputs (see Terry, 2020b). In my case, these getaways were not so much for the need to "go out to survive," but rather for leisure or research reasons, as an ethnographer eager to document COVID-19 and its effects.

Auto-ethnographic accounts show the limits of the #YoMeQuedoEnCasa government's call, even for those, like me and my family, who have the privilege of being able to do so. When I mentioned in the stories the word "lucky" (in quotation marks), my intention was to emphasize the privilege of having grown up and lived in a family and social environment that has the material and economic resources to study, work, travel, eat, and today, to better bear the pandemic. I received the social, cultural and economic capital (in the sense of Bourdieu)[13] to lead a privileged life. In these conditions, the #YoMeQuedoEnCasa is easier to respect and implement, although not always to comply fully, as seen in auto-ethnographic accounts (see also Chaparro, 2020). This without mentioning the clandestine parties, governors uncovering curfew, football matches between friends, fanatical fans celebrating in crowds the anniversary of their team, among other events that one sees in the news, sitting at home quietly in front of the television. These actions demonstrate the limits of #YoMeQuedoEnCasa by those who do not have the need to leave home to survive. For some it is *#YoMeQuedoEnCasa, if I want*; for others it is *#YoMeQuedoEnCasaYMueroDeHambre* (I stay home and starve to death).

The stories told here allow us to reflect precisely on the privilege of being able to stay at home in times of pandemic, a privilege that is not given to all, even less to those most in need, who were already deprived before the arrival of the coronavirus. In *Crónicas del gran encierro: Pensando el Perú en tiempos de pandemia* (Asensio, 2020a), a number of authors emphasize the fact that COVID-19 has particularly affected vulnerable and poor populations, despite government efforts and measures, such as the "Yomequedoencasa" bonus (see Barrantes, 2020; Trivelli, 2020), which would have benefited only 19% of those in need (see survey in Aragón, 2020). As Raúl Asensio points out:

> The confinement has highlighted the precariousness in which a large percentage of the Peruvian population lives, condemned to fight day by day for their livelihood. [...] Large population groups have been forced to resume their daily activities in precarious conditions in the face of the need to generate income to support their families. (Asensio, 2020b, pp. 16–17)

The "Yomequedoencasa" bonus has effectively had its limits, sometimes reaching the less needy people (as it was the case of my cousin Talus). Added to this are the acts of corruption reported by the press, for example baskets that should have reached poor families, but which went to others less in need (Oxenford, 2020). These commendable government measures were thus short-circuited, forcing many people out to survive. In the news, you could hear it recurrently: "I didn't get the bonus. I have to go out. I need to eat."

According to a national survey conducted by the Institute of Peruvian Studies (Instituto de Estudios Peruano, IEP) in April, "51 percent claim to be more afraid of starvation than coronavirus" (Amaya, 2020, p. 79). "There is an important section of the population that would like to be able to stay at home, but that is a luxury that those who live off the day by day cannot afford, because if they do not work, they do not eat" (Amaya, 2020, p. 80; see also Comaroff, 2020). Indeed, it is a luxury

---

[13] See Bourdieu (1980, 1984, 1994).

of some, those who have time even to worry about other matters: marriages, field trips, recreational walks in the city, delivery food sent home, etc. I do not try here to make an auto-criticism or criticize acts that concern my family and other privileged families. Above all, I would like to emphasize that social differences and inequalities (precedent to the pandemic) unequally affect people,[14] being the most disadvantaged, the most vulnerable, those who should have been supported before COVID-19 by creating favorable conditions to improve their quality of life. And this weighs hard today because:

> [...] A good part of the population does not respect the epidemic (*epidemia*) because they are not in a position to do so: it is lived in overcrowded conditions, no state aid has been available, no income, savings or ability to make purchases in greater volume, there are not many options for reaching points of purchase, and they go to those they find, even if they provide services in a disorderly manner, while people are forced to go out to obtain resources and be transported in crowded means. (Tanaka, 2020b, p. 95)

Similarly, Sharon DeWitte (2020) claims that the poor are more exposed to COVID-19, for example in the inability to access water that facilitates frequent hand washing. Also, without money, how can they buy soap, alcohol, face masks, and other important items to prevent contagion?

Coronavirus today brings to light these social inequalities that have characterized Peruvian history (Contreras & Cueto, 2013), and that of other Latin American countries, marked by a strong social injustice of colonial origin, according to Laura Loeza Reyes (2015). It is these inequalities that made Latin America the new global focus of COVID-19 during the so-called first wave, where pandemic and social inequality form an evil marriage, whose desired but complicated divorce would avoid so much cost in human lives and the spread of the pandemic.

8.4 Recommendations

This chapter invites us to think about a new social pact, more equitable and fairer, that divorces the pandemic -social inequality marriage, observed in different parts of the planet, as shown here in Peru. I thus subscribe to the call for a "new social pact" (*nuevo pacto social*) that guarantees the "exercise of rights and access to basic services" (Tanaka, 2020a, p. 84), quality public health (Vich, 2020), the right to good education (Carrillo, 2020) and equal opportunities, "in a country subject to three successive decades of accelerated neoliberal growth without equivalent social democratization" (Pajuelo, 2020, p. 182), growth that has benefited mostly large entrepreneurs (Vich, 2020). And the Peruvian case illustrates well the inequalities and social injustice that are observed today with the pandemic, for example in Argentina (Gerbaudo Súarez et al., 2020), Brazil (Abrahão, 2020), and the United States (Blow, 2020;

---

[14] Going back to the auto-ethnographic story, one can also see the intra-family differences, for example my case and my sister's, she was more affected and concerned about the pandemic and its economic impacts.

Low & Maguire, 2020; Vesoulis, 2020). This new social pact is necessary to avoid future problems of equal or greater magnitude that often take their bills to vulnerable populations that tend not to have what to pay with, or that pay by risking their lives. This chapter was written before the beginning of vaccination against COVID-19. However, social inequalities are still valid today in terms of access to vaccination. Peru was one of the lastest countries in South America kicking off the vaccination program. Well-off people could afford to travel abroad to be vaccinated while the rest could not. If it is true that there are debates about the use of these vaccines and several people are not willing to be vaccinated, this example simply points out current social inequalities shown here through auto-ethnographic stories. Other issues like climate change are particularly affecting vulnerable people in the Peruvian Andes (Cometti, 2015) as elsewhere (Godber & Wall, 2014; Leary et al., 2008; Monge-Barrio & Sáchez-Ostiz Gutiérrez, 2018). And the future climate change situation does not seem to improve, which more likely will reinforce pre-existing social inequalities.

Perhaps COVID-19 will make us aware of the inequalities of the world in which we live, inequalities we observe through auto-ethnographic stories that show the privilege of some. #QuedándomeEnCasa (by staying home), writing these lines, I try to use that privilege to make anthropology "a professional tool of commitment to social justice" (Gerbaudo Súarez et al., 2020, p. 177).

References

Abrahão, J. (2020, April 1). Um vírus democrático que evidencia a fragilidade da democracia. *Folha de S. Paulo*. https://www1.folha.uol.com.br/colunas/jorge-abrahao/2020/04/um-virus-dem ocratico-que-evidencia-a-fragilidade-da-democracia.shtml

Ahílesva. (2020, July 28). *El país más golpeado de América: ¿En qué falló Perú ante el coronavirus?* https://www.youtube.com/watch?v=dWEpl9qnAbw

Amaya, L. (2020). No solo un tema de salud pública. In R. H. Asensio (Ed.), *Crónicas del gran encierro. Pensando el Perú en tiempos de pandemia* (pp. 79–80). IEP. https://iep.org.pe/wp-con tent/uploads/2020/06/Cr%C3%B3nica-del-Gran-Encierro-1.pdf

Anderson, L. (2013). Analytic autoethnography. In P. Sikes (Ed.), *Autoethnography* (Vol. II, pp. 69–89). Sage.

Aragón, J. (2020). No solo un tema de salud pública. In R. H. Asensio (Ed.), *Crónicas del gran encierro. Pensando el Perú en tiempos de pandemia* (pp. 77–78). IEP. https://iep.org.pe/wp-con tent/uploads/2020/06/Cr%C3%B3nica-del-Gran-Encierro-1.pdf

Asensio, R. H. (Ed.). (2020a). *Crónicas del gran encierro. Pensando el Perú en tiempos de pandemia.* IEP. https://iep.org.pe/wp-content/uploads/2020/06/Cr%C3%B3nica-del-Gran-Encierro-1.pdf

Asensio, R. H. (2020b). Introducción. In R. H. Asensio (Ed.), *Crónicas del gran encierro. Pensando el Perú en tiempos de pandemia* (pp. 11–18). IEP. https://iep.org.pe/wp-content/uploads/2020/ 06/Cr%C3%B3nica-del-Gran-Encierro-1.pdf

Atkinson, P. (1997). Narrative turn or blind alley? *Qualitative Health Research, 7*(3), 325–344. https://doi.org/10.1177/104973239700700302

Aylesworth-Spink, S. (2017). The failure of public relations during a pandemic outbreak: Using actor-network theory to highlight the news media as a complex mediator. *Public Relations Journal, 11*(2), 1–17. https://prjournal.instituteforpr.org/wp-content/uploads/Failure-of-PR-in-Pandemic-2-2.pdf

Barrantes, R. (2020). Para la lista de prioridades. In R. H. Asensio (Ed.), *Crónicas del gran encierro. Pensando el Perú en tiempos de pandemia* (pp. 33–34). IEP. https://iep.org.pe/wp-content/upl oads/2020/06/Cr%C3%B3nica-del-Gran-Encierro-1.pdf

Benites Alvarado, A. (2020, May 26). ¿Es el COVID-19 un virus democrático? *Instituto de Derechos Humanos – Pontificia Universidad Católica del Perú.* https://idehpucp.pucp.edu.pe/notas-inform ativas/es-el-covid-19-un-virus-democratico/

Bidegain, N., Sabatini, S., & Iwasaki, F. (2020, June 25). *Conversatorio ¿Cómo afecta la pandemia a Latinoamericana?* [Conferencia organizada por la Swiss School of Latin American Studies (SSLAS)], Universität Zürich.

Blow, C. M. (2020, April 5). Social distancing is a privilege. *The New York Times.* https://www.nyt imes.com/2020/04/05/opinion/coronavirus-social-distancing.html

Bourdieu, P. (1980). Le capital social. *Actes de la Recherche en Sciences Sociales, 31*(1), 2–3. https://www.persee.fr/doc/arss_0335-5322_1980_num_31_1_2069

Bourdieu, P. (1984). Espace social et genèse des "classes." *Actes De La Recherche En Sciences Sociales, 52–53*, 3–14. https://doi.org/10.3406/arss.1984.3327

Bourdieu, P. (1994). *Raisons pratiques. Sur la théorie de l'action.* Seuil.

Brougère, G. (2014). Soi-même comme touriste apprenant – Essai d'autoethnographie. In G. Brougère & G. Fabbiano (Eds.), *Apprentissages en situation touristique* (pp. 155–180). Presses universitaires du Septentrion.

Burneo, M. L., & Castro, A. (2020). Movilidad y retorno frente al Covid-19 en el contexto de una ruralidad transformada. In R. H. Asensio (Ed.), *Crónicas del gran encierro. Pensando el Perú en tiempos de pandemia* (pp. 136–141). IEP. https://iep.org.pe/wp-content/uploads/2020/06/Cr% C3%B3nica-del-Gran-Encierro-1.pdf

Carrillo, S. (2020). ¿Qué debería pasar con la educación pública después del Covid-19? In R. H. Asensio (Ed.), *Crónicas del gran encierro. Pensando el Perú en tiempos de pandemia* (pp. 142–146). IEP. https://iep.org.pe/wp-content/uploads/2020/06/Cr%C3%B3nica-del-Gran-Encierro-1. pdf

Centro Bartolomé de las Casas (CBC). (2020, June 16). *Testimonio de retornantes* [Conferencia organizada por el grupo Martes Campesino del CBC]. https://www.facebook.com/watch/live/? v=686365822209678&ref=watch_permalink

Chaparro, H. (2020). Los que ni acatan ni cumplen. In R. H. Asensio (Ed.), *Crónicas del gran encierro. Pensando el Perú en tiempos de pandemia* (pp. 42–43). IEP. https://iep.org.pe/wp-con tent/uploads/2020/06/Cr%C3%B3nica-del-Gran-Encierro-1.pdf

Coffey, A. (1999). *The ethnographic self: Fieldwork and the representation of identity.* Sage.

Comaroff, J. (2020). When the virus makes the timeline. *Social Anthropology, 28*(2), 245–246. https://doi.org/10.1111/1469-8676.12811

Cometti, G. (2015). *Lorsque le brouillard a cessé de nous écouter.* Peter Lang.

Cometti, G., Fabio, E., Terry, C., & Mathieu, U. (2018, August 12). *Il Signore di Quyllurit'i.* Iceberg. https://ethnologie.unistra.fr/institut/conferences-et-films-en-ligne/docume ntaires-ethnographiques/le-seigneur-de-quylluriti-2018/

Contreras, C., & Cueto, M. (2013). *Historia del Perú contemporáneo: Desde las luchas por la independencia hasta el presente* (5ta ed.). IEP.

Cuenca, R. (2020). El covid-19 y el examen al sistema educativo. In R. H. Asensio (Ed.), *Crónicas del gran encierro. Pensando el Perú en tiempos de pandemia* (pp. 54–56). IEP. https://iep.org.pe/ wp-content/uploads/2020/06/Cr%C3%B3nica-del-Gran-Encierro-1.pdf

Delamont, S. (2013). Arguments against auto-ethnography. In P. Sikes (Ed.), *Autoethnography* (Vol. II, pp. 95–100). Sage.

DeWitte, S. N. (2020, June 19). Social inequality in times of pandemics. *Anthropology News Website.* https://www.anthropology-news.org/index.php/2020/06/19/social-inequality-in-times-of-pandemics/

Dijstelbloem, H. (2014). Missing in action: Inclusion and exclusion in the first days of AIDS in The Netherlands. *Sociology of Health & Illness, 36*(8), 1156–1170. https://doi.org/10.1111/1467-9566.12159

El Peruano. (2020, July 21). *Decreto Supremo que establece las medidas que debe observar la ciudadanía en la Nueva Convivencia Social y prorroga el Estado de Emergencia Nacional por las graves circunstancias que afectan la vida de la Nación a consecuencia del COVID-19-DECRETO SUPREMO-N° 116-2020-PCM*. http://busquedas.elperuano.pe/normaslegales/decreto-supremo-que-establece-las-medidas-que-debe-observar-decreto-supremo-no-116-2020-pcm-1869114-1/

Ellis, C., & Bochner, A. P. (2013). Autoethnography, personal narrative, reflexivity: Researcher as subject. In P. Sikes (Ed.), *Autoethnography: Vol. I* (pp. 125–173). Sage.

Essén, A., & Winterstorm Värlander, S. (2012). The mutual constitution of sensuous and discursive understanding in scientific practice: An autoethnographic lens on academic writing. *Management Learning, 44*(4), 395–423. https://doi.org/10.1177/1350507611431529

Figueroa, A., Altamirano, T., & Sulmont, D. (1996). *Exclusión social y desigualdad en el Perú*. OIT (Oficina Regional para América Latina y el Caribe).

Franco, S. (2007). Poverty in Peru: A comparison of different approaches. In F. Stewart, R. Saith, & B. Harriss-White (Eds.), *Defining poverty in the developing world* (pp. 160–197). Palgrave Macmillan.

García-Sayan, D. (2020, March 19). Virus no tan "democrático." *El País*. https://elpais.com/elpais/2020/03/19/opinion/1584627363_620196.html

Gerbaudo Suárez, D., Golé, C., & Pérez, C. (2020). Diario etnográfico de tres becarias en cuarentena: Entre el aislamiento y la intimidad colectiva. *Perifèria. Revista de Recerca i Formació en Antropologia, 25*(2), 167–178. https://doi.org/10.5565/rev/periferia.756

Godber, O. F., & Wall, R. (2014). Livestock and food security: Vulnerability to population growth and climate change. *Global Change Biology, 20*(10), 3092–3102. https://doi.org/10.1111/gcb.12589

Lancaster, R. N. (2011). Autoethnography. When I was a girl (notes on contrivance). In F. E. Mascia-Lees (Ed.), *A companion to the anthropology of the body and embodiment* (pp. 46–71). Wiley-Blackwell.

Leary, N., Conde, C., Kulkarni, J., Nyong, A., & Pulhin, J. (Eds.). (2008). *Climate change and vulnerability*. Routledge.

Loeza Reyes, L. (2015). Desigualdad e injusticia social: Los núcleos duros de las identidades sociales en México. *Sociológica, 30*, 181–206.

Low, S., & Maguire, M. (2020). Public space during COVID-19. *Social Anthropology, 28*(2), 309–310. https://doi.org/10.1111/1469-8676.12885

Macher, S., Ugarteche, O., Paz, R., Pariona, T., & McEvoy, C. (2020, August 8). *Perú, 30 años después: Del shock de la pandemia a la urgencia de diálogo* [Conferencia organizada por la Coordinación Nacional de Derechos Humanos (CNDDHH Perú)]. https://www.facebook.com/cnddhh/videos/291722855452450

Mayer, E. (2018). *The articulated peasant: Household economies in the Andes*. Routledge.

Méndez, M. (2013). Autoethnography as a research method: Advantages, limitations and criticisms. *Colombian Applied Linguistics Journal, 15*(2), 279–287. http://www.scielo.org.co/pdf/calj/v15n2/v15n2a10.pdf

Monge-Barrio, A., & Sánchez-Ostiz Gutiérrez, A. (2018). *Passive energy strategies for mediterranean residential buildings: Facing the challenges of climate change and vulnerable populations*. Springer.

Morgan, N., & Pritchard, A. (2005). On souvenirs and metonymy: Narratives of memory, metaphor and materiality. *Tourist Studies, 5*(1), 29–53. https://doi.org/10.1177/1468797605062714

Morlon, P. (1992). *Comprendre l'agriculture paysanne dans les Andes centrales: Pérou-Bolivie*. Institut National de la Recherche Agronomique.

Noy, C. (2008). The poetics of tourist experience: An autoethnography of a family trip to Eilat. *Journal of Tourism and Cultural Change, 5*(3), 141–157. https://doi.org/10.2167/jtcc085.0

Oxenford, J. (2020, July 9). *Trabajadores de municipio de Independencia recibieron canastas*. https://www.youtube.com/watch?v=gcFCSr9TnUs

Pajuelo, R. (2020). Pandemia y conocimiento: Visibilizando un desafío pendiente en Perú. In R. H. Asensio (Ed.), *Crónicas del gran encierro. Pensando el Perú en tiempos de pandemia* (pp. 178–184). IEP. https://iep.org.pe/wp-content/uploads/2020/06/Cr%C3%B3nica-del-Gran-Encierro-1.pdf

Pink, S. (2009). *Doing sensory ethnography*. Sage.

Popkewitz, T. S. (2013). What's in a research project: Some thoughts on the intersection of history, social structure and biography. In P. Sikes (Ed.), *Autoethnography* (Vol. I, pp. 87–107). Sage.

Radio ambulante. (2020, May 15). *La paradoja peruana—[El hilo]*. NPR.Org. https://www.npr.org/2020/05/15/856687290/la-paradoja-peruana-el-hilo]

Reátegui, L. (2020). La desigualdad educativa en tiempos del covid-19. In R. H. Asensio (Ed.), *Crónicas del gran encierro. Pensando el Perú en tiempos de pandemia* (pp. 50–51). IEP. https://iep.org.pe/wp-content/uploads/2020/06/Cr%C3%B3nica-del-Gran-Encierro-1.pdf

Reed-Danahay, D. E. (2013). Introduction to auto/ethnography: Rewriting the self and the social. In P. Sikes (Ed.), *Autoethnography* (Vol. I, pp. 3–12). Sage.

Sikes, P. (Ed.). (2013a). *Autoethnography: : Vol. I–IV*. Sage.

Sikes, P. (2013b). Editor's introduction: An autoethnographic preamble. In P. Sikes (Ed.), *Autoethnography: Vol. I* (pp. xxi–lii). Sage.

Stanley, L. (2013). On auto/biography in sociology. In P. Sikes (Ed.), *Autoethnography* (Vol. I, pp. 67–78). Sage.

Tanaka, M. (2020a). Estado y necrosis (2). In R. H. Asensio (Ed.), *Crónicas del gran encierro. Pensando el Perú en tiempos de pandemia* (pp. 83–84). IEP. https://iep.org.pe/wp-content/uploads/2020/06/Cr%C3%B3nica-del-Gran-Encierro-1.pdf

Tanaka, M. (2020b). La culpa es de la gente. In R. H. Asensio (Ed.), *Crónicas del gran encierro. Pensando el Perú en tiempos de pandemia* (pp. 94–95). IEP. https://iep.org.pe/wp-content/uploads/2020/06/Cr%C3%B3nica-del-Gran-Encierro-1.pdf

Terry, C. (2011). *Tourisme et réduction de la pauvreté: Études des impacts socio-économiques de l'agro-écotourisme du Parque de la Papa (Cusco-Pérou)* [Mémoire de Master, Institut des Hautes Etudes Internationales et du Développement]. https://repository.graduateinstitute.ch/record/14084

Terry, C. (2017). Turismo Rural Comunitario: ¿Una alternativa para las comunidades andinas? El caso del agro-ecoturismo del Parque de la Papa (Cusco, Perú). *PASOS. Revista de Turismo y Patrimonio Cultural, 18,* 139–159. http://www.pasosonline.org/Publicados/pasosoedita/PSEdita18.pdf

Terry, C. (2019). *Tisser la valeur au quotidien. Une cartographie de l'interaction entre humains et textiles andins dans la région de Cusco à l'heure du tourisme du XXIe siècle* [Thèse de Doctorat, Université de Lausanne]. https://serval.unil.ch/resource/serval:BIB_61191E671028.P002/REF

Terry, C. (2020a). Weaving social change(s) or changes of weaving? The ethnographic study of Andean textiles in Cusco and Bolivia. *Artl@s Bulletin, 9*(1), 68–89. https://docs.lib.purdue.edu/artlas/vol9/iss1/6/

Terry, C. (2020b, June 15). En voyage à deux pas de chez soi. Balade d'un touriste clandestin à Cusco. *Co-vies20.Vivre (dé)confiné-e-s, penser en commun*. https://covies20.com/2020/06/15/en-voyage-a-deux-pas-de-chez-soi-balade-dun-touriste-clandestin-a-cusco/

Terry, C. (2020c, December 15). Does the new coronavirus has soroche? Controversy over high altitude effects on Covid-19: The case of Cusco (Peru). *Viral. Les multiples vies du Covid-19*. https://wp.unil.ch/viral/le-nouveau-coronavirus-a-t-il-du-soroche-controverse-sur-les-effets-de-laltitude-sur-le-covid-19-le-cas-de-cusco-perou/

Terry, C. (2020d, December 17). L'invité invisible. Mariage à l'heure du Covid-19: Un récit auto-ethnographique à Cusco (Pérou). *Viral. Les multiples vies du Covid-19*. https://wp.unil.ch/viral/linvite-invisible-mariage-a-lheure-du-covid-19-un-recit-auto-ethnographique-a-cusco-perou/

Terry, C. (2021). "Catch me if you can". Récits de voyage et de confinement. In A. Lya (Ed.), *Echos vides—La poétique du coronavirus* (pp. 214–221). Editions Let-Know Café.

Trivelli, C. (2020). ¿Cobertura universal o focalizada? In R. H. Asensio (Ed.), *Crónicas del gran encierro. Pensando el Perú en tiempos de pandemia* (pp. 60–62). IEP. https://iep.org.pe/wp-content/uploads/2020/06/Cr%C3%B3nica-del-Gran-Encierro-1.pdf

Vesoulis, A. (2020, March 11). Coronavirus may disproportionately hurt the poor—And that's bad for everyone. *Time.* https://time.com/5800930/how-coronavirus-will-hurt-the-poor/

Vich, V. (2020). Comenzar a salir del capitalismo: Arriesgar lo imposible. In R. H. Asensio (Ed.), *Crónicas del gran encierro. Pensando el Perú en tiempos de pandemia* (pp. 185–190). IEP. https://iep.org.pe/wp-content/uploads/2020/06/Cr%C3%B3nica-del-Gran-Encierro-1.pdf

Vionnet, C. (2018). *L'ombre du geste: Le(s) sens de l'expérience en danse contemporaine* [Thèse de Doctorat, Université de Lausanne]. https://core.ac.uk/download/pdf/156954768.pdf

Voirol, J. (2013). Récit ethnographique d'une expérience partagée de la fête de San Juan/Inti Raymi à Otavalo (Andes équatoriennes). *Ethnologies, 35*(1), 51–74. https://doi.org/10.7202/1026451ar

Worldometers. (2020, August 8). *Coronavirus update (Live): 19,697,932 cases and 726,948 deaths from COVID-19 virus pandemic—Worldometer.* https://www.worldometers.info/coronavirus/

Cristian Terry has a Master in Development Studies from the Graduate Institute of International and Development Studies (Geneva) and a PhD in Social Sciences from the University of Lausanne (Switzerland). His fieldwork studies focus on tourism dynamics and effects in the Cusco region, especially among Andean rural populations working on Community-based tourism. He also worked as coordinator of the agro-ecotourism program in the Potato Park (five Andean communities of the Pisaq district, Cusco). He is currently doing ethnographic research on the COVID-19 pandemic, its evolution and its effects in Peru. He particularly pays attention to its impacts on people's daily life and on economic activities like gastronomy and tourism sectors during and after the lockdown.

Chapter 9
Koro ti Lo: Popular Deconstruction of the COVID-19 Pandemic in Southwestern Nigeria

Mofeyisara Oluwatoyin Omobowale, Olugbenga Samuel Falase, Olufikayo Kunle Oyelade, and Ayokunle Olumuyiwa Omobowale

Abstract The emergence of the COVID-19 pandemic and its persistence are global phenomena, that greatly impact human life and existence. In Nigeria, the incidence and prevalence of the COVID-19 has attracted various interpretations and actions across cultures and spaces. While many people accept the reality of the deadly virus, many others still live in the denial of its existence and persistence. In the recent times, Nigeria seemed to experience a decline in the daily incidence rate of infected people partly due to mass education and the enforcement of preventive protocols. Subsequently, many Nigerians have thrown caution to the wind celebrating the supposed decline of the pandemic with a popular slogan: Koro ti lo (COVID-19 has gone). Preventive measures were largely abandoned and interactions in public spaces returned to pre-COVID-19 social and spatial relations. The consequence of this is the second wave of the pandemic. Therefore, this chapter examines the (1) socio-cultural deconstructions of the COVID-19 pandemic, (2) probes the second wave of the pandemic and (3) makes post-COVID-19 public health policy recommendations viz-a-viz prevalent relational cultures.

Keywords COVID-19 · Pandemic deconstruction · Pandemic denial · Public health

---

M. O. Omobowale (✉)
Social and Behavioural Health Unit, Institute of Child Health, College of Medicine, University of Ibadan, Ibadan, Nigeria

O. S. Falase
Department of Sociology, Lead City University, Ibadan, Nigeria

O. K. Oyelade
Emmanuel College of Theology and Christian Education, Ibadan, Nigeria

A. O. Omobowale
Department of Sociology, University of Ibadan, Ibadan, Nigeria

© The Author(s), under exclusive license to Springer Nature Singapore Pte Ltd. 2022
S. Roy and D. Nandy (eds.), *Understanding Post-COVID-19 Social and Cultural Realities*, https://doi.org/10.1007/978-981-19-0809-5_9

9.1 Introduction

The COVID-19 pandemic has proven to be one of the greatest public health challenges of the twenty-first Century. The COVID-19 was first reported in China in December 2019 as a variant of the Coronavirus. Aided by highly contagious nature and international travels, COVID-19 has spread to over 223 countries and dependencies, and resulted in over 92 million confirmed cases and about 2 million confirmed deaths by January 2021 (WHO, 2021). By January 2021, Nigeria has recorded a hundred thousand confirmed cases and more than 1300 deaths as community transmission rages (Nigeria Centre for Disease Control, 2021a). COVID-19 is one of the most contagious diseases and it is no respecter of international boundaries and races, ethnicity and/or social class barriers. Yet, in Nigeria, COVID-19 is popularly deconstructed by myths and denials, and subsisting social interactions indicate popular disregard for social distancing and other protocols aimed at preventing the coronavirus (Omobowale et al., 2020). Hence it is pertinent to ask: how do people in Ibadan, Nigeria interpret Covid-19 incidence, spread and seemingly reduction in its recent incidence? This chapter, therefore, examines the popular deconstruction of COVID-19 pandemic in Southwestern Nigeria by (1) discussing the socio-cultural deconstruction of the COVID-19, (2) examining the second wave of the pandemic and (3) making post-COVID-19 public health recommendations.

Early research on the COVID-19 pandemic in Nigeria indicates an initial rejection that such a deadly virus existed and many others opined it affected only the elite class (Omobowale et al., 2020). Whereas, COVID-19 is now largely recognized as a deadly virus and through ethnographic study, it was indicated that many across the mass population assume its severity among the privileged and the economically challenged that are relatively less exposed to the deadly virus. Nigeria is not currently among the most COVID-19 affected countries, yet, the country is experiencing community transmission and public disposition to the pandemic is an indicator that the nation may be a major COVID-19 affected country if care is not taken. Poor public disposition to the curtailment of the pandemic is not unconnected to the poverty statuses of the majority and the assumptions that it could be easily remedied by herbs. More than 80 million Nigerians live below the poverty line $1.9 per day while 20 to 30 million others live at the borderline of poverty earning just a little above the poverty line to provide for themselves and their dependents (Danaan, 2018; Olutayo & Omobowale, 2008). Poverty limits access to modern healthcare services; thus, the majority of the poor primarily patronizes herbal medicine practitioners and spiritualists, and readily assumes that herbs and spirituality cure all illnesses (Omobowale, 2020). These are some factors that deconstruct the virus and may make the pandemic difficult to curtail.

The COVID-19 pandemic attracted public deconstruction across many nations. Uscinski et al. (2020) posited that many Americans attributed conspiracy constructions to the COVID-19 pandemic due to denialism and conspiracy thinking. Many Americans just reject expert findings on the virus based on political constructions related to the contentions between Republicans and Democrats, and support for President Donald Trump (see also Kemp et al., 2020). Romer and Jamieson (2020)

9 *Koro ti Lo:* Popular Deconstruction …

rightly posits that the conspiracy theories are impediments to curtailing the spread of COVID-19 in the USA, irrespective of the nation's vibrant and advanced health care and public health systems. Also, Jolley and Paterson (2020) examined how 5G conspiracy theories fueled COVID-19 violence in Great Britain. Many conspiracy theorists across the world claimed that the 5G technology was the cause of the COVID-19 pandemic and some protesters violently damaged 5G masts within their vicinities (see also BBC, 2020b; Waterson & Hern, 2020). Such is the power of unfounded conspiracy theories at driving people's actions. The research of Clark et al. (2020) confirms that belief in government recommended precautions and readiness to protect one's health is pivotal at avoiding COVID-19. The research also concluded that females are more careful to protect themselves against COVID-19 than males.

Allington et al. (2020) also rightly confirm the contribution of the social media to the dissemination of misinformation on COVID-19 and discouragement of self-protective behaviour. Conspiracies, ideas and misinformation regarding COVID-19 on social media is going on which significantly threaten public health and safety. In Africa, Rutayisire et al. (2020) and Iwuoha et al. (2020) posit that people rejected COVID-19 curtailment protocols of social distancing and movement restrictions due to religious and cultural beliefs. Furthermore, people who are endemically poor are more concerned about earning daily income to survive than to be concerned about coronavirus that they cannot see (George, 2020; Nkengasong & Mankoula, 2020). Despite the popular deconstruction of COVID-19, it remains a public health threat in Nigeria. This chapter, therefore, examines the popular deconstruction of the COVID-19 pandemic in Southwestern Nigeria. This section introduces the chapter, the next section presents the methodology and the third section discusses the second wave of COVID-19 pandemic in Nigeria. Furthermore, the fourth section gives post-COVID-19 public health recommendations and the fifth section presents the conclusion.

9.2 Methodology

This research adopted a contextual reflective approach. The approach allows contextual reflections on the subject matter, based on experience of existing social realities that shape constructions, understandings and people's reactions to prevailing realities such as the COVID-19 pandemic (Nowacek et al., 2019; Hallo, 2020; Omobowale et. al., 2020). Data were drawn from observations in Ibadan, Nigeria. The observations included those on refusal to adhere to COVID-19 preventive protocols and made comments at informal conversations, communications and interactions claiming that COVID-19 affected the elite class more and the pandemic was gone. The observation lasted between May and December 2020 COVID-19 statistical data were sourced from the COVID-19 websites of the Nigeria Centre for Disease Control (https://covid19.ncdc.gov.ng/) and the World Health Organisation (https://www.who.int/emergencies/diseases/novel-coronavirus-2019). Media data were sourced from the BBC, The Guardian (UK), The Guardian (Nigeria), Inter Press Service, The Punch and Premium Times. Data were subjected to contextual reflective analysis. The findings offer important insights into the contextual interpretations and understanding that deconstruct COVID-19 pandemic in everyday interactions.

9.3 Socio-Cultural Deconstructions of the COVID-19 Pandemic

The COVID-19 remains a major global public health challenge. Its emergence, rapid spread and government response to curtail the pandemic through prevention protocols have culminated in socio-cultural shocks and reactions that advance disbelief and deconstruction in many societies and local communities (Omobowale et al., 2021). COVID-19 spreads through droplets from saliva and nose discharge when talking, coughing or sneezing, and transmits at a fast rate to reach thousands and millions of people over a short period of time (WHO, 2020, Seminara, 2020). In another recent study conducted by the United State National Academy of Sciences, Engineering and Medicine, it has also been confirmed that a new that the virus can spread is through breathing and talking (Ningthoujam, 2020). Against this contagious reality, there was a global campaign for the use of facemasks, social distancing, avoidance of public gatherings, avoidance of handshakes and practice of respiratory etiquettes (among others) as ways of combatting COVID-19 pandemic. In many embedded societies, as the case in Africa in general and Nigeria in particular, these protocols have severe implications for the value of social and inter-personal relations that require physical closeness and gathering of people for interactions.

In Nigeria, the COVID-19 pandemic was initially received with some disbelief that it does not exist and cannot survive under hot weather (Muaya, 2020; Obinna, 2020). As the virus continued to spread and cases mounted in Nigeria, the disbelief gradually transformed to misconceptions, which were also accompanied by various conspiracy theories to discountenance the existence of COVID-19 (Azuh, 2020). It was observed that many people among the mass public described COVID-19 as an elite disease transported to the country by international travelers. There is also an assumption that a regular intake of hot water and spirits with at least 40% alcoholic content prevents the novel coronavirus. However, having realized the existence of the virus and the weirdness of its mode of transmission, which is alien to the people and their health belief system, it was ethnographically observed that the COVID-19 pandemic was contextually interpreted and culturally constructed in various ways as *ako iba* (chronic malaria), *igbona* (fever), and *ajakalearun* (epidemic) (see also Jegede, 2002). Others gave interpretations based on religious orientations, thus claiming that the COVID-19 was a demon or spirit and it penetrated the world by sin. Some prominent religious leaders also dismissed COVID-19 as mere threats of the devil that they would dispel by religious rituals (Augoye, 2020; Oyero, 2020).

Nigeria started a gradual lifted of lockdown in the Federal Capital Territory-Abuja, Lagos and Ogun States on 4 May 2020, the gradual process of the removal of lockdown went on till 1 June 2020 while schools resumed on 21 September 2020 for the 2020/2021 academic year in Oyo State (BBC, 2020a; Ibrahim et al., 2020). Of course, the government encouraged the public to abide by prevention protocols. The easing of the lockdown and a noticeable decline in daily active cases from about the second week of August up to mid-November 2020 (see Nigeria Centre for Disease Control, 2021b; Our World in Data, 2021; Worldometer, 2021) gave a false assurance among the mass public that the COVID-19 pandemic had gone (*koro ti lo*) for good and that normalcy in everyday activities should be brought back. Hence, many people increasingly practiced limited personal protection measures lost their guards. Large gatherings resumed in parties and religious places, handshaking and hugs were once again normalized, wearing of facemasks, hand-sanitising and washing observably declined, and many Nigerians in diaspora who travelled back home for end of year festivities from about November 2020 refused to self-isolate and conduct mandatory COVID-19 tests among other COVID-19 protocol failings. Some who strive to abide by the pandemic protocols were dismissed as faithless, weak and snubbish and reminded on the normative code that *ara o ki nsa fara* (human beings should not run away from human beings).

With the relaxation of COVID-19 rules, Nigerians believe that the pandemic period is short-lived. Perhaps, this is linked to the presumptions of Nigerians about China that anything that comes from China does not last, hence, koro was a *chinco* virus, which is ephemeral and has returned to its base. As interactions reconnect people again, the social distancing rule was deconstructed. As George (2020) notes, for some societies, physical interaction and closeness are parts of their national culture deeply rooted in their heritage, hence, maintaining social distancing in such society with a culture of social interaction, may be difficult. Nigeria is like such a society, where personal and public spaces are always contested for interactions to take place (see Omobowale, 2019), and as such, social distancing may seem impracticable. As people interact and believe that *koro ti lo* (COVID has gone), the COVID-19 slogan turns to COVID-money, denoting that the lockdown period that characterized COVID-19 pandemic has ended, and now that the society has returned to normalcy, Nigerians will make COVID-money. The assumed COVID-money is drawn from the adverse economic effects of COVID-19 pandemic, which has increased the prices of goods. Thus, money lost during the pandemic is expected to be regained during the COVID-money period. Also, the refusal in shaking of hands as a form of discreet salutation during the pandemic has also produced some social implications for respect reciprocity. As a pandemic rule, greetings become through feet, elbow or fist. This change in regular greetings was seen as a disrespect to some people who always feel insulted whenever they received an elbow or fist in return for their stretched hand for greetings.

The resumption of churches and schools have also deconstructed the existence of the COVID-19 and contributed to the second wave of the pandemic. Churches are places for religious activities that accommodate thousands of believers. With the social deconstruction that *koro ti lo*, people put their faith in church doctrine and appreciate God for putting an end to the pandemic. Although they are reminded to use their facemasks and comply with the COVID-19 protocols, the general belief among members is that coro period is over. With this, many religious gatherings are observed to be found wanting in strict observance of physical distancing and proper use of face mask. Many congregants turn their face mask to chin mask with a view to satisfying their spiritual yearning, especially in terms of singing and fervent prayer. What also strengthens the popular deconstruction is the misleading statement by pastors and religious leaders to convince the congregation that COVID-19 was a battle, which had been won and defeated, and 'now that the koro period is over', people are urged to remain steadfast and pray against its recurrence.

Be that as it may, social gathering of wedding, naming, funerals parties etc., resume. Although planners, celebrants and guests at these occasions claim to observe the pandemic protocols, in the course of eating, drinking and dancing, people are carried away seen flouting the pandemic protocols. The opening of borders, land, airport and seaports, also depicts the general belief of the public and the government that COVID-19 is gone. With this new development, many government officials compromise the rules and guidelines against the spread of the disease for money making. Besides, the local transportation, both intra and interstate, has resumed their normal duty prior to the COVID-19 pandemic, as transporters care less about overloading, knowing full well that they would always have their ways at the instance of bribing the law enforcement agents. It is important to mention that all these have serious health implications within the context of the second wave of COVID-19.

The sum of all the aforementioned easing resulted in sharp increase in daily confirmed cases of the COVID-19 as from the end of November 2020. Observations of communications in everyday social relations and on social media indicate that many people initially dismissed the increase as a deliberate official inflation of data to justify acceptance of COVID-19 vaccines which were coincidentally approved especially in the USA and Great Britain in November 2020. Recent reports however, reveal that the Nigerian health sector is undergoing COVID-19 pandemic stress; an increasing number of patients require hospital admission, available beds are declining, there is oxygen crisis due to high demand for patients and both low- and high-profile deaths due to COVID-19 are on the rise (Njoku et al., 2021; *The Guardian*, 2021).

9.4 The Second Wave of COVID-19 in Nigeria

The advent and continued spread of the COVID-19 pandemic has called for the attention of the entire global community by many, while some others still deny its existence. Despite drastic efforts to curtail the spread of the pandemic, cases and deaths due to COVID-19 has substantially increased in Nigeria. The 'second wave' of a disease as described by expert explains the initial phenomenon of a pandemic, its reduction and the sudden increase (see Sheil, 2018). The second wave of the COVID-19 in Nigeria cannot be dissociated from the nonchalant attitude of citizens and residents to COVID-19 protocols. A seemingly initial decline of daily active cases gave a false impression that the pandemic was gone as mentioned above, hence, many people who were initially cautious lost their guards and encouraged others to do so. It was common for people to say, *koro ti lo, e nilo facemask* (the novel coronavirus has gone, you do not need face mask). In relational terms, this was a process of stigmatizing those who actively strived to maintain the COVID-19 protocols. Notwithstanding, overall confirmed COVID-19 cases and mortality in Nigeria reveal an upward gradient as the below Charts. 9.1 and 9.2 show:

Furthermore, Table 9.1 below gives the actual figures of the confirmed cases, discharge and mortality due to COVID-19 from February to December 2020.

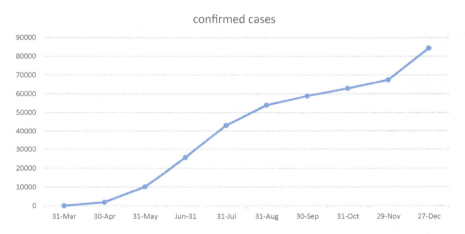

Chart 9.1 Confirmed cases March–December 2020. *Source* Nigeria Centre for Disease Control (2020a) Situation Reports

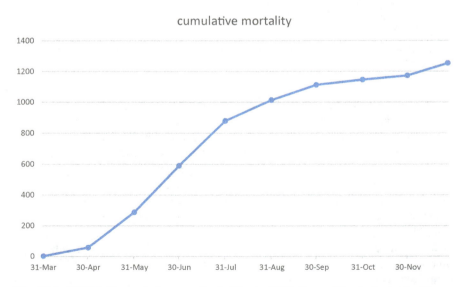

Chart 9.2 COVID-19 cumulative mortality in Nigeria, 2020. *Source* Nigeria Centre for Disease Control (2020a) Situation Reports

Table 9.1 COVID-19 cumulative confirmed cases, discharge mortality and percentage increase of cases from February, 2020 to June, 2021

Date	Confirmed cases (Cumulatively)(Morbidity)	Percentage increase in cases (%)	Number discharged (Cumulatively)	Mortality (Cumulatively)
29 February 2020	1	0	0	0
31 March 2020	139	–	9	2
30 April 2020	1932	128.9	319	58
31 May 2020	10,162	425.9	3007	287
30 June 2020	25,694	152.8	9746	590
31 July 2020	43,151	67.9	19,565	878
31 August 2020	54,008	25.2	41,638	1013
30 September 2020	58,848	8.9	50,358	1112
31 October 2020	62,964	(6.9)	58,790	1146
28 November 2020	67,412	(7.1)	63,055	1172
27 December 2020	84,414	(25.2)	71,034	1254
January–February 2021	131,242	18.6	94,150	133,742
February–March 2021	162,593	4.4	150,308	2048
March–April 2021	165,181	1.63	155,361	2063
April–May 2021	166,019	0.5	156,476	2067
May–June 2021	167,467	0.9	163,949	2119

Source Nigeria Centre for Disease Control (2020a) *Situation Reports: Nigeria Centre for Disease Control* (2021c)

Starting with the record of the first case of COVID-19 on 27 February 2020 (Nigeria Centre for Disease Control, February 28, 2020b), the number of confirmed cases rose to 139 by 31 March 2020. Nine (9) were discharged and mortality has set in with 2 cases. As of April 31, 2020, the cases confirmed rose to 1,932 with 128.9% rate of increase, the number of persons discharged was 319 while the mortality increased to 58 deaths. By May 31, 2020, the number of COVID-19 cases confirmed was 10,162 with 425.9% rate of increase compared with that of April; the number discharged was 3,007 while the mortality was 287 deaths. As of June 30, 2020, the confirmed cases were 25,694 with 152.8% rate of increase compared with that of May, 2020. Hence, as from June 2020, the increase in daily rate of confirmed cases started falling. The number of confirmed cases as at July 31, was 43,151 with 67.9% rate of increase compared with that of May, 2020. The number of cases confirmed as at August 31 was 54, 008 with 25.2% rate of increase compared with that of July 2020. As of

September 30, 2020, the rate of increase further reduced to 8.9% with 58,848 number of confirmed cases. By October, 31, 2020 the rate of increase of confirmed cases of COVID-19 reduced further to 6.9% with 62,964 in number. However, the data further reveals that the rate of increase of confirmed cases significantly increased to 67,412 cases signifying an increase of 7.1% compared to that of October, 2020, and further increased by 25.2% as of December 27, 2020 with 84, 414 confirmed cases. The confirmed cases in Nigeria as of 23 January 2021 was 118,969 representing 40.94% surge in less than a month. Hence, indicating the occurrence of the second wave of COVID-19 in Nigeria.

Analytically, the rate of increase in infection reduced consistently between March and October, 2020, but began to increase again in November 2020. This is an indication that Nigeria entered the second wave of the infection about November 2020, but people initially paid little attention to the gradual increase of the daily reported cases of COVID-19. From January to June 2021 the percentage increase in the cases indicates that there is decrease in the incidence of cases but the number of people tested also decreased. This is not unconnected to the wrong popular assumption that the novel coronavirus had been defeated despite the regular warnings from government health and pandemic management agencies. People just generally had a false conviction that COVID-19 had been conquered. Religious leaders attributed victory over the virus to prayers and other religious rituals while many among the populace gave the credence to the efficacy of Nigerian herbs, hot weather conditions and the supposed natural immunity of the African biological system. The second wave with its rapid infection rates, hospital admission and consequent reported shortage of essential treatment resources, such as beds and oxygen in public hospitals, has proven that COVID-19 is yet to be conquered.

9.5 Post-COVID-19 Public Health Policy Recommendations

The COVID-19 is a highly contagious and deadly disease with enormous global, national and local impacts. Yet, the understanding of COVID-19 pandemic in Nigeria is still wrapped with misinformation, misinterpretations, myths, mistrust, denial and insufficient public contextualized pandemic preparedness education. The following recommendations are therefore suggested to address the misinformation and other social challenges associated with COVID-19:

1. **Contextualization of Pandemic in Community Engagement, Education and Intervention**: All information and mis-information about COVID-19 were disseminated and circulated via social relations and through agents of socializations. It is therefore, important to annex same social processes and their agents in disseminating the right information about COVID-19. Community leaders, religious leaders, gate keepers, market leaders, youth leaders and other significant others in the society should be civically recruited to participate actively

in teaching and spreading evidence-based COVID-19 information: existence, prevention and control, within their immediate social environment. Contextualizing COVID-19 pandemic information will address the challenges of misinformation, misinterpretations, mistrust and denial of the existence of the novel coronavirus.

2. **Access to Information**: All citizens must be reached with appropriate messages on the emergence, persistence and prevention of COVID-19. COVID-19 information should be easily accessible and not sophisticated. Available information and findings on COVID-19 should be interpreted into local languages and contents with the aim of leaving no one behind. Information on COVID-19 should be accessible to all classes of citizens in their local parlances and sub-cultural codes.

3. **Pandemic Preparedness Education**: Despite previous epidemics/pandemics that have been experienced in Nigeria, the current disposition to the COVID-19 pandemic especially by the public shows that many citizens are not educated on and prepared for a pandemic like COVID-19. It is therefore important to include pandemic history and preparedness into education pedagogy across all levels: kindergarten, primary, secondary and tertiary. In addition, the mass media should be encouraged and mandated to adopt pandemic history and preparedness education into their programmes to advance mass education across socio-economic groups and literacy contexts, such that the un-educated too could have access to pandemic education through popularly available mass media sources. COVID-19 education should particularly emphasise facemask wearing in public places, observance of good hand and respiratory hygiene, and keeping a distance of 2 m from other people for personal and communal good.

4. **De-stigmatising COVID-19 and its survivors:** Governments and non-governmental organisations should create platforms for the public to locally discuss the issues of COVID-19. COVID-19 survivors should be encouraged to speak on their experiences of the infection. Both known and unknown citizens that have survived the pandemic should be given a platform and be allowed to share their views and experiences. Open disclosures of COVID-19 experiences and admonishments for others to take personal responsibility for safety would enhance the adoption of safe relational lifestyles to stay protected from the COVID-19 and other pathogens.

9.6 Conclusion

Nigeria reported the first case of COVID-19 in February 2020. The number of confirmed cases has reached over 100 thousand and Nigeria is clearly in the second wave of the pandemic. The huge surge of cases in the second wave of the pandemic is not unconnected to a social perception that COVID-19 had been conquered, subsequently the few who adhered to COVID-19 prevention protocols lost their guards. Yet, many people within the low socio-economic range assume that COVID-19 is not really infectious and deadly to the poor, because they erroneously assume that they are immune, and if infected, herbs would effectively dispel the virus. These social constructions make COVID-19 a constant threat to public health in Nigeria and if care is not taken, Nigeria may remain in the COVID-19 entanglement as other nations where citizens are better educated about the pandemic and its prevention exits the pandemic trap. This chapter therefore recommends that a contextualised approach to community engagement, education and intervention to involve primary stakeholders, opinion leaders and gate keepers in the dissemination of COVID-19 information. Also, update and empirical information on COVID-19 should be communicated in local languages and sub-cultural codes to ensure that the information reach the door steps of the most vulnerable populations. Furthermore, pandemic preparedness education should be integrated in curricula and pedagogy across all education levels and finally, de-stigmatisation strategies should be adopted by particularly creating platforms for COVID-19 survivors to render their views and experiences and advise on prevention protocols. This study is limited in terms of geographical coverage, it applicable to situation in the South Western Nigeria and may not be generalizable.

References

Allington, D., Duffy, B., Wessely, S., Dhavan, N., & Rubin, J. (2020). Health-protective behaviour, social media usage and conspiracy belief during the COVID-19 public health emergency. *Psychological Medicine, 1–7*. https://doi.org/10.1017/S003329172000224X

Augoye, J. (2020, 30 August). I'll lay my bare hands on COVID-19 patient, breathe into them—Oyedepo. *Premium Times*, Accessed 16 January 2020 from https://www.premiumtimesng.com/entertainment/naija-fashion/411625-ill-lay-my-bare-hands-on-covid-19-patient-breathe-into-them-oyedepo.html

Azuh, C. (2020). *Standing up to myths and misinformation in Nigeria during the pandemic*. Accessed 8 January, 2021 from Retrieved from www.ipsnews.net/2020/08/standing-myths-misinformation-nigeria-pandemic/.

BBC. (2020a, 21 July). Nigeria schools resumption date and WAEC latest: Oyo cancel third term, release calendar for reopening of classes. *BBC.*, Accessed 16 January 2021 from https://www.bbc.com/pidgin/tori-53494846

BBC. (2020b, 24 May). Coronavirus: Derby 5G phone mast set on fire. *BBC*, Accessed on 16 January 2021 from https://www.bbc.com/news/uk-england-derbyshire-52790399

Clark, C., Davila, A., Regis, M., & Kraus, S. (2020). Predictors of COVID-19 voluntary compliance behaviors: An international investigation. *Global Transitions, 2*, 76–82.

Danaan, V. V. (2018). Analysing poverty in Nigeria through theoretical lenses. *Journal of Sustainable Development, 11*(1), 20–31.

George, M. (2020). Socio-cultural determinants of the spread of Covid 19. *Health and Primary Care, 4*, 1–2. https://doi.org/10.15761/HPC.1000189

Hallo, W. (2020). The book of the people. *Providence, RI: Brown Judaic Studies* (pp. 23–34). https://doi.org/10.2307/j.ctvzgb9g4

Ibrahim, R. L., Ajide, K. B., & Julius, O. O. (2020). Easing of lockdown measures in Nigeria: Implications for the healthcare system. *Health Policy and Technology, 9*(4), 399–404. https://doi.org/10.1016/j.hlpt.2020.09.004

Iwuoha, V. C., Ezeibe, E. N., & Ezeibe, C. C. (2020). Glocalization of COVID-19 responses and management of the pandemic in Africa. *Local Environment, 25*(8), 641–647.

Jegede, A. S. (2002). The Yoruba cultural construction of health and illness. *Nordic Journal of African Studies, 11*(3), 322–335.

Jolley, D., & Paterson, J. L. (2020). Pylons ablaze: Examining the role of 5G COVID-19 conspiracy beliefs and support for violence. *British Journal of Social Psychology, 59*(3), 628–640.

Kemp, E., Price, G. N., Fuller, N. R., & Kemp, E. F. (2020). African Americans and COVID-19: Beliefs, behaviors and vulnerability to infection. *International Journal of Healthcare Management, 13*(4), 303–311.

Muaya, C. (2020, 25 March). Nigeria's high temperature, humidity capable of reducing spread of virus. *The Guardian.*, Accessed on 16 January 2020 from https://guardian.ng/news/nigerias-high-temperature-humidity-capable-of-reducing-spread-of-virus/

Nigeria Centre for Disease Control. (2020a). *First case of Corona Virus disease confirmed in Nigeria.* Accessed 16 February, 2021 from https://ncdc.gov.ng/news/227/first-case-of-corona-virus-disease-confirmed-in-nigeria#:~:text=The%20Federal%20Ministry%20of%20Health,in%20China%20in%20January%202020

Nigeria Centre for Disease Control. (2020b). *Situation Reports.* Accessed 7 January 2021 from https://ncdc.gov.ng/diseases/sitreps/?cat=14&name=An%20update%20of%20COVID-19%20outbreak%20in%20Nigeria

Nigeria Centre for Disease Control. (2021a). *COVID-19 Nigeria.* Accessed 14 January 2021 and November 25, 2021 from https://covid19.ncdc.gov.ng/; https://ncdc.gov.ng/diseases/sitreps/?cat=14&name=An%20update%20of%20COVID-19%20outbreak%20in%20Nigeria

Nigeria Centre for Disease Control. (2021b). *Epicurve by State: Confirmed COVID19 cases—Nigeria 2020.* Accessed 16 January 2021 from https://covid19.ncdc.gov.ng/state/

Nigeria Centre for Disease Control. (2021c). *COVID-19 Nigeria.* Accessed 23 January 2021 from https://covid19.ncdc.gov.ng/

Ningthoujam, R. (2020). COVID 19 can spread through breathing, talking, study estimates. *Current Medicine Research and Practice, 10*(3), 132–133. https://doi.org/10.1016/j.cmrp.2020.05.003

Njoku, L., Daniel, E., & Edward, O. (2012, 7 January). Oxygen crisis hits Nigeria's COVID-19 response scheme. *The Guardian*, Accessed 16 January 2021 from https://guardian.ng/news/oxygen-crisis-hits-nigerias-covid-19-response-scheme/

Nkengasong, J. N., & Mankoula, W. (2020). Looming threat of COVID-19 infection in Africa: Act collectively, and fast. *The Lancet, 395*(10227), 841–842. https://doi.org/10.1016/S0140-6736(20)30464-5

Nowacek, R., Hoffmann, A., Hurlburt, C., Lamson, L., Proodian, S., & Scanlon, A. (2019). Everyday reflective writing: What conference records tell us about building a culture of reflection. *The Writing Center Journal, 37*(2), 93–126. https://doi.org/10.2307/26922019

Obinna, C. (2020, 17 March). COVID-19: Effect of weather, race not proven scientifically—Experts. *Vanguard.* Accessed 16 January 2021 from https://www.vanguardngr.com/2020/03/covid-19-effect-of-weather-race-not-proven-scientifically-experts/

Olutayo, A. O., Olutayo, M. A. O., & Omobowale, A. O. (2008). 'TINA', Aids and the underdevelopment problem in Africa *Revista De Economia-Brazilian Journal of Political Economy, 28*(2), 239–248.

Omobowale, A. O., Oyelade, O. K., Omobowale, M. O., & Falase, O. S. (2020). Contextual reflections on COVID-19 and informal workers in Nigeria. *International Journal of Sociology and Social Policy, 40*(9/10), 1041–1057. https://doi.org/10.1108/IJSSP-05-2020-0150

Omobowale, M. O. (2019). Class, gender, sexuality and leadership in Bodija Market, Ibadan, Nigeria. *Journal of Anthropological Research, 75*(2), 235–251.

Omobowale, M. O. (2020). "You Will Not Mourn Your Children": Spirituality and child health in Ibadan Urban markets. *Journal of Religion and Health, 60*, 406–419. https://doi.org/10.1007/s10943-020-01032-5

Omobowale, M. O., Bamgboye, E. A., Akinyode, A., Falase, O. S., Ladipo, T. O., Salami, O., & Adebiyi, A. O. (2021). Contextual interpretation of COVID-19 pandemic among public space users in Ibadan Metropolis, Oyo State, Nigeria: An ethnographic review. *Plos one, 16*(11), e0259631.

Our World in Data. (2021). *Nigeria: Coronavirus Pandemic Country Profile.* Accessed 16 January 2020 from https://ourworldindata.org/coronavirus/country/nigeria?country=~NGA

Oyero, K. (2020, 31 December). COVID-19: Any system the church attacks will crash, says Oyedepo. *Punch.* Accessed 16 January 2021 from https://punchng.com/covid-19-any-system-the-church-attacks-will-crash-says-oyedepo/

Romer, D., & Jamieson, K. H. (2020). Conspiracy theories as barriers to controlling the spread of COVID-19 in the US. *Social Science & Medicine, 263.* https://doi.org/10.1016/j.socscimed.2020.113356

Rutayisire, E., Nkundimana, G., Mitonga, H. K., Boye, A., & Nikwigize, S. (2020). What works and what does not work in response to COVID-19 prevention and control in Africa. *International Journal of Infectious Diseases, 97,* 267–269.

Seminara, G., Carli, B., Forni, G., Fuzzi, S., Mazzino, A., & Rinaldo, A. (2020). Biological fluid dynamics of airborne COVID-19 infection. *Rend. Fis. Acc. Lincei, 31,* 505–537. https://doi.org/10.1007/s12210-020-00938-2

Shiel, W. C. (2018). *Medical definition of second wave.* Accessed 16 February, 2021 from https://www.medicinenet.com/second_wave/definition.htm

The Guardian. (2021). Bed occupancy level in Lagos COVID-19 care centres increases to 51%. Accessed 10 January, 2021 Retrieved from https://guardian.ng/news/bed-occupancy-level-in-lagos-covid-19-care-centres-increases-to-51/

Uscinski, J. E., Enders, A. M., Klofstad, C., Seelig, M., Funchion, J., Everett, C., Wuchty, S., Premaratne, K., & Murthi, M. (2020). Why do people believe COVID-19 conspiracy theories?. *Harvard Kennedy School Misinformation Review, 1*(3), https://doi.org/10.37016/mr-2020-015.

Waterson, J., & Hern, A. (2020, 6 April). At least 20 UK phone masts vandalised over false 5G coronavirus claims. *The Guardian,* Accessed 16 January 2021 from https://www.theguardian.com/technology/2020/apr/06/at-least-20-uk-phone-masts-vandalised-over-false-5g-coronavirus-claims

World Health Organisation. (2020, 20 October). *Coronavirus disease (COVID-19): How is it transmitted?* Accessed 16 February, 2021 from https://www.who.int/emergencies/diseases/novel-coronavirus-2019/question-and-answers-hub/q-a-detail/coronavirus-disease-covid-19-how-is-it-transmitted.

World Health Organisation. (2021). *Coronavirus disease (COVID-19) pandemic.* Accessed 14 January 2021 from https://www.who.int/emergencies/diseases/novel-coronavirus-2019

Worldmerter. (2021). *Coronavirus: Nigeria.* Accessed 16 January 2021 from https://www.worldometers.info/coronavirus/country/nigeria/

Mofeyisara Oluwatoyin Omobowale holds a PhD in Anthropology. She is a recipient of the American Council of Learned Societies–African Humanities Programme (ACLS-AHP) Doctoral Fellowship 2012, the Cadbury Fellowship (Department of Anthropology and African Studies, Birmingham University) 2014 and ACLS-AHP Post-Doctoral Fellowship 2016. Her interests lie in medical anthropology, cultural studies, sexuality issues and maternal, child and adolescent studies. Mofeyisara is a research Fellow/Lecturer at the Institute of Child Health, College of Medicine, University of Ibadan, Nigeria.

Olugbenga Samuel Falase got a PhD from the Department of Sociology, University of Ibadan, Nigeria in 2018. He is a recipient of the Next Generation, Social Science Research Council (SSRC) fellowship in 2014, 2016, 2017 and 2020, and an awardee of the Life Above Poverty Organisation (LAPO) Doctoral Research Support Grant in 2015. His doctoral research titled 'The Politics of Forest Governance in South-Western Nigeria' explored the everyday "taken-for-granted" nuances in forest governance. He specialises in Development and Rural studies and 'sociology of forest'. He is a lecturer at the Department of Sociology, Lead City University, Ibadan Nigeria.

Olufikayo Kunle Oyelade obtained a PhD degree in Sociology, with special bias for Development and Religion, at the University of Ibadan in 2018. He serves as an adjunct lecturer at the Emmanuel College of Theology and Christian Education (affiliated to the University of Ibadan). He won International Sociological Association (ISA) PhD Students' Laboratory Award, 2015. His research interest includes sociology of religion with bias for symbolism of religion in everyday taken-for-granted reality, development sociology, social ethics, globalisation, religion and development. He is currently the Chaplain of Chapel of the Resurrection, University of Ibadan.

Ayokunle Olumuyiwa Omobowale is a Professor of Sociology. He has won the University of Ibadan Postgraduate School Award for scholarly publication, 2007, IFRA (French Institute for Research in Africa) Research Fellowship 2009, American Council of Learned Societies–African Humanities Programme Post-Doctoral Fellowship 2010 and African Studies Association (USA) Presidential Award 2014. He teaches Sociology at the University of Ibadan, Ibadan, Nigeria. Dr Omobowale was also a visiting scholar at the Centre for African Studies, Rutgers University, New Jersey, USA in November 2014. He served on the Board of Editors of International Encyclopedia of Revolution and Protest (2009), and he is the author of The Tokunbo Phenomenon and the Second-hand Economy in Nigeria (2013).

Chapter 10
COVID-19 and Decline of Multilateralism

Khushnam P N

Abstract Multilateralism and multilateral diplomacy have been the most desired vision for a peaceful and stable global system with capacity to deal with challenges and streamline the deviations as and when it comes on the way. As the system of multilateralism is devised and sustained by the by the nation's desire to ensure and secure their national interests, its capacity to measure up to its aims is directly proportional to the level the great power relations and cooperation. The changes in the structure of international system must be reflected by the commensurate reforms in the multilateral institutions like United Nations Organizations. There is a growing concern about unilateral actions and withdrawal by powers in the recent years and the changing power landscape of the globe is not appropriately reflected in the existing multilateral institutions and mechanism. Such withdrawal syndrome led to the ultimate breakdown of the post-WWI system. Our current scenario is far from such alarming stage as multilateralism is still in consonance with most of the nations of the globe. The COVID-19 with its global spread has impacted heavily on the multilateral institutions as never before. But is its very transnational implications impacting on the global supply chain and economic process have been pushing the nations for multilateral and global cooperation to deal with such impending pandemic. The mini-lateralism and regional multilateralism has shown greater pandemic outreach diplomacy and cooperation but their effective functioning needs an inclusive global multilateral structure. India with its global aspiration must work as an emerging world leader to shape a robust multilateral world with its pandemic measures, outreach and diplomacy.

Keywords Multilateralism · Covid-19 · Pandemic diplomacy · Mini-lateralism · Regional multilateralism

---

Khushnam P N (✉)
Independent Researcher, Bangaluru, India

© The Author(s), under exclusive license to Springer Nature Singapore Pte Ltd. 2022
S. Roy and D. Nandy (eds.), *Understanding Post-COVID-19 Social and Cultural Realities*, https://doi.org/10.1007/978-981-19-0809-5_10

10.1 Research Questions

1. What has been the performance of Multilateralism and multilateral institutions so far, in light of its intended goals?
2. How has the COVID-19 pandemic underway impacted the process and institutions of multilateralism?
3. What would be the implications of COVID-19 for future course and role of multilateralism?

10.2 Methodology

- Historical analysis of independent variable of of multilateral institutions and its performance in terms of attainment of its intended goal.
- Qualitative analysis of the changes (independent variables) envisioned in the concept and vision of multilateralism.
- Descriptive method to explain the outcomes (dependent variables) in light of COVID-19 pandemic underway.
- Application of 'globalization' concept and framework to explain the changes envisioned in the multilateralism, global aspirations and prospects during pandemic.
- Use of Primary and Secondary sources for the requisite analysis and explanation.

10.3 Introduction

Multilateralism and multilateral diplomacy have been the most desired vision for a peaceful and stable global system with capacity to deal with challenges and streamline the deviations as and when it tries to disrupt the system. In international relation, multilateralism refers to mutually coordinated alliance of nations in pursuit of their common goal and shared peace, security and prosperity. In the post-World War II liberal world order, multilateralism assumes crucial role in for peace, crisis management and prosperity. There is a growing concern about unilateral actions and withdrawal by powers in the recent years and the changing power landscape of the globe is not appropriately reflected in the existing multilateral institutions and mechanism. The COVID-19 with its global spread has further impacted heavily on the multilateral institutions as never before. The closing of national boundaries and sudden disruption of global network of transport and supply chain has led to skepticism about the capacity of multilateralism and multilateral institutions. But the very transnational implications of the pandemic and multilateral cooperation in responses, sharing of pandemic information and research cooperation signifies that world needs the multilateral cooperation and enhanced institutional capacity more than before to deal with impending pandemic which are going to recur more frequently as per the medical research and predictions. The intent of the chapter is to understand the broad trends of multilateralism and its performance so far. The central concern of the study is to examine and analyze the impact and implications of the pandemic underway on multilateral institutions, their responses and approach of the powers and other countries. The study would involve the methodology of historical analysis of independent variable of multilateral institutions and its performance in terms of attainment of its intended goal. A qualitative descriptive analysis of independent variables would be adopted to explain the outcomes (dependent variables) with the use of appropriate primary and secondary sources.

10.4 COVID-19 and Its Impact on Multilateralism

The apparent syndrome of national responsibility and global movement is part of immediate response. The world is already faced with numerous challenges of transnational nature like climate change, terrorism, geopolitical tension, and migration-crisis. Besides, unprecedented headways in science and technology like space technology, cyber space and weapons of mass destruction. All these developments have altered the inter-state relations in such a way that no country, irrespective of their power, will not be able to stand alone and manage alone. The pandemic has exposed our shared vulnerability. "The COVID-19 pandemic is a tragic reminder of how deeply connected we are. The virus knows no borders and is a quintessential global challenge. Combatting it requires us to work together as one human family" (United Naions, 2020, April 24).

Besides, the contemporary world is extremely networked and interdependent place which cannot be dismantled by any means. In the so-called 'Multilateralism 2.0' state is no more sovereign actor in international relations. There are many non-governmental organizations, multinational institutions and networks and regional organization. Though they have been created by the states themselves, once created, they have a life of their own and not always regulated and controlled by their creators-the states (Langenhove, 2011). In such a scenario, multilateralism and multilateral process cannot be done away with by the states.

The pandemic underway has made it apparent that virus has impacted the life across the national boundaries. The whole world is under the catastrophic tentacles of the crisis. The scale of the crisis and its debilitating impacts and implications points to the global extent and nature of the consequences. Thus, the national governments are in active mode to engage in minimizing the risks and arresting the spread. But the sheer scale of the pandemic is beyond the ambit of states and need of stronger spirit of multilateralism and functioning multilateral institutions are need of the hour. The multilateralism is based on the fact that it minimizes the cost of negative actions and maximizes the positive actions of other countries as well as shared benefits of global public goods. The contemporary multilateral institutions are based on pragmatic and realist benefits and clearly weakened by geopolitical contest and great power rivalry. The pandemic and its scale has strained it to the bottom and exposing its utilitarian nature. The present crisis has emphasized the moral imperative that one is safe when all other is safe. Thus multilateralism needs to infuse the ethical content and moral ethos to the realist approach of verified dividend based cooperation (Dervis, 2020).

The most devastating consequences of the COVID-19 are in the arena of international trade. Barring the essential goods and services associated with health, food and housing other necessary utilities, all other sectors of the economy are either closed or extremely down. There is increasing return of the state and its machinery in economies of the countries. There is growing syndrome of protectionism and isolation. The debate around reduction on dependence and urge for self-reliance are the pattern towards de-globalisation. The protectionism bids are especially stronger in the advanced economies which have been further complicated by the spiralling US-China trade war. Still the course of multilateralism is an integral part of resilient pandemic response in international trade as well to beat the economic implications of the crisis. Building resilient multilateral structure, expanding transformative capacity and economic diversification is vital to overcome the fractured global landscape by the pandemic. The new multilateralism must be dynamically resilient to deal both the pandemic damages and the negative forces of globalization causing inequality and vulnerability of large sections of people and countries (UNCTAD, 2020, December 17). The signing of the Regional Comprehensive Economic Programme (RCEP) by ASEAN plus Australia, Japan New Zealand and South Korea are positive development besides the Trans Pacific Partnership (TPP) and the African Continental Free Trade Area (ACFTA) of 55 countries with 1.3 billion population (Dollar, 2020).

10.5   Multilateralism and Arms Control

The pandemic has caused tremendous loss to life and trade and commerce. It has created an unprecedented spectre of fear and skepticism in the normal pace of life and thinking of whole generation. Still the human civilization runs higher hazards and risk of catastrophic proportion from our accelerating technological prowess to produce and amass sophisticated weapons of mass destruction. The cooperative arms control architecture which were playing decisive role in managing the insecurity and avoiding miscalculations are crumbling fast leaving the world to a dangerous syndrome catastrophic suspicion and arms race. Security dilemmas are aggravated by new disruptive technology of competitive weapon industries. The security concerns of the nation, therefore, cannot be ensured merely by principle of 'deterrence' in such emerging scenario. The pandemic has generated intense inward nationalistic tendencies across the world. These propensities have produced fast-paced geopolitical competition as well pushing the world towards a dangerous edge (Petricek, 2020). Hence there is an increasing need for stronger common platform and institutions with set of rules and regulation to manage this dangerous pattern through the pandemic into the post-pandemic world of peace, security and shared prosperity.

Given the possibility of the New START lapsing owing to the ongoing suspicion and skepticism of Russia and USA, the last President of the erstwhile USSR, Mikhail Gorbachev urged the US president and Russia to consider seriously and renew the treaty for the better security of the world. Regarding insisting others to join, mainly China, the leader remarked that it appears difficult at the moment. If Russia and US take it on, others can be made to join later on (Gorbachev, 2021). Thus a major multilateral Arms control mechanism can be sustained and the world can be saved from intensified spectre of nuclear arms race and its attendant impending catastrophic consequences.

The spectre of violence and destruction of men and materials with ever increasing production of weapons of mass destruction and their unprecedented sophistication is on pillaging rampage to disrupt structure of peace and stability. The UN Secretary General stressed the need to prepare the future generation to face the global challenges with appropriate structure of multilateralism and multilateral cooperation. The nuclear race and chemical weapons production have made it more important than ever to build robust multilateral mechanism to strengthen the system of international peace and security (Secretary-General, 2016, November 22).

The technological advances have enhanced the lethality of the weapons beyond imagination. The cooperation among nations is a necessary step to arrest expansion of these weapon which has the potential to destroy the planet and the human civilization altogether. The former Soviet leader once again reiterated the need to renew the New START hours before Joe Biden was about to enter the White House (Al Arabia, 2021). The stalled talk needed to be resumed so that the treaty acquires the true spirit of multilateral cooperation and other parties like China can join at later stage. The issue is the concern of whole humanity and security of the planet with sustainable cooperation and multilateral platform and mechanism. The change of US administration is also marked by the change of approach the US sees the multilateralism as part of international relations and interaction. The emphasis of the new US President on diplomacy, rebuilding alliances and reengaging the world has boosted the sagging confidence of global community in 'multilateral' institutions and practices. By signing the extension of the New START has signaled a powerful message of renewed confidence in international agreements and their enhanced role in the post-Covid-19 world. This is amply manifest when it reads that "President Biden has made clear that the New START Treaty extension is only the beginning of our efforts to address twenty-first century security challenges (State Department, 2021, February 3). The treaty extension can be utilized to persuade allies to join to deal with the catastrophic nuclear race and pursue disarmament to make the planet safer and better. The extended period will provide space to bring China into its ambit and making the agreement, true multilateral fora to overcome our common threats and shared hazards.

10.6 New Urge for Capable and Resilient Multilateralism

The pandemic has produced a strong current of nationalistic wave of concerns but this is not anti-globalization or against the interdependent world rather short-term responses to the sudden scourge of the pandemic. The process of globalization and its interdependent webs has brought numerous issues and challenges of global nature which no single sovereign entity on the planet can deal with alone. Thus, multilateralism is fundamental to the contemporary stage of human civilization for a sustainable peace and security. We are witnessing several kinds of dissatisfaction and disillusionment with the exiting multilateralism. These are manifestation of unproductive rigidities of the present multilateral system and the growing chasm between the demands of nations and the response capacity of these multilateral institutions. Thus, it has led to multitudes of bilateral engagement and regional mechanism to serve their specific interests. So, the need of the hour is to make the necessary reform and reset of the multilateral institutions which are able to reflect the contemporary demands and requirements. The past half a century has brought about profound synergies in multifarious ways. But there are still substantial different and opposing views and opinion about building multilateral institutions and framework for desirable performance and sustainable architecture catering the needs of diverse political culture and national aspirations (Kharas, 2020).

The pandemic has hit hard the very way of life and the way we earn our livelihood in our well-connected world. Trade and travel have been the yardstick of our level of development and dynamic prospect. The pandemic and its fast spread were blamed on these fundamental features of globalization. But given the history of pandemics these are largely a short term and social reflex action behavior. The pandemic has put on test the health preparedness and infrastructure of the countries and the policy vision of the governments. Thus, with the passage of time and better understanding the evolving perception are rather hinting towards more collaborative approach and stronger multilateral framework to deal with such pandemic and other common dangers (Shrestha, 2020). The multilateralism needs to address these issues and concerns keeping in mind the global goods and challenges for a sustainable future role in consonance with the national interests of the countries and the people across the board. The withdrawal of US from many multilateral institutions and forums under the President Donald Trump had created an atmosphere of skepticism and increasing loss of trust around the globe. When the most powerful country leaves the multilateral platform it not only causes harm to the existing state of affair rather it dents the very relevance of the idea of multilateralism and its sustainability. But President Biden has infused a new hope with his remarks in his inaugural address. In his message to the world, he said that "we will repair our alliances and engage with the world once again. We will be a strong and trusted partner for peace, progress and security (White House, 2021a, January 20).

10.7 Health Security and Multilateralism

The pandemic has produced a deeper sense among the people and leadership in the world about need of Multilateralism and sustained efforts to buttress their performance as an effective means to fight the health hazards and keep the world healthier and safer. The letter of President Biden to UN expressing US intention to remain member of WHO with clear words of appreciation of the organization and its fights against the pandemic is the telling testimony of renewed global understanding and recognition of the power of multilateral institutions to deal with crisis of such unprecedented global scale. The return of US with assurances will surely spur the pursuit of global health and health security (White House, 2021b, January 20). UN Secretary General welcomed the US rejoining with the statement that the step is absolutely critical to support the organization for coordinated fight against the COVID-19. He added "Now is the time for and for the international community to work together in solidarity to stop this virus and its shattering consequences" (United Nations, 2021a, January 20). The presence of United States and its support will give momentum to the efforts to ensure equitable access to vaccine across the world.

There was a positive development China allowed WHO team to investigate into the virus origin in Wuhan. Last week a WHO team has visited Wuhan and the Wuhan market as well as the Wuhan medical laboratory which has been the centre of the Covid-19 virus. In a virtual meeting for the World Economic Forum, the Chinese President has called on the governments world to cooperate in the fight against the pandemic and work for the early repair of the pandemic-damaged world economy. At this juncture, these appear to be a positive measure towards the new post-pandemic architecture of multilateralism. The UN Secretary-General, Mr Antonio Guterres has reiterated the points before that "COVID-19 is not only a wake-up call; it is a dress rehearsal for the world of challenges to come. The pandemic has taught us that our choices matter. As we look to the future, let us make sure we choose wisely" (UNGA, 2020, September 22). The choice referred was building a robust structure and network of multilateralism keeping an eye on the impending future pandemic and crisis.

10.8 Climate Change and Need of Multilateral Response

Climate is the most important global common. The climate change and its implications cannot be limited within the national boundaries. Given the scope and extent of the challenge of the climate change only a practice and process of multilateralism can lead us to the desired path to face it and overcome it before it goes to the state of beyond repair. A multilateral international climate regime is the necessary option and its relevance and centrality cannot be reduced by the pandemic underway. Rather, the common vulnerability of the pandemic has underlined the need of a common mechanism to deal such challenge to such global common as climate. The Paris Agreement 2015 has been significant international action and multilateral process of cooperation in this regard (Biniaz, 2020). The issue of 'multilateralism' and its relevance for dealing with contemporary challenges and crisis also found ample echo in US Presidential election and its campaign. Throughout his campaign candidate Joe Biden put it emphatically that if elected he will bring the United States back into multilateral institution the Trump administration had left, the important ones being the Paris Climate Agreement and the World Health Organization. This symbolizes, in the thick of the pandemic that the climate is changing so far as the 'multilateralism' and its continued importance as global mechanism and process in the post-Covid-19 world (Akbaruddin, 2020). The victory of Joe Biden in November, 2020 has thus produced strengthening ripples of support and re-emergence of 'multilateralism' as a driving tool for international relations. The re-engagement of US as a strongest nation surely infuses enthusiasm, requisite support from others and necessary direction. Thus, the change of guard in the United States with declared commitment is a profound endorsement of the 'multilateralism.

The US election campaign was full of talk of diplomacy, rebuilding alliances and reengaging the world with responsibility created a renewed sense of enthusiasm to 'multilateralism' which was in a state of demoralization. On the day inauguration, the new President sent a letter of acceptance to the Paris Climate Agreement on behalf of the United States of America (White House, 2021c, January 20). The moment has heralded a new journey of 'multilateralism' as a well-considered strategy to meet the global challenges with renewed commitment of the most powerful nation. It has generated a new energy of policy-pursuance towards multilateralism as an international process for shared strategy for global common and shared challenges. The potential outcome of this US decision is evidenced by the warm welcome by the UN Secretary General to the ambitious strategy and action to confront and overcome the climate crisis which entails disastrous impending implications for the planet and the very survival of the human existence (United Nations, 2021b, January 20). The US leadership with commitments will take the Agreement to achieve its 2030 targets and the world can breathe healthy to direction of development with assured sustainability.

The new Secretary of State, Antony J Blinken, talked to his counterparts of France, Germany and United Kingdom and exchanged views on several pressing issues of global importance, strategy to deal with them. They all expressed their willing cooperation and affirmed the centrality of transatlantic relationship in dealing with such global challenges as security, climate and health and other challenges. The secretary underscored the US commitment to all efforts of coordinated action to overcome the challenges (State Department, 2021, February 5). These are sure patterns of renewed commitments and endorsements of the idea and practice of 'multilateralism. These are profound evidence of multilateral approach and its unbending relevance which are not bound by the exigencies of the pandemic.

The COVID-19 has brought tremendous strain on the governments around the world. The initial responses of the governments to safeguard its citizenry led to closing of borders and restrictions on travel as an immediate measure to stem the spread of the virus and its debilitating consequences. This led to growing perceptions that nations are turning inward and their trust in the multilateral institutions are on the sharp wane. But soon this perception is in clear retreat as the world has been in sincere contemplation and realization that no country alone can deal with this niggardly and menacing virus. The mettle of the multilateral strategy and institutions became clear when the new US Secretary of State said that 'Domestic policy is Foreign Policy' and vice versa. Because our strength at home determines our strength in the world and our policies and performance in the world determines our safety and security at home. He further added that "At this moment of unprecedented global challenge it's more important than ever that US show up and lead, we need diplomacy to get the pandemic under control worldwide" (State Department, 2021, February 4). These are powerful endorsement of multilateralism and indication of its accelerating march ahead in the post-pandemic world.

10.9 Geopolitical Competition: Multilateralism

Multilateralism has been envisioned and designed based on shared principles of conduct for nations in pursuit of avoiding dangerous reciprocity and escalation of tension and crisis as well as to promote cooperative behaviour and coordinated action for shared benefits and protection of global common. The post-World War II period witnessed considerable progress in the rise and growth of multilateral concepts, institutions and their spread in the different sphere of life and pursuits of nations. However, the multilateral architecture grew into a confusing network of numerous frameworks in different arenas-development, health, environment, international security and socio-political demands like human rights. There was significant momentum in the multilateral system with participation of government, civil society bodies and non-governmental organization (Eggel, 2020).

However, the multilateral frameworks and architecture could not transcend the Great power interests and their pursuits. The major powers used the institutions for their own agendas behind the high value goals of these frameworks. As a result, multilateralism could not develop collective decision-making capacity in consonance with the changing magnitude of global common demands and shared responsibility. Finally, the first two decades have witnessed fast decline in the normative content of the multilateral structures marred by intensifying geopolitical competition, protectionist policies, unilateral military action and sanctions. The unilateralism has become a common practice mainly by the powerful countries. It seems that very foundation and capacity of the multilateralism is in shambles. The pandemic in its initial impacts seems to have accelerated the syndrome. But slowly the pandemic and its challenges is generating a new sense cooperation building into revised form and framework of multilateralism which now appears to far more salient than before. The UN General Assembly president put it emphatically that United Nations has become more important in the face of the COVID-19 pandemic. It appears to have become more crucial as a multilateral platform to international peace and security. But it must respond to the changing realities in its intent and structure. There is a corresponding need to reform the UN Security Council and its functioning to reflect the twenty-first century realities. "The implementation of the Council's decisions and its very legitimacy could be enhanced if the Council was reformed to be more representative, effective, efficient, accountable and transparent," he said (United Nations, 2021, January 26).

The special session of the United Nation General Assembly was dedicated to the Covid-19 crisis. All the delegates expressed their solidarity and stressed the need for multi-lateral approach to mitigate the impact of the pandemic world-wide and ensure equitable distribution of vaccine all across the nations (UNGA, 2020, December 14). There was an identical expression by the majority of the delegates that given the nature of the pandemic and its spread across the boundaries of the nations, there must be a coordinated multilateral action to ensure that every country get access to the vaccines. There was call for non-partisan approach without any political and financial considerations so that pandemic can be arrested and overcome at the earliest and a normal process can be resumed soon benefitting one and all. Such an expression for collective initiative and action is a strong sign of resurgence of trust in multilateralism and its reliability as a future of international relations and cooperation.

In the recent years, Joint Comprehensive Plan of Action (JCPOA) or the Iran Nuclear Deal has been an important success of multilateral diplomacy and mechanism. The withdrawal of the US from the Deal has weakened the intended process and the prospect of attaining the goal. European Union is at work to stich back the differences between Iran and US and its allies in the region. The diplomatic engagements have gained steam with the change of US administration as the new president has repeatedly talk about return to the deal as better option to ensure peace and better chance of containing Iranian nuclear ambition. The diplomatic engagement in this multilateral framework has the potential to reach to an amicable solutions and tension can be reduced substantially in this crisis-ridden region. Besides it will embolden the diplomacy and enhance trust in the multilateralism as mechanism to deal with contemporary challenges for promoting and ensuring security and making and building peace (Agence France Presse, 2021).

In his address to the General Assembly, United Nations, the Secretary General remarked that "the pandemic is the human tragedy- but it can also be an opportunity. I our interconnected world, we need a networked multilateralism so that the global and regional organizations communicate and work towards common goal. We must transform our global system into a global partnership. At the international level I have called for a new global deal. Together, I am confident that we can emerge from Covid-19 and lay the foundation for a cleaner, safer and fairer world for all and for generations to come" (UNGA, 2021, January 10). These are the powerful expression for a better and stronger multilateral architecture and structure to deal with the COVID-19 pandemic and prepare the world for future global threats in front of the world leaders. Therefore, the dominant sentiment remains in favour of multilateralism and the pandemic rather spurred the sense of urgency.

The 75th General Assembly focussed its main session on "The future we want; the United Nations we need: Reaffirming our collective commitment to multilateralism- Confronting Covid-19 through effective multilateral action." The Declaration stressed: "we have the tools and now we have to use them. Urgent efforts are required. Therefore, we are not here to celebrate. We are here to take action" (UNGA, 2021, January 5). The pandemic has caused many-sided havoc but the crisis has pushed the world to a new level of realisation and a very strong sense of commitment towards multilateralism and its role in the face of unprecedented nature and content of such crisis as the COVID-19 underway.

10.10 Challenges Ahead

The assumption behind the multilateralism has been that peace and prosperity goes hand in hand. The shared purpose would hold the members and the increasing economic engagement would produce shared prosperity and shared stakes. This in turn would usher in peace and stability. But practically all the multilateral forums and institution fail to qualify by these assumptions and has been marred by national interests of powerful countries, the Great powers. No multilateral institution could grow into a genuine forum with the underlying idea of well-being for all and shared peace and prosperity. The Secretary-General, United Nations has already reminded about challenges and required actions in the very beginning of 2020 when he said in his remark that we achieved tremendous strength together, "Yet anniversaries are not about celebrating the past; they are about looking ahead. We must cast our eyes to the future with hope" (UNGA, 2020, January 22). Then he enumerated the challenges and how to grapple with these with the strength of togetherness.

The onset of COVID-19 with its devastating global spread has imposed unexpected number of loads on the existing multilateral structures and therefore caught unprepared. The World Health Organization faced the blistering strain and attack with the pandemic enveloping the globe fast. Like all other multilateral organization, it was also suffering from same malaise- absence of requisite cooperative members, transparency, negotiation capacity and hold on members to carry out its instruction in a time-bound manner, the essential ingredients felt with the pandemic. Its weaknesses on these counts dented its credibility further and all other existing structures.

Nevertheless, the pandemic has not only exposed weakness of our multilateral architecture, it has also produced a new urgency in the global community to create credible network of multilateralism with requisite capacity, resources and support structure and spirit to render the desired services in a fair manner. The President of the UN General Assembly remarked that, "Not only do we need a multilateral system, we need a system that is relevant for our increasingly globalized and interconnected world: a system that is flexible and able to adapt quick to react to multiple challenges at the same time, to be responsive to the needs of people everywhere, ensuring that none are left behind" (UNGA, 2020, December 10). There is an urgent introspection to make necessary reform and restructuring of institutions and process of multilateralism based on new vision of shared responsibility and shared security and prosperity. Following are few potential ways and means to redesign and rebuild new network of robust system and structure of multilateralism.

First, an informed cooperation and commitment is the foremost requirement and challenge. The withdrawal of the US from various crucial multilateral forums had been a very negative impact on the idea and goals of multilateralism. The return of US to WHO and Paris Agreement has instilled the multilateral zeal at an appropriate time.

Second, Great Power Competition has been a constant factor of weakness and failure of the multilateral movement and institutions. Biden administration's emphasis on 'diplomacy' and rebuilding alliances is boding well for calming geopolitical rivalry and tension is the much-desired course for stronger foundation multilateralism.

Third, building capacity of the new and revised multilateral structure is another urgent need which requires greater willingness of nations to share responsibility and commitments. This can be attained only by making the institutions representative in content and reflective of the share goal of the members.

Fourth, necessary reform of the existing structure reflecting the contemporary realities of the world and shared responsibility.

Fifth, the rules and regulation must be qualified by fair play and transparency in consonance with goals and its values.

10.11 Conclusion

Multilateralism is not merely for confronting the common threats, rather an unavoidable path for a shared peace and progress of humanity. The pandemic is a reminder of this shared opportunity to mobilise the common pool of human intelligence and attainments to build sustainable economies and inclusive societies. The COVID-19 has forced an unprecedented coordination of different stakeholders, communities, government, business and scientific community and their research. The shared vulnerability of the pandemic has activated inclusive responses and can be utilized for building capacities for shaping an inclusive and sustainable global society and order. There are numerous challenges on the way. The COVID-19 has dented heavily our contemporary global structure, exacerbated the geopolitical trends, sharpened the rise in nationalism and protectionism even the great power competition making effort difficult to resuscitate the already multilateral structure and spirit. But the extent and spread of the vulnerability the pandemic has thrown up make the multilateral frameworks more relevant as a source of assured safety against such crisis in the future. Thus, it can be said that the COVID-19, irrespective of its devastating impacts has raised the importance of the multilateral processes and actions which can be understood with the growing cooperation in sharing of pandemic information, the ongoing researches, and vaccine development. There is a strong momentum for value-based cooperation and global civics. Sustainable Development Goals (SDGs) and Agenda 2030 have substantial component of value-based cooperation. The pragmatic treaties and agreements with equitable responsibility and burden sharing can ensure the desired momentum to multilateral process. The US-China rivalry and competition is again dragging the world towards bipolar division. There is an important opportunity for countries like India to take an increasing role and responsibility at the global stage. This will arrest the bipolar syndrome and produce a multi-polar global landscape, a better stage for multilateral cooperation with resilient institutions. The prediction of future virulent pandemic X is making the multilateralism increasingly integral to the future course of health security and economic stability. In brief, multilateralism is no more an option but an inseparable part of an assured path of life and progress.

References

Agence France Presse (AFP). (2021, February). EU Working 'Extremely Hard' To Revive Iran Deal. *Agence France Presse*. https://www.barrons.com/news/eu-working-extremely-hard-to-rev ive-iran-deal-01612278005?tesla=y

Akbaruddin, S. (2020, November 16). For multilateralism, a change in climate. *Hindustan Times*. https://www.hindustantimes.com/analysis/for-multilateralism-a-change-in-climate/story-ZeENji3KRR2KSzJSoIB6rJ_amp.html

Al Arabia. (2021, January 20). Mikhail Gorbachev calls on Russia and US to mend ties under Biden. *Al Arabiya*. https://english.alarabiya.net/News/world/2021/01/20/US-foreign-policy-Mik hail-Gorbachev-calls-on-Russia-and-US-to-mend-ties-under-Biden

Biniaz, S. (2020, September 30). *Multilateralim*, the Climate Challenge, and the (Greater Metropolitan) Paris Agreement, Wilson Center. https://www.wilsoncenter.org/article/multilate ralism-climate-challenge-and-greater-metropolitan-paris-agreement

Dervis, K. (2020, November 17). Multilateralism: What policy options to strengthen international cooperation. *Brookings*. https://www.brookings.edu/research/multilateralism-what-policy-options-to-strengthen-international-cooperation/

Dollar, D. (2020, November 17). The Future of Global Supply Chains: What are the implications for international trade. *Brookings*. https://www.brookings.edu/research/the-future-of-global-sup ply-chains-what-are-the-implications-for-international-trade/

Eggel, D. (2020, April). Multilateralism Is in crisis-or is it? *Global Challenges*. https://globalchalle nges.ch/issue/7/multilaterism-is-in-crisis-or-is-it/

Gorbachev, M. (2021, January 11). Gorbachev Expects Biden to Extend US-Russia Arms Curbs. *The Moscow Times*. https://www.themoscowtimes.com/2021/01/11/gorbachev-expects-biden-to-extend-us-russia-arms-curbs-a72575

Kharas, H., Snower, D. J., & Strauss, S. (2020). The Future of multilateralism, Global Solution Initiative, *Global Solutions*, The World Policy Forum. https://www.global-solutions-initiative. org/press-news/the-future-of-multilateralism/

Langenhove, L. V. (2011, May 31). *Multilateralism 2.0: The Transformation of international relations*. United Nations University. https://unu.edu/publications/articles/multilateralism-2-0-the-tra nsformation-of-international-relations.html

Petricek, T. (2020, June 19). Strengthening Arms Control Through Multilateralism Through Arms Control, Commentary, *UK Integrated Review*, United States, Russia, proliferation and Nuclear Policy, RUSI. https://rusi.org/commentary/Strengthening_Arms_Control_Through_Mul tilateralism

Secretary-General. (2016, November 22). *Secretary-General's remarks on "Future of Multilateral Disarmament" at New York University*, United Nations Secretary-General. https://www.un.org/ sg/en/content/sg/statement/2016-11-22/secretary-generals-remarks-future-multilateral-disarm ament-new-york

Shrestha, N., Yousaf, M., Ulvi, O., Hossain, M., Wardrup, R., Aghamohammadi, N., ... & Haque, U. (2020, December 20). The impact of COVID-19 on Globalization. *One Health* (Vol. 11). https:// www.sciencedirect.com/science/article/pii/S2352771420302810

State Department. (2021, February 3). Blinken, Antony J. (2021). *On Extension of, the New START Treaty with the Russian Federation*, Press Statement, State Department, United States. https:// www.state.gov/on-the-extension-of-the-new-start-treaty-with-the-russian-federation/

State Department. (2021, February 4). *Secretary Antony J. Blinken Introductory Remarks for President Biden—United States Department of States*. https://www.state.gov/secretary-antony-j-bli nken-introductory-remarks-for-president-biden/

State Department. (2021, February 5). *Secretary Blinken's Call with French Foreign Minister Le Drian, German Foreign Minister Mass, and UK Foreign Secretary Raab*, Readout, United States department of State. https://www.state.gov/secretary-blinkens-call-with-french-foreign-minister-ledrian-german-foreign-minister-maas-and-uk-foreign-secretary-raab/

United Nations. (2020, April 24). *The Virtues of Multilateralism and Diplomacy*, International Day of Multilateralism and Diplomacy for Peace, Guterres, Antonio United Nations. https://www.un.org/en/observances/Multilateralism-for-Peace-day#:~:text=The%20Virtues%20of%20Multilateralism%20and%20Diplomacy&text=Preserving%20the%20values%20of%20multilaterali sm,security%2C%20development%20and%20human%20rights

Uinted Nations. (2021a, January 20). *UN Secretary General welcomes US joining back WHO, Secretary General*, Statements and Messages, SG/SM/20546. https://www.un.org/press/en/2021/sgsm20546.doc.htm

United Nations. (2021b, January 20). *Statement by the Secretary-General—On US steps to re-enter the Paris Agreement on Climate Change*. https://www.un.org/sg/en/content/sg/statement/2021-01-20/statement-the-secretary-general-%E2%80%93-us-steps-re-enter-the-paris-agreement-cli mate-change

United Nations. (2021, January 26). *Security Council reforms must reflect 21st century realities*, 75th Year UN Assembly President, UN News. https://news.un.org/en/story/2021/01/1082962

UNGA. (2020, January 22). *Secretary-General's remarks to the General Assembly on his priorities for 2020, United Nations*. https://www.un.org/sg/en/content/sg/statement/2020-01-22/secret ary-generals-remarks-the-general-assembly-his-priorities-for-2020-bilingual-delivered-scroll-down-for-all-english-version

UNGA. (2020, September 22). *Address to the Opening of the General Debate of the 75th Session of the General Assembly"*, United Nations. https://www.un.org/sg/en/content/sg/speeches/2020-09-22/address-the-opening-of-the-general-debate-of-the-75th-session-of-the-general-assembly

UNGA. (2020, December 10). *Statement by H.E. Volkan Bozkir, President of the 75th session of the United Nations General Assembly*, "The Need for Multilateralism in a changing world". https://www.un.org/pga/75/2020/12/10/the-need-for-multilateralism-in-a-changing-world/

UNGA. (2020, December 14). Thirty-First Special Session. *Cautiously Optimistic about COVID-19 Vaccine, Speakers in General Assembly Say Multilateral Approaches Key for Ensuring Unhindered, Equitable Distribution*. General Assembly, Meetings Coverage and Press Releases, United Nations. https://www.un.org/press/en/2020/ga12302.doc.htm

UNGA. (2021, January 5). *Seventy-Fifth Session Highlights "Heeding COVID-19 'Wake-Up Call', General Assembly Urges Collective Action to Tackle Global Crisis, Marks Seventy-Fifth Year of United Nations*, Meetings Coverage and Press Releases, GA/12308. https://www.un.org/press/en/2021/ga12308.doc.htm

UNGA. (2021, January 10). *Remarks at the Commemoration of the 75th Anniversary of the First Meeting of the United Nations General Assembly*, United Nation Secretary-General, UN Headquarters. https://www.un.org/sg/en/content/sg/speeches/2021-01-10/remarks-commem oration-of-75th-anniversary-of-first-meeting-of-un-general-assembly

UNCTAD. (2020, December 17). *Transforming trade, backing productive capacities is key to fixing global economy*, United Nations Conference on Trade and Development. https://unctad.org/news/transforming-trade-backing-productive-capacities-key-fixing-global-economy

White House. (2021a, January 20). *Inaugural Address by President Joseph R. Biden, Jr, Speech*, White House. https://www.whitehouse.gov/briefing-room/speeches-remarks/2021/01/20/inaugu ral-address-by-president-joseph-r-biden-jr/

White House. (2021b, January 20). *Biden letter to UN General Secretary to rejoin WHO, Letter His Excellency Antonio Guterres*, Statements and Releases, White House, United States of America. https://www.whitehouse.gov/briefing-room/statements-releases/2021/01/20/letter-his-excellency-antonio-guterres/

White House. (2021c, January 20). *Biden letter to join Paris Climate Agreement, Acceptance on behalf of the United States of America*, White house, United States of America. https://www.whi tehouse.gov/briefing-room/statements-releases/2021/01/20/paris-climate-agreement/

Khushnam P N, PhD is an Independent IR and Regional Security Researcher & Analyst at Bangaluru, India. His research interest includes Iran, US & Gulf Security.

Chapter 11
COVID-19 and Its Impact on Culture: The Experience of Nepal

Shree Prasad Devkota and Laxmi Paudyal

Abstract With the subsequent rise of the COVID-19 cases worldwide and the declaration of Public Health Emergency of International Concern (PHIEC) by WHO, every country has realized increase public health concerns. The uncertainty of the availability of the vaccine to every people again leads to a panic situation among the public. Different non-pharmaceutical preventive techniques are adopted by most countries, including nationwide complete and partial lockdown, physical distancing, and giving awareness and encouraging people to practice hygienic measures such as wearing a protective mask, frequent hand washing, using alcohol-based hand sanitizer, etc. Nepal government has adopted a complete nationwide lockdown for almost six months with shut down of all cinema halls, gyms, health clubs, and museums as well as banned the gathering of people for cultural, social, and religious activities including temples, monasteries, churches, and mosques and partial lockdown for next two months. Still, yet many of the public places are not open. Although these measures have been taken to prevent this contagious disease, the fear, anxiety, panic situation, and uncertainty created in the people are in ruins. The psychological and socio-cultural effects of the illness and its mitigation measures are significantly higher than the actual physical health effect due to COVID-19, which are in the shadow and not noticed. Moreover, the indirect impact on the economy, social harmony, religious and cultural beliefs, and processes, and others so many sectors are beyond the fact seen on the face of this pandemic.

Keywords Psychological · Socio-cultural · Religious · Culture · Social harmony

---

S. P. Devkota (✉)
Tribhuvan University, Kathmandu, Nepal
e-mail: spdevkota@kusoed.edu.np

L. Paudyal
Gandaki Medical College Teaching Hospital and Research Center, Pokhara, Nepal

© The Author(s), under exclusive license to Springer Nature Singapore Pte Ltd. 2022
S. Roy and D. Nandy (eds.), *Understanding Post-COVID-19 Social and Cultural Realities*, https://doi.org/10.1007/978-981-19-0809-5_11

11.1 Methodology

The descriptive study was carried out to explore the unseen impacts of COVID-19 on culture. The objective of the study was to identify the direct and indirect impact of COVID-19 on different aspect of culture and its process. Different published articles were reviewed systematically and published data were used as reference. Various research were conducted concerning the direct physical effect from the COVID-19 but present study light to focus on the hidden impact of COVID-19 on culture which is un noticed but is major area of concern for today's scenario.

11.2 Introduction

A new genus of Coronavirus, named Severe Acute Respiratory Coronavirus 2 (SARS-Cov-2), was first identified in Wuhan one of the cities of China at the end of December 2019. Thus, this contagious respiratory illness was named Coronavirus disease 19 or COVID-19 (Zhu et al., 2020). This disease is so infectious that within two months of the outbreak, cases of COVID-19 are found across most of the countries of Europe, the USA, Australia, Asia, and Africa, affecting 213 countries around the globe. In Nepal, the first confirmed case was a 31-year-old Nepali student of Wuhan University who had returned home on January 5th from China. He was confirmed positive for COVID-19 on January 23rd, and it was the first-ever reported case in South Asia (NDTV, 2020). With the World Health Organization (WHO) declaration of Public Health Emergency of International Concern (PHIEC) for the 6th time on January 30th, the various countries have adopted non-pharmaceutical mitigation measures such as physical distancing, lockdown, safety precautions, etc. Hence country lockdown is considered an effective measure in slowing the spread of this virus; many countries imposed various degrees of lockdown to stop the spread of the virus. Nepal imposed a complete nationwide lockdown from March 24th, 2020, to June 10th, 2020 (Poudel & Subedi 2020).

The COVID-19 response has generally been based on physical detachment, albeit this has unfortunately been referred to as social distancing in formal and informal language. However, there are notable similarities between the two conceptions, with physical distances not always implying social connectedness, whereas social distancing invariably means disconnectivity. The problems of social and economic inequalities are amplifying the challenge of managing the spread of COVID-19 globally. Yet, arguably one of the pandemic's primary ironies is that, in the face of physical separation and interruption to regular service delivery systems, solidarity, both local and international, has risen to the forefront of our coordinated responses (UNESCO, 2020a). The pandemic has made physical distancing a catchphrase and an essential ingredient to deal with it. Indeed, social distancing, though, does not mean keeping away from social connections and bonding. It instead means physical distancing to limit the transmission of the virus in social interactions (Kafle, 2020). The COVID-19 pandemic, on the other hand, emerges as a stressful, even painful event that demands people to make sense of their new position and develop suitable coping strategies (Guan et al., 2020).

Aside from the economic impact, the social implications for countries like Nepal, which can be foreseen given its variety and history of armed conflict and disaster, can be widespread, long-lasting, and devasting. Many cultural events were canceled, cultural institutions were closed, community cultural practices were ceased, the risk of plundering cultural sites and poaching and looting in natural areas increased, artists could not make ends meet, and the cultural tourism sector was seriously hit. Since then, the COVID-19 has influenced the cultural industry, affecting the fundamental right to culture, the social rights of artists and creative workers, and the protection of a diverse range of artistic manifestations. Civil society organizations, particularly sector-specific associations (such as music or cinema), professional networks, or city-based organizations, began analyzing the impact within days of the lockdown. According to one survey, cultural items are at the top of the list of critical activities for French internet users during this time of confinement.

The most important cultural challenges presented at the national level are the loss of tourism earnings, the social security of artists and cultural professionals, art and culture in detention, and guaranteeing culturally appropriate pandemic awareness (UNESCO, 2020b). Some of the impacts of COVID-19 concerning culture, cultural practices, cultural heritages, and ultimately to society are as follows.

11.3 Religious Hit by COVID-19

Simply religion is a specific fundamental set of beliefs and practices generally agreed upon by several persons. People have their shared ideas, values, and opinions, and their faith and trust with their religion and religion give way to the people to deal with ultimate concerns about their lives and fate after death. COVID-19 and its mitigation measures had affected religious practice and beliefs in several ways.

11.3.1 People Struggling to Find Faith and Internal Peace

With the implementation of lockdown and closure of all holy places to maintain physical distance between people, the entry of devotees to different pilgrimages was restricted. Due to that, the people get challenging to find faith in their god, and the internal peace them get disturbed. Entry of devotees to the Pashupatinath temple, which has continued regularly since ancient times, was prohibited during this pandemic. People visiting temples, churches, and the mosque are for their religious belief and internal comfort and peace. Many people find confidence and get strong faith in visiting those holy places, but they get suffered due to the pandemic and its mitigation measure. Due to closure of the temple many people have lost their one of the palliative measure as well as Pashupati Area Development Trust (PADT) has suffered losses around 5000–6000 devotees who visited the temple premise daily especially during the month of Shrawan, Teej and other festival and around 700 million income from the devotees (The Himalayan Times, 2021).

11.3.2 Affected religious tourism

The COVID-19 pandemic has impacted religion in various ways, including the cancellation of the worship services of different faiths and the closure and cancellation of all pilgrimages in temples, churches, mosques, and revocation and restriction to ceremonies and festivals. Nepal is also regarded as a religious tourist destination and adventure, culture, and nature. Nepal was enjoying the Nepal 2020 campaign as the year 2020 approached. Still, due to the Coronavirus pandemic, the religious tourism sector of the country has been adversely affected. Various religious institutions, as well as the government and commercial sector, were planning for significant festivities. Generally, Hindu and Buddhist tourists travel to Nepal for pilgrimage, but due to this pandemic country had lost millions of religious tourists and billions of rupees income from them, as stated by Achyut Guragain, President of Nepal Association of Tour and Travel agents (*Nepali Times*, 2020).

11.3.3 Shaken Religious Cohesion

The country was put under lockdown as the virus spread (in March), and the government tested 75 persons for COVID-19. Because some of them are Muslims, the religious minority has been singled out for contact tracing, particularly in the places where the cases were discovered in Nepal. During that time, it was the festive time of Ramadan, which has always meant a time of joyous celebration with friends and family. Still, this year there was anxiety and fear among Nepali Muslims because of worries that they will be blamed for the virus. In Nepal, however, Muslims are in the minority. They have happily coexisted for generations, but there is fear for the future as xenophobia and intolerance expand across the border due to this circumstance. With the different Indian News media spreading rumors and at the same time, 11 out of 13 Tablighi Jamaat who are Indian and had come for religious instructions living in a mosque of Udayapur district of Nepal tested positive for COVID-19, the fear and anxiety among other people becomes exacerbated. With that, the Muslim people find themselves bearing stigma from other religious groups (*Nepali Times*, 2020). The news media sensationalized a report alleging that certain religious groups were trying to spread the Coronavirus throughout the community. It was soon reinforced by hundreds of thousands of social media messages, inciting religious violence. Although the news report was finally found fake, the very fabric of social cohesion was shaken.

The epidemic can worsen existing inequity and spark conflict, particularly in areas where specific communities and groups are stigmatized and discriminated against. While Nepali society is generally considered accepting of religious variety, religious disputes have occasionally turned violent in the past. These crises and disasters fuel existing frustrations created from unequal access and opportunities among different personnel and religious groups. This puts some communities and groups at risk of discrimination. This leads to a lack of knowledge and regard for one another's cultures, religions, lifestyles, and worldviews. (Kafle, 2020).

11.3.4 Economic Loss

The devotee's faith and trust towards religion are affected due to this pandemic. Still, the economic gain and donation by the devotees to different temples and other holy places have been lost. As per the figure released by PADT, Pashupatinath temple, which stands as the highest-earning temple in the nation, has lost around half a million rupees as offering to Lord Shiva from the devotees daily due to lockdown. Apart from the offering to Lord Shiva, tourists entrance fee of Nepali rupees 3 to 4 lakh which use to contribute 10 million rupees in a month to the fund of PADT. Again, special puja arranged for devotees on specific days of a week used to stand at around Nepali 7 million a month. This suggests that around 700 million lost was figured during this lockdown and closure of the Pashupatinath temple. These losses cause vital conservation and restoration work to those sites to withhold or cancel, adversely affecting the preservation of such cultural and religious properties.

11.4 Impact on Tourism

The outbreak of the COVID-19 pandemic has brought uncertainty and spillover impact on almost all the sectors, but its enduring crisis on global tourism is a burning issue. The travel restrictions to and from different international destinations were put into action to prevent the spread of COVID-19 infection, which massively affected the tourism sector. According to the United Nations World Tourism Organization (UNWTO), 96% of all global locations have imposed total or partial restrictions, with some countries continuing to do so. In some parts of the world, the role of culture for identity building, social cohesion, dialogue, and reconciliation is paramount, while its economic contribution may be underestimated. Yet, cultural heritage and tourism and the cultural and creative industries represent a large portion of the cultural sector. Again, culture plays a vital role as 1 in 3 tourists cite culture as a reason for choosing their destination. The tourism industry is gigantic, global business accounting for 10.4% of GDP, 10% global employment, and contributes $225 BN to the global economy (UNESCO, 2020i).

11.4.1 Great Economic Recession

For some countries, tourism and related sectors are equivalent to up to 70% of the national economy. According to preliminary OECD estimates, each government expects a 2% drop in GDP for each month of confinement with a 50–70% drop in tourist flows for 2020. Nepal is the fifth most remittances dependant country, sends millions of labor migrants abroad every year for international labors. While remittances range up to 25% of the GDP, migrant remittances may decline during this pandemic, limiting the income of households in Nepal, which cause the families too hard to get out of poverty, paying off unscrupulous loans, and investment in education, health, and land. Similarly, Nepal has also been affected adversely by the pandemic, and its preliminary impact recorded a 14.37% loss to the Nepalese economy as a repercussion of travel restrictions and flight cancellations (Shrestha, 2020). Nepal's tourism industry generated NRs. 240.7 billion in 2018 that stood at 7.9% GDP (Prasain, 2019). Millions of people who are directly employed in hotels, restaurants, trekking, mountaineering, airlines, and other tourism subsectors in Nepal are significantly affected by the pandemic. This is not the first crisis that Nepal's tourism industry has experienced at this level. The sector was hard-hit by catastrophic earthquake & trade disruptions along the southern border in 2015, which had resulted in a 33% tourism decline. Now it is a COVID-19 pandemic. According to Nepal Tourism Statistics (2019), there are 1254 registered hotels (star and tourist standard categories), 29 international airlines that fly to Nepal, 20 domestic airlines, and 2649 registered trekking agencies and various subsectors that are struggling to stay afloat. There is an estimated loss of 10 billion Nepali Rupees (83 million U.S. dollars) each month during the lockdown (Xinhua, 2020). Compared to the previous year, 2019, the declining rate of the tourist was 1.96% in January, 1.00% in February, and 73.26% in March. This is a precipitous drop of more than 99.9% in tourist numbers compared to the same month in 2019, as there were 70,000 arrivals (Ulak, 2020a).

Tourism is a seasonal industry, April–March is the highest tourist season of Nepal, but the industry has gone into a coma because of COVID-19. The significant effect of this situation is devasting, and it requires a long time to cure. Nepal's tourist sector has been consistently rising, adding NRs.45.7 billion to the country's GDP, according to the Travel and Tourism Economic Impact (2019) research. The international recession again will hit the country very hard as the country is highly dependent on remittance (Ulak, 2020b).

11.4.2 Job Loss

By 2020, the travel and tourism industry might lose up to 75 million jobs, resulting in a $2.1 trillion loss in GDP, according to the World Travel and Tourism Council. This is equivalent to an astounding 1 million jobs being lost every day in travel and tourism, which is an area of concern and worry for many countries. It has a spillover impact on almost every sector. Postponing of visit Nepal 2020 and suspension of on-arrival visas, and the countrywide lockdown have led to a loss of thousands of jobs. In all, 20,000 tours trek and guides, and porters lost their livelihood when mountaineering was suspended (The Kathmandu Post, 2020). People, who rely on tourism, both directly and indirectly, are hurting. Nepal's tourism industry also represents small operators, souvenir shops, ground handlers like tourist bus and car services, drivers, and others dependent on tourism are severely affected. Around 10,000 were collapsed in Nepal as they have had to survive through a daily transaction. Still, because of no prospect of tourist arrivals, they cannot pay even monthly rent to their landlords.

11.4.3 Impact Intercultural Exchange

Travel, once again, facilitates international communication and leads to a better understanding of our standard human narrative. Given the global scope of the COVID-19 epidemic, it is becoming increasingly clear that no single country can effectively combat its effects on its own. International cooperation is critical in UNESCO's mission as an UN-mandated organization for culture, and on April 22nd, nearly 130 ministers met in Paris to discuss strategies to preserve the cultural sector. To enhance and unite their efforts, they reiterated their commitment to intergovernmental discussion and worldwide solidarity (UNESCO, 2020d). It is known that Nepal is a landlocked country and largely depends on India and China for its trade. But as mitigation measures to stop the spread of this virus, Nepal Government has closed the border of China on January 28th and the edge of India on March 22nd (*The Economic Times*, 2020). This closure leads to limited availability of materials used to come from China and India, which causes severe effects in importing and exporting goods. The WHO is encouraging people to use safety behaviors such as frequent washing hands with soap and water, using alcohol-based hand sanitizers, and proper usage of facial masks for protecting spreading of the Coronavirus ignited panic-buying and hoarding of these goods leading to shortages in the majority of cities in Nepal leading to mental stress among health care workers, hygienic staff and the public (The Kathmandu Post, 2020).

11.5 Closed World Heritage Sites

Social distancing measures the hardest hit the venue-based sectors (such as museums, performing arts, live music, festivals, cinema, etc.). World Heritage Sites are a source of cultural and natural diversity with cultural, historical, scientific, or other significance. The sites are judged to contain cultural and natural heritage worldwide, considered outstanding value to humanity. These sites are more importantly cared for and protected to preserve the cultural diversities for future generations, and they also serve as the learning place. But due to the current pandemic and its mitigation measures, about 89% of countries worldwide have closed or partially closed their world heritage sites to the public. This leads to an abrupt drop in revenues, puts their financial sustainability at risk, and has resulted in reduced wage earnings and lay-offs with repercussions for the value chain of their suppliers, from creative and non-creative sectors alike. As experienced in several countries, reduced security due to its closure had elevated the risk of theft of artifacts in cultural sites and illegal activities in natural heritage areas (UNESCO, 2020e).

11.5.1 Permanent Closure of Some Museums

Museums play a fundamental role in societies' resilience; again, museums have played an integral role in preserving the history of our organization. It exhibits the stories about how our nation, our communities, and our cultures came to be, and without them, those stories could be forgotten. Hence, since 2012 UNESCO had pointed out that the number of museums globally should be increased by almost 60%, demonstrating how important they have become in national cultural policies over the past decade. But now, already existing museums face difficulty sustaining and continuing due to this pandemic and lockdown. According to the International Council on Museums (ICOM), 95% of the estimated 60,000 museums worldwide have closed due to the pandemic, with some (13%) closing permanently due to the significant financial losses sustained during this time(UNESCO, 2020e).

11.5.2 Increased Risk of Animal Poaching

During the lockdown, poaching was at an all-time high in numerous countries. There has been an increase in the risk of poaching at other natural areas, including world heritage holdings, partly due to the reduced presence of tourists and employees in the park. Images of smog-free skies and films of tigers and deer strolling over fairways may easily lead us to assume that nature is prospering amid the pandemic; so, while lockdown may be good news for some species, the situation is far worse for many others. It provides optimal living space because there is less traffic on the roads and fewer people in wealthy countries' cities. However, neither the wildlife nor the people are in the same situation. Poaching is driving some people to extremes to support themselves. Millions of individuals have been laid off without warning, and they have nothing to fall back on. Huge urban to rural migration where people have lost their jobs in cities overnight now have to depend on poaching, logging, or other degrading nature activities because they have no other option. Bushmeat poaching has reportedly increased in Kenya and other countries of Africa, as well as Cambodia. Bushmeat hunters aren't the only ones at peril; the Rhino, which is poached for its horn, is also at risk. Park closures, the redirection of law enforcement to COVID-19-related activities, and fewer ranger patrols have all been considered by poachers as ideal opportunities for exploitation. Poaching is an issue for those who care about wildlife and the environmental and economic benefits it delivers, but it's also an issue for individuals who care about the environment. It also a concerns since it increases the likelihood of future pandemics. We have lost 60% of our natural habitat in the previous 50 years, while the number of new infectious diseases has quadrupled. It is no coincidence that the destructions of ecosystems have coincided with a sharp increase in such conditions. Natural habitats are being reduced, causing species to live in closer quarters than ever one another and to humans (BBC, 2020).

A species-group comparison during pre lockdown and post lockdown reveals that the most significant increase in reported poaching was related to ungulates. The percentage jumped from 22% of total reported cases during pre-lockdown to 44% during the lockdown period. The poaching of wild animals and birds, including the endangered Chinkara or Indian gazelle, has registered a sharp increase across Rajasthan during the lockdown. The hunters took advantage of slack monitoring and sparse public movement in remote areas (*The Hindu*, 2020). According to reports, poaching of birds and endangered animals increased in Pakistan and Nepal in April and May. Despite efforts by authorities to limit illegal wildlife hunting and selling, poaching is a lucrative business in the region. The rules also concentrated on implementing the lockdown limits. The circumstance was used by criminals involved in the illicit wildlife trade, who increased their activity. Furthermore, economic costs imposed by the lockdown also pushed some people to poach to support themselves (DW, 2020).

11.6 Hit Livelihood of Artists

Governments are putting in place widespread confinement or mobility restrictions on an unprecedented scale. Many countries have closed down their cultural institutions. In these circumstances, billions of people turn to culture as a source of comfort, well-being, and connection, mainly affecting artists and their work. Canceled concerts, postponed festivals, delayed album launches, suspended film production, and closed cinemas, all of which are having a devasting impact on the livelihoods of artists, many of whom are independent workers or who work in small and medium-sized enterprises, which are particularly vulnerable to financial shocks. Nearly two-thirds of artists and creative work industry workers have lost their jobs due to this pandemic. A survey done between April 8 and 21, 2020, the COVID-19 Impact Survey for Artists and Creative Workers, found that 62% of respondents have become fully unemployed, and 95% have experienced income loss (UNESCO, 2020e). Folk performers, ritual dancers, theatre artists, dancers, people working in the handicraft sector, etc., have all been seriously affected by the lockdown. This includes stage artists, dance school teachers, makeup artists, and costume rental people, pageantry artists, wedding dancers and musicians, classical and folk, and tribal artists who have lost their income.

Channapatna, popularly known as Toy Town in Karnataka, has long been noted for its wooden lacquered handicrafts. However, during the last few years, demand for these products has been progressively declining. The situation worsened this year due to the COVID-19 pandemic since tourists stayed away and bulk orders were cut, making it difficult for handcraft artists to sustain their daily lives (NDTV, 2020). According to surveys performed since the epidemic, the lockdown period cost at least half of all visual artists' money due to the loss of contracted work and the cancellation of regular and forward expectations. This research quantifies the direct economic impact of market volatility on artists in the face of unforeseen shocks that influence both the private and public sectors. For artists, the most pressing worry is income. The livelihoods of artists are reliant on locations remaining open and activities taking place. Around 60% of those polled expect a drop in revenue of more than 50% this year. Those who work in craft applied arts, performance, and those who live in rural areas expect the most substantial loss. Also essential are commissions, grants, and awards. Evidence suggests some uncertainty on the impact of COVID-19 on gifts and prizes—some artists are unsure if awards will be honored when activities are no longer possible due to COVID-19 (COVID-19 Impact Survey, 2020).

11.7 Interrupted Living Heritage Practices

Communities and their social fabric and cohesion have been directly harmed by the cancellation of national and local cultural and religious events such as festivals, ceremonies, and many forms of traditional customs. Many intangible cultural heritage traditions, such as rites and rituals, have been placed on hold due to COVID-19 affecting communities worldwide.

11.7.1 Cancellation of Traditional Festivals

Due to the pandemic, living heritage practices and expressions such as Norwuz celebrations in Central Asia and the Middle East, Buddhist Vesak celebrations in Southeast Asia, Christian holy week celebrations While some of the impacts of the COVID-19 for some aspects of the cultural sector can be quantified, such as the closure of several institutions or sites, loss of revenue for cultural and creative industries, and so on, other facets of culture are not necessarily prioritized in terms of urgent response measures in several countries, Carnivals in Latin America and the Caribbean, Dashain and Dipawali celebrations in Nepal and India, and countless other festivals, celebrations, and community performances around the world have been disrupted (UNESCO, 2020e). The survey and web platform on living heritage and the COVID-19 pandemic, launched by UNESCO, show the effects on bearers and practitioners of living heritage worldwide. In Japan, for example, the Yamahoko floats procession at the Kyoto Gion Festival, which has been held sincethe ninth century, was canceled (UNESCO, 2020f). Spring was the season for Kathmandu Valley's traditional festivals like Bhaktapur's Bisket Jatra, Machhindranath, Ram Navami, and Chaite Dasain. But the Coronavirus lockdown means many of the celebrations were muted or canceled. The old palace courtyard packed with hundreds ofthousands of people each year during the Indra Jatra festival is deserted. The temples are locked, and the government bans all public celebrations to curb the Coronavirus. The cancellation of Rato Machhindranath Jatra (a chariot procession in honor of the god of farming) involving large crowds to honor different deities causes people to become angry towards the government and fearfulness about god's anger. Autumn was the festival season in predominantly Hindu Nepal, where religion, celebrations, and rituals are significant parts of life. Still, people, this year, had to scale down their rituals within their homes. This year, the Coronavirus has taken a heavy toll on the health and wealth of many Nepal people. People have less money to spend, and for health reasons, many people are not celebrating the holiday with friends or extended family. In many places of the city, a collective uneasiness hangs in the air, which even Dashain and Tihar festivities also can't seem to cover up.

11.7.2 Impact on Major Social Ceremonies

Not only the festivals, different ceremonies like marriage and other rituals got affected. Many couples throughout the world have shared memories of postponed weddings because many people decided it was best to cancel celebrations and stay at home with their loved ones to ride out the pandemic. But, as the months have turned into a year, and lockdowns have been lifted and re-imposed, the pair has chosen to get on with it. The majority of people seem to have grown bored of holding their breath and waiting for the pandemic to end. While some people may still like to wait things out, others have adopted a new standard for marriages. They aren't grumbling because they are saving money by not holding extravagant week-long celebrations.

11.7.3 Affect Solidarity and Cultural Transmission among People

At the same time, living heritage practices, festivals, and ceremonies can be a source of resilience in such difficult circumstances. People continue to draw inspiration, joy, and solidarity from practicing their cultures. The survey also shows that transmission of living heritage to younger generations in crises help to boost mental health in the immediate term and benefit the longer-term recovery of communities (UNESCO, 2020g).

11.7.4 Hit Livelihood of Indigenous People

The cancellation of living heritage and such events not only has an impact on communities' social and cultural lives, but it can also result in a loss of revenue for many bearers and practitioners. Those who work in the performing arts and traditional crafts, which are predominantly in the informal sector, have been affected particularly hard. In Botswana, for example, earthenware pottery is still being manufactured, but the pandemic has disrupted the employees' ability to sold (UNESCO, 2020f).

11.8 Impact on Underprivileged Cultural Group

In almost every country, cultural life has taken a hit in one way or another in terms of social and economic impact. The pandemic has exposed some structural vulnerabilities and inequalities within and between countries. Within countries, the pandemic has further revealed inequalities facing vulnerable groups, particularly women, indigenous peoples, migrants and refugees, and LGBTI groups, including access to culture. The need for a greater understanding of cultural diversity and more excellent dialogue to build cohesive societies has also been thrown into stark relief. A recent report by human rights watch has shown that there has been a sharp global increase in Antiracism and Xenophobia around the world (UNESCO, 2020c).

11.8.1 Worsen Already Existing Discrimination Within Society

COVID-19 and the societal changes that have resulted from social distancing measures have revealed gaps in access to good work and discrimination, affecting many of society's most vulnerable groups, including racial/ethnic minorities, those from low socioeconomic backgrounds, and women. Racial, gender, and social class disparities have been well documented in educational and work opportunities for a decade. Again, with this pandemic, the individuals from vulnerable and marginalized backgrounds got hit most with discrimination. Individuals ranging from pop artists to legislators dubbed the COVID-19 a "great equalizer" in the early days of the global response. Yes, all rich and poor are asked to shelter at home (lockdown and social distancing); liberals and conservatives may acquire the virus. But that commonality is a veneer, making underlying social and economic inequalities that make some populations more vulnerable and affected by the disease and its mitigation measures than others and that vulnerable groups are typically those who have experienced a history of discrimination and marginalization (Jane Addams College of Social Work, 2020). Discrimination against affected people has increased at alarming rates as a result of the spreading of fear, rumors, and stigmas. COVID-19 survivors and their families, returnee migrant laborers, health workers, and other vulnerable groups have encountered substantial discrimination. When social distancing measures are implemented in countries like Nepal, where caste-based discrimination is prevalent, their unintended consequences may reinforce and legitimize existing social distancing practices, further reinforcing and legitimizing social, cultural, and gender-based discrimination against the marginalized population. Furthermore, economically deprived groups will incur a more significant price due to social distancing measures since they will have fewer options for surviving in daily life. As the economy and services become increasingly digitized, they are also becoming victims of the new digital divide. This perpetuates poverty, widens inequality, and puts more individuals in danger of social prejudice (Kafle, 2020).

11.8.2 Poor and Transportation

With the implications of nationwide lockdown on March 24th, the international flight ban resulted in the stranding of thousands of Nepalese in different parts of the world. Many Nepalese labor migrants and students could not return to their destinations abroad from Nepal, resulting in severe ruins in daily public life. Even thousands of Nepalese who wanted to return to Nepal got stuck at India Border points (Al Jazeera, 2020). The people within the country also face challenging to survive due to job loss, not only from abroad. They wish to migrate from urban to rural for survival, but due to imposed lockdown and travel restrictions, they find it challenging to return home. When they returned with lots of difficulties again, they are faced with social stigma and discrimination. The stories of thousands of people, including small children, mothers returned home by walking hundreds kilometer for many days without proper food, water, shelter is heartbreaking.

11.9 Positive Impact

COVID-19 and the preventive measures adopted by the countries to avoid transmission have affected peoples adversely, so the consequences of this cannot be overcome very soon and easily. However, within the worse outcome of this pandemic for almost one year, we can also find some of the positive sides.

11.9.1 Digitalization of Cultural Material

Measures of confinement around the world have demonstrated the relevance of culture in connecting with one another. For the 1.57 billion children and youth in 190 countries, accounting for 90% of the world's student population, who have had their schools closed for extended periods in recent months, art and culture have demonstrated an effective practical approach to keep youngsters engaged and learning at home. Several schools have modified their curriculum, while cultural institutions such as galleries, museums, and theatres have rapidly developed educational material and made them available online. According to recent research by a network of European museum groups, educational resources were the most requested service by internet visitors after social media content. These activities also aid in the reduction of emotions of isolation and the healing of trauma and loss, and the development of resilience. However, such cultural materials for educational purposes are not available in all parts of the world (UNESCO, 2020i). Despite the issues facing the environment and the oceans, some positive outcomes have arisen from the lockdown. Increased use of virtual platforms has expanded access to knowledge about natural world heritage sites and mixed world heritage sites. These platforms have raised awareness of the importance of cultural heritage for preserving natural world heritage sites and underwater archeological sites. Many communities worldwide have found digital solutions to share an intangible cultural heritage by social distancing measures. For example, the government in Czechia organized the Prague Spring festival to be celebrated in virtual form; traditional music groups in Costa Rica, the United Kingdom, and France have been rehearsing or performing online (UNESCO, 2020h).

11.9.2 Healing Nature

Biological diversity is intimately linked to cultural diversity. Humans have always adapted to the particular environment they found themselves in, leading to the flourishing of societies, cultures, and languages that have developed throughout human history. At the same time, according to the international energy agency, the health crisis and lockdown of countries are projected to reduce greenhouse emissions by 8% this year, according to the global energy agency, which is a positive sign to nature.

11.9.3 Cultural Practices and Solidarity

Many aspects of intangible cultural heritage are being repurposed to enhance public health responses in the pandemic's wake. Traditional strong puppet play in Sri Lanka conveys stories of imprisonment and social estrangement. In some cases, people respond by creating new rituals. E.g., In Europe, people applaud healthcare workers at the same time every night for their tireless service, and teddy bears appear in the windows for children to point out along walks around the neighborhood. These collective rituals give meaning in uncertain times and are a powerful tool for resilience and solidarity during a crisis (UNESCO, 2020f).

11.9.4 Emphasis on Local Food Resource to Sustain

Another consequence of the pandemic has been on the global supply chains. In some parts of the world, this means that local food from the sea and land and local, traditional recipes are more important than ever as local food chains can provide food for communities when sustainably managed. According to a survey carried out by UNESCO on the impact of the pandemic on intangible cultural heritage, there has been a resurgence in interest in traditional farming and local ingredients and recipes. In Lebanon, for example, there has been a return to healthier and organic agriculture and animal husbandry and the harvesting of wild plants that can be consumed, prepared or used for healing purposes among the younger generations (UNESCO, 2020i). This can be taken as a positive part of this pandemic and preparedness for a similar situation in the future.

11.10 Conclusion

Culture is crucial for identity formation, social cohesion, discourse, and healing and contributing significantly to the economy. At the same time, culture contributes to the gross domestic product by creating jobs, generating income, and generating revenue (GDP). A significant portion of the cultural sector, represented by natural and cultural heritage, heritage-based tourism, and cultural and creative industries, was negatively affected by the COVID-19 pandemic. The sudden closure of these landmarks, museums, and cultural events has unhappily resulted in a drop in national and international tourism. Overseas travelers consider cultural heritage to be a key element when selecting tourist destinations. Not only that, the loss of tourists, fewer people movement, and decreased security and supervision to world heritage sites causes looting of property of heritages and poaching of animals. Many people in the cultural and creative spheres have lost their contract or employment temporarily or permanently with varying degrees of warning and financial support. Again, tourist deficits lead to catastrophic high-income shortages, so significant protection and this cutback hampered restoration of cultural and natural heritage sites in finance. Religious sites and pilgrims are closed, ceremonies and festivals are canceled, held, or postponed, which causes frustration among people; people felt less confident and have difficulty finding inner peace and comfort. The positive cohesiveness among the different religious groups is shaken, and the harmony among people is disturbed due to false news and belief during this pandemic.

Similarly, the rise in xenophobia, racism and discrimination during this pandemic and lockdown within groups is havoc. The culture and creative field are not only for entertainment, but it also embodies educational, historical, and social identities and values. As a result, assessing COVID-19's impact on culture and, ultimately, society is critical to comprehend the scope of the problem and develop immediate solutions to protect and promote the nation's unique identity.

References

Adhikari, B. A. (2020, June 12). *Income of Pashupatinath temple dives down as it remains closed over two months.* Available from https://www.aninews.in/news/world/asia/income-of-pashupatinath-temple-dives-down-as-it-remains-closed-over-two-months20200612121357/

Al Jazeera. (2020, April 1). *Hundreds of Nepalese stuck at India border amid COVID-19 lockdown.* https://www.aljazeera.com/news/2020/04/hundreds-nepalese-stuck-india-border-covid-19-lockdown-200401031905310.html

BBC. (2020). *Wild animal at risk in lockdown.* Available from: https://www.bbc.com/future/article/20200520-the-link-between-animals-and-covid-19

COVID-19 impact Survey: An Artists information Company. (2020). https://static.a-n.co.uk/wp-content/uploads/2020/04/Covid-19-impact-survey-2020.pdf

DW. (2020). *Coronavirus: South Asia sees rises in Poaching during Lockdown.* Available from: https://www.dw.com/en/coronavirus-south-asia-sees-rise-in-poaching-during-lockdowns/a-54090081

Guan, Y., Deng, H., & Zhou, X. (2020). Understanding the impact of the COVID-19 pandemic on career development: Insights from cultural psychology. *Journal of Vocational Behavior, 119,.* https://doi.org/10.1016/j.jvb.2020.103438

Jane Addams College of Social Work. (2020). *COVID-19: The disproportionate impact on Marginalized populations.* Available from: https://socialwork.uic.edu/news-stories/covid-19-disproportionate-impact-marginalized-populations/

Kafle, B. (2020). *Social Cohesion in the context of COVID-19 in Nepal.* Available from: https://www.np.undp.org/content/nepal/en/home/blog/2020/Social-cohesion-in-the-context-of-COVID19-in-Nepal.html

Khadka D, Pokhrel GP, Thakur MS, Magar PR, Bhatta S, Dhamala MK, Aryal PC, Shi S, Cui D, & Bhuju DR. (2020). Impact of COVID-19 on the tourism industry in Nepal. *Asian Journal of Arts, Humanities and Social Studies*, 3(1), 40–48. http://www.ikprress.org/index.php/AJAHSS/article/view/5089

NDTV. (2020). *Nepal reports South Asia's first confirmed case of deadly coronavirus.* https://www.ndtv.com/world-news/nepal-reports-south-asias-first-confirmed-case-of-deadly-coronavirus-2169362

Nepali Times. (2020). Nepal's Muslims face stigma after COVID-19 tests. Available from https://www.nepalitimes.com/banner/nepals-muslims-face-stigma-after-covid-19-tests/

Poudel, K., & Subedi, P. (2020). Impact of COVID-19 pandemic on socioeconomic and mental health aspects in Nepal. *International Journal of Social Psychiatry., 66,* 002076402094224. https://doi.org/10.1177/0020764020942247

Prasain, S. (2019). *Nepal tourism generated Rs.240b and supported 1m jobs last year: Report.* Available from https://kathmandupost.com/money/2019/05/26/nepal-tourism-generated-rs240b-and-supported-1m-jobs-last-year-report

Shrestha, P. M. (2020). *Nepali economy starts to feel the pinch as coronavirus spreads.* Available from https://kathmandupost.com/national/2020/03/04/nepalieconomy-starts-to-feel-the-pinch-as-coronavirus-spreads

The Economic Times. (2020, March 23). Nepal seals border with India, China to prevent Coronavirus outbreak. https://economictimes.indiatimes.com/news/politics-and-nation/coronavirus-nepal-seals-borders-with-india-china/articleshow/74771722.cms?from=mdr

The Himalayan Times. (2021). COVID impact on religious tourism overlooked. Available from: https://thehimalayantimes.com/business/covid-impact-on-religious-tourism-overlooked/

The Hindu. (2020). Poaching double during Coronavirus Lockdown, says wildlife group. Available from: https://www.thehindu.com/news/national/poaching-doubled-during-coronavirus-lockdown-says-wildlife-group/article31768167.ece

The Kathmandu Post. (2020). Hand sanitizers in short supply due to buying rush sparked by outbreak fears. https://kathmandupost.com/money/2020/03/04/hand-sanitisers-in-short-supply-due-to-buying-rush-sparked-by-outbreak-fears

Ulak, N. (2020a). A preliminary study of novel Coronavirus disease (COVID-19) outbreak: A pandemic leading crisis in tourism industry of Nepal. *Journal of Tourism and Hospitality Education, 10*, 108–131. https://doi.org/10.3126/jthe.v10i0.28763

Ulak, N. (2020b). COVID-19 pandemic and its impact on tourism industry in Nepal. *Journal of Tourism & Adventure, 3*(1), 50–75. https://doi.org/10.3126/jota.v3i1.31356

UNESCO. (2020a). *The Socio-cultural implications of COVID-19.* Available from https://en.unesco.org/news/socio-cultural-implications-covid-19

UNESCO. (2020b). *Culture and COVID-19. Impact and response tracker.* Available from: https://en.unesco.org/sites/default/files/issue_1_en_culture_covid-19_tracker.pdf

UNESCO. (2020c). *Culture and COVID-19. Impact and response tracker.* Available from https://en.unesco.org/sites/default/files/issue_2_en_culture_covid-19_tracker-4.pdf

UNESCO. (2020d). *Culture and COVID-19. Impact and response tracker.* Available from https://en.unesco.org/sites/default/files/issue_3_en_culture_covid-19_tracker-5.pdf

UNESCO. (2020e). *Culture and COVID-19. Impact and response tracker.* Available from https://en.unesco.org/sites/default/files/issue_4_en_culture_covid-19_tracker-6.pdf

UNESCO. (2020f). *Culture and COVID-19. Impact and response tracker.* Available from https://en.unesco.org/sites/default/files/issue_5_en_culture_covid-19_tracker-7.pdf

UNESCO. (2020g). *Culture and COVID-19. Impact and response tracker.* Available from https://en.unesco.org/sites/default/files/issue_8_en_culture_covid-19_tracker-10.pdf

UNESCO. (2020h). *Culture and COVID-19. Impact and response tracker.* Available from https://en.unesco.org/sites/default/files/issue_9_en_culture_covid-19_tracker-11.pdf

UNESCO. (2020i). *Culture and COVID-19. Impact and response tracker.* Available from https://en.unesco.org/sites/default/files/issue_10_en_culture_covid-19_tracker-12.pdf

Xinhua. (2020). *Nepal's tourism sector faces loss of around 300 mln USD due to COVID-19.* http://www.xinhuanet.com/english/2020-07/04/c_139187827.htm

Zhu, N., Zhang, D., Wang, W., Li, X., Yang, B., Song, J., & Tan, W. (2020). A novel coronavirus from patients with pneumonia in China 2019. *The New England Journal of Medicine, 382*, 723–733. https://doi.org/10.1056/NEJMoa2001017

Shree Prasad Devkota, Chairperson, Sustainable Development and Empowerment Forum, Nepal. PhD, Scholar, Conflict, Peace and Development Studies, Tribhuvan University, Kathmandu, Nepal.

Ms Laxmi Paudyal is a Lecturer at Gandaki Medical College Teaching Hospital and Research Center, Nepal.

Chapter 12

Pandemic Within a Pandemic: Gendered Impact of COVID-19 in Bangladesh with a Focus on Child Marriage and Domestic Violence

Nazmunnessa Mahtab and Tasnim Nowshin Fariha

Abstract This chapter aims to provide an explanation for the observed increase in VAWG during COVID-19 pandemic in Bangladesh with a focus on child marriage and domestic violence—two of the widespread forms of gender-based violence in the country. The study has been conducted based on data derived from secondary sources, focusing on both qualitative as well as quantitative studies. By applying the social ecological framework, the study identifies a number of factors represented at individual, familial, community, and societal levels and how these factors interact with each other and result in an increased prevalence of VAWG in a pandemic context. Increased poverty at family level, prolonged school closures, girls pursuing positive attitude towards child marriage, the urge to save family honor, inadequate state laws and community breakdown have been identified as the main factors behind the increased risk of child marriage, especially in urban slums and rural areas. Whereas widespread poverty and unemployment, movement restrictions, overwhelmed health care system, breakdown in legal system and police, and shifting gender roles and relationship dynamics are all amplifying the stress and tensions at personal, household and community levels leading up to increased prevalence of domestic violence. Finally, the chapter recommends a few pathways to avert the alarming surges in child marriage and domestic violence across the country with regard to mitigating their detrimental effects on the lives of women and girls.

Keywords COVID-19 · Pandemic · Lockdown · VAWG · Child marriage · Domestic violence

12.1 Introduction

World Health Organization (WHO) declared the novel Coronavirus disease-2019 (COVID-19) as a public health emergency of international concern on 30th January 2020, and later a pandemic on 11th of March. 2020. Bangladesh, a middle-income country situated in South Asia, is among the top 33 countries which accounts for

---

N. Mahtab (✉) · T. N. Fariha (✉)
Department of Gender and Women Studies, University of Dhaka, Dhaka, Bangladesh

© The Author(s), under exclusive license to Springer Nature Singapore Pte Ltd. 2022
S. Roy and D. Nandy (eds.), *Understanding Post-COVID-19 Social and Cultural Realities*, https://doi.org/10.1007/978-981-19-0809-5_12

199

0.50% of the COVID-19 cases of the world. Between 8 March 2020 and 2 May 2021, according to the DGHS the country had 761,943 confirmed COVID-19 cases including 11,579 related deaths (CFR 1.52%) (WHO, 2020). To tackle the epidemiological emergency, Bangladesh Government issued a lockdown order—known as 'general holiday'—remained in place from March 26 to May 30, 2020 (Shawon, 2020). Later, when the country experienced a second wave of COVID-19 infections in 2021, lockdown measures were reintroduced from April 5 extended unto May 16 (Bhattacharjee & Palma, 2021).

Public health measures such as lockdown, stay at home orders, business shutdowns, school closures or channeling resources towards emergency service provision, while essential for disease control, often disproportionately impact the lives of women as existing gender inequalities exacerbate gender-based disparities between women, men, girls and boys. Movement restriction, economic strains, food insecurity, growing household level tension and individual vulnerabilities, often instigate miscellaneous and compounding forms of discrimination, inequality, and maltreatment against women and girls in home setting, including domestic violence [DV], child marriage, abuse or exploitation. Their sufferings are further aggravated due to lack of access to their regular social networks, sources of social support, health and other support services.

Child, early or forced marriages are particularly high in insecure environments (Tembon & Fort, 2008), such as natural disasters, health emergencies or conflict affected areas. West Africa's Ebola outbreak is a major example as it caused a massive surge in child marriage, exploitation and sexual abuse (John et al., 2020; Onyango et al., 2019). Not surprisingly, evidence indicates child marriages have escalated during COVID pandemic too. The consequences of COVID pandemic however seem to be unprecedented and way more harmful than any other time. Unlike regional epidemics, the global pandemic has led to school closures on a global scale, that is estimated to affect at least 800 million girls who are potential victims of an additional 13 million child marriages between 2020 and 2030 (UNFPA, 2020). Bangladesh, a country already burdened with 59% of girls being married before attaining majority (18 years) (MICS, 2019), saw a 44% spike in child marriage compared to previous year (Antara, 2021). Currently, 40 million students are out of schools in Bangladesh (Emon et al., 2020) and half of them are girls. As coronavirus continues to spread, it will push more families into poverty, placing these girls at high risk of child marriage, with almost non-existent chances of ever returning to school.

Women and girls, who constitute half of the world's population, remain at high risk of gender-based violence both during and post a crisis time (Akel et al., 2021; Sánchez et al., 2020), including natural disasters, health outbreaks, war and conflict situations. Evidence from previous health crises predict that COVID pandemic is likely to leave an ever-lasting legacy of gender inequality and violence against women and girls [VAWG] on our planet (UN Women, 2020). DV, already an underreported social pandemic, exacerbate in emergency circumstances because of no and/or limited prevention measures, inadequate support services and potential social instability. In absence of vaccination, staying at home is considered as the safest option to avoid the virus. However, not always a home is the safe heaven to live in.

Globally, 1 in every 3 women at some points of their lives have been inflicted with physical and/or sexual violence by an intimate partner or husband (WHO, 2021), while it is 1 in 2 married women in Bangladesh (BBS, 2016). Security and health concerns as well as money problems elevate the level of household tensions along with confined living conditions further magnify women's encounter with DV. During lockdown, women were trapped in home with their abusers and the safest heaven turned to a prison of continuous physical, psychological and sexual violence with no place to escape. Reports all around the world hint at a global raise in DV. Countries where 'stay at home' measures were in place to curb coronavirus saw consequential increase in violence within home setting (UN Women, 2020). A global 20% increase was recorded in just fees days of lockdown (UN ESCAP, 2020), while Europe Union alone saw a 60% increase in emergency calls from female victims of spousal violence (Mahase, 2020). Within just a few days since the virus broke out in Wuhan, the hashtag #antidomesticviolenceduringepidemic was trending in Chinese social media with more than 3000 searches. Moreover, some 4249 women in Bangladesh suffered from DV and their sufferings continue to exacerbate in post lockdown era too (MJF, 2020).

Therefore, the context of women and girl's lives need to be addressed in talks of public health measures. Yet, there is a lack of research and studies focusing on how women and girls face discrimination, inequalities, and exploitation differently than men during any disaster, emergency and afterwards. Consequently, those responding to disasters or in the current situation those who are responsible for COVID management might not be fully aware of the possibility of a second pandemic triggered by the surges in gender-based maltreatment or violence. Due to lack of proper understanding on such issues, they are hardly prepared to deal with them, which in turn make the situation worse. For example, tackling violence within home, child marriage or teen pregnancy remain the least discussed areas of concern in Bangladesh's response to the pandemic. Since the outbreak of novel coronavirus, Bangladesh government has proposed two fiscal budgets. None of them however have specified any allocation to tackle the gendered challenges faced by women during a pandemic such as violence or child marriage. John et al. (2020) have identified such laxity as the "lessons never learnt". We thereby outline the gendered impact of COVID-19 pandemic as to how the pandemic exacerbate pre-existing inequalities and disparities. By applying the social ecological framework, this chapter aims to explore the link between COVID-19 pandemic and VAWG in Bangladesh, with regard to identifying the factors leading up to the risk of child marriage and DV, which are two of the prevalent forms of gender-based violence in the country.

12.2 Research Questions

The major research question is: How do COVID-19 pandemic elevate the risk of VAWG?

The specific research questions are:

What factors do lead up to the risk of child marriage during a pandemic? and

What factors do lead up to the risk of DV during a pandemic?

12.3 Conceptual Framework

This study adopts social-ecological model as the conceptual framework as it allows to analyze the risk factors of VAWG from multiple domains. The model describes the sphere of influence in multiple layers, typically represented as individual, relationship (familial), community and societal factors (Bronfenbrenner & Morris, 1998; Heise, 1998)—and regards VAWG as resulting from the interaction of factors at each level of the social environment. First developed by Bronfenbrenner in the 1970s, this theory-based framework has been used by many researchers in explaining various issues, such as family violence, VAWG, IPV, child abuse, and sexual and reproductive health (Bronfenbrenner & Morris, 1998; Fulu & Miedema, 2015; Gashaw et al., 2018; Marcell et al., 2017). By applying this framework, this chapter tends to provide an explanation for the increase in VAWG during COVID-19 pandemic with regard to exploring the contributing factors in multiple layers of influence.

12.4 Methodology and Data Collection

The study has been conducted based on data derived from secondary sources, focusing on both qualitative as well as quantitative studies. The chapter attempts to explain the observed increase in child marriage and DV in Bangladesh in the context of COVID pandemic. Considering the contagious nature of coronavirus, the option of primary field investigation didn't appear to be safe. Instead of primary data collection, the authors decided to review the appropriate and credible sources of literature. Interweb resources and websites such as Springer, JStor, Social Science Research Network (SSRN), Elsevier, SAGE Publications and various other research and journal portals were searched for relevant materials and information. A series of key search terms was used in the process including COVID-19, Coronavirus, COVID-19 Outbreak, COVID-19 Pandemic, health crisis, SARS-CoV-2, gender impact, VAWG, DV, child marriage, epidemic, lockdown, social distancing, quarantine, and Bangladesh etc. This review incorporates all types of publications reporting information related to VAW in the COVID-19 context, including original articles, opinion papers, commentaries, letters, and editorials. The review also includes articles from both national and international newspaper, relevant reports from government and non-government organizations, periodic situation reports, working papers, policy briefs, webpages, blogs etc.

The authors have conceded all the ethical bindings ought to be acknowledged. Every source of information used in this study was referenced and accredited. All collected information has been analyzed and interpreted in a manner which reflects the chapter in terms of relevance. As the pandemic is still evolving, the authors don't claim this study to be an exact manifestation of the magnitude of changes in the prevalence of VAWG as a result of the pandemic. Moreover, the scale of violence related issues is difficult to be measured as they are often underreported, the number of available protection services is limited, and the ability to record such incidents is also limited. The study simply offers an insight into the gendered problems emerging as a consequence of COVID-19 pandemic in Bangladesh context.

12.5 COVID-19 and Child Marriage: A Pandemic's Untold Consequences

Child marriage or early marriage is known as formal marriage or informal union between a child under the age of 18 and an adult or another child (Unicef, 2020a). It is a social evil and a harmful cultural practice which can be a precursor to death sentence. Child marriage is one of the worst manifestations of gender-based violence as it contravenes the human rights of young girls. It usually means an end to formal education. Every year, around 12 million girls fall victims of child marriage under the age of 18 (Unicef, 2020b) who consequently face life time threats of poor health, lack of autonomy and dignity. Child marriage puts women and girls at high risk of DV including sexual, physical and psychological, by their partners and partner's families for the rest of their lives.

There is clear literature on the effect of disasters on poor families, which in times of crisis end up marrying their underage daughters (Rahiem, 2021). Natural disasters, droughts, earthquakes, conflicts, public health crises, and outbreaks historically appear to exacerbate existing gender inequality, making girls disproportionately affected by forced marriages (Neumayer & Plumper, 2008; Paul & Mondal, 2021). As a result of breakdown in family and community structures, many of the complex factors that drive up child marriage in stable environments are exacerbated in emergency settings. Ebola outbreak (2014–2016) in West Africa is a glaring example of how young girls are disproportionately affected by the effects of emergency situation. There was a massive increase in child labor, child marriage, teenage pregnancies, and sexual exploitation due to staggering hikes in school dropout rates for girls during the epidemic period (Fraser, 2020). In Nepal, child marriages reportedly rose as destruction of houses and property and interruption of livelihoods from the 2015 earthquake resulted in additional financial strain (Logan & Maharjan, 2020). COVID-19 pandemic is no different. Though it puts everyone at risk, the social consequences on girls have been particularly devastating.

COVID pandemic poses unique challenges for the society, including loss of livelihood means and income, higher risk of violence in private sphere and lack of access to schooling; all of which elevate the risk of child marriage both in acute and recovery phases (Bellizzi et al., 2021; Paul & Mondal, 2021; Rahiem, 2021). Unicef (2021) has identified five main reasons behind the spike of child marriage during pandemic; these include interrupted education, economic shocks, pregnancy, death of a parent, and disruption to programmes and services aiming to prevent child marriage. Child marriage and its drivers however are complex and vary within and across countries. Given the adverse implications of COVID-19 on the global economy, the girls in low-income countries and mainly living in vulnerable and poor communities are at higher risk of child marriage. Contextual factors also play a role in affecting child marriages in certain settings: these include gender and social norms, the prevalence of child marriage, the amount and direction of marriage payments, the availability of social protection, the availability of poverty alleviation programmes and the presence of displacement, ongoing conflict and forced migration (Alqahtani & Alqahtani, 2021; Bellizzi et al., 2021; Kamal, 2010).

Unicef (2021) report titled "COVID-19: A Threat to Progress Against Child Marriage" indicates that the total number of girls at risk, or affected, is significant. Numerous reports from different sources have already confirmed that child marriages are rising appallingly in different countries around the world (Frayer & Pathak, 2020; Jones et al., 2020). World Vision (2021b) revealed that between March and December 2020 child marriages more than doubled compared to 2019 in several communities in Afghanistan, Bangladesh, Senegal and Uganda. In India, child marriages reportedly increased by more than 33% between June and October 2020, compared to the same period in 2019 (Bellizzi et al., 2021). Yet, there is not enough evidence on the exact impact of the pandemic on child marriage globally. Some predictions have been made based on evidence from past pandemics. Save the Children (2020) predicted that an additional of 1.3–2.5 million girls can fall victim to child marriage between 2020 and 2025 with South Asia topping the list as nearly 200,000 more girls at risk of child marriage in 2020, including Bangladesh, which is among the top-10 countries in the world for rates of child marriage. Unicef (2021) predicted that 10 million more child marriages may take place between 2020 and 2030; which places 100 million girls at risk of child marriage by 2030.

12.5.1 COVID-19 and Child Marriage: Bangladesh Context

Despite the significant progress in recent years, Bangladesh was already burdened with curse of child marriage. Even before COVID-19 showed up, the country ranked 4th globally (Arnab & Siraj, 2020) with 51.4% of women married before reaching the age of 18 and 15.5% before even reaching 15 (MICS, 2019). The COVID outbreak has intensified many social and economic drivers including poverty, lack of security of girls, risk of violence, risk of early pregnancy and the mindset of families considering their daughters as burden, that further accelerate child marriage. When children are unable to continue their education, families struggle to make ends meet and access to basic services like reproductive health are reduced, the risk of child marriage significantly increases.

Due to a lack of country-wide surveillance or data gaps, there is no actual statistics of child marriage in Bangladesh. We here rely on different media reports, government and NGO's data collation to understand the trend of child marriage during COVID-19 pandemic in Bangladesh. According to a survey conducted in 11 districts of Bangladesh, incidence of child marriage has increased by 13% during the COVID pandemic, making this the highest rate of child marriage in the country in the past 25 years (Dhaka Tribune, 2021a). Another study shows that Bangladesh experienced a spike by 44% in 2020 with 101 girls falling victim (Antara, 2021). Manusher Jonno Foundation (MJF) reported at least 13,886girls in 21 districts were victims of child marriages between April and October of 2020; 48% out of the total were between 13 and 15 years old (Sakib, 2021). While BRAC (international development organization) counted, a total of 778 child marriages were reported between January to September of the same year (Brac, 2020). Women and Children Affairs ministry has identified the districts of Kurigram, Natore, Jessore, Kushtia, Narsingdi and Jhalokati with highest increase in pandemic induced child marriages. The northern district of Kurigram encountered the highest spike in under aged marriages (Dhaka Tribune, 2021b). In this district alone, child marriages have shot up from 8% in March to over 11% in July (Uttom & Rozario, 2020). The figures mentioned above provide us with an indication that COVID-19 pandemic works as a predictor of child marriage. Though they might fail to represent the wholesome picture, as underreporting of child marriage has always been a common problem in Bangladesh.

Below, we will outline a number of factors at individual, familial, community, and societal levels and how the different level factors interact with each other and contribute to the observed increase in child marriage prevalence in the pandemic context of Bangladesh.

12.5.1.1 Family Poverty

Social distancing requirements, business closures and travel restrictions associated with COVID-19 have all led to a drop in economic activity, the loss of livelihoods, and household poverty. Households tend to respond to economic insecurity in two ways: cutting spending (such as education costs) and cutting household size. Both can lead to child marriage (Dewi & Dartango, 2019). There is evidence that, marriage timing of daughters is an important household coping strategies in the face of aggregate shocks in developing countries (Dercon, 2002). The pandemic can reportedly drive Bangladesh's poverty rate up to 40.9%, with 16.4 million new poor in the country (Dhaka Tribune, 2020). Pre-COVID, child marriage was more widespread among poor families in Bangladesh (Unicef, 2020c), therefore, the growing impoverishment due to pandemic along with school closures is likely to magnify the child marriage rates in poor communities. Among one-third of vulnerable households in South West of Bangladesh, the risks of child marriage and other forms of gender-based violence have increased significantly and 4% of families already had to marry off one of their children since the start of the crisis (World Vision, 2021a).

Poor families seem to be more affected by pandemic of hunger than pandemic of coronavirus disease. The resulting economic insecurity may limit the ability of parents to provide for their children. Reduced family income puts poor parents in a fix where they have to choose whether to invest in boys or girls. Driven by son preference, they always consider saving money for son more sensible than investing in daughters (Uttom & Rozario, 2020). Family income has a 32% impact on child marriage for the poorer quintiles, and only a 5% impact on richer income quintiles (Paul, 2019). Girls from poor families are three-times more likely to marry before the age of 18 than girls from wealthier families (World Vison, 2021a). The COVID-19 pandemic has seen many families face food shortages and decreases in household income and resources; the threat of child marriage has become even more imminent (Paul & Mondal, 2021; Rahiem, 2021). Deepening poverty has led to a huge financial burden on families, so parents see the option of marrying off their underage daughters, or sold them off to rich families as domestic workers, as one of the easiest ways to reduce their economic burden and get rid of more mouths to feed.

Marrying an under aged daughter, moreover, allows parents to wipe off their responsibilities with lower dowry payments (Monsoor, 2003). The time of COVID-19 is also suitable for a simple wedding where poor people do not need to spend a lot of money for the dowry. Lower dowry demands and lower marriage expenses due to the lockdown further incentivized families who were already considering child marriage as a coping strategy.

The positive relationship between increased poverty and child marriage, leads the girls in poor rural households or urban slums towards greatest risk of child marriage where the rates are already worrisome (Kamal et al., 2014). A study in rural Bangladesh reports, the likelihood of marriage/engagement and marriage-related discussions increased steadily for girls aged 15 or above (Makino et al., 2021). Not to forget the costal girls who faced a triple disaster of COVID, cyclone (e.g. Amphan) and floods. They are not only at risk of child marriage but also of trafficking, displacement and transactional sex.

12.5.1.2 School Closures

Year-long school closures are likely to create a long-lasting impact on futures of girls—particularly those in poorer and more remote families—as many of them might not return to school after being forcefully married or pregnant. World Bank (2017) advocates that "keeping girls at school is one of the best and most effective ways to end child marriage". According to Unicef (2021), school closures increase marriage risk by 25% per year and 2% of girls will never return to school, bringing the risk of marriage due to school closures and dropout to 27.5%. School closures in

West Africa contributed to massive spikes in child marriage during Ebola outbreaks (Davies & Bennett, 2016). In patriarchal societies, it is often an "either/or" option between getting married or remaining in school (World Bank, 2020). Moreover, as girls don't need to go to schools, parents or family members force them to help with care or housework.

Parents are tended to marry their daughters off at an early age out of fear that, as girls were sitting idle amid school closures, they could begin romantic relationships, attempt to elope from home or be subjected to sexual harassment; all of which could harm the family's image in the community (Raha et al., 2021). If girls do not attend school, it is difficult for them to reject the marriage arranged by their guardians; however, when in school, they can oppose and take the help from friends and teachers to avoid being into forced marriage (Jones et al., 2020). Evidence demonstrated that 71% of underage marriages in Bangladesh occurred due to the school closure amid the ongoing COVID-19 pandemic (Afrin & Zainuddin, 2021). Moreover, as schools are closed, girls are not getting stipends and other financial incentives which used to work as strong motivators for parents to continue their daughters' education.

12.5.1.3 Individual (Girl) Attitudes Towards Child Marriage

In humanitarian contexts, young girls tend to grow a positive attitude toward child marriage. They often perceive the option of marriage as the easiest way out of their problems or a way to relieve the expenses for parents who do not have enough money to cover their food or other basic needs and expenses (Freccero & Taylor, 2021). Due to the prolonged school closures, child marriage which previously was typically been encouraged by only struggling parents, is now also being encouraged by struggling rural girls. Nearly 40 million students are out of classrooms education in Bangladesh (Emon et al., 2020), including a huge section constituted of rural girls. Many of the girls are at high risk of dropouts due to almost non-existent accessibility to distant learning. Moreover, their freedom and mobility have also been curtailed. Unlike boys, rural girls are generally not allowed to go anywhere without being escorted by male family members. While at home, they don't have access to enough means of entertainment. Altogether, rural girls are becoming frustrated and see no future for themselves. Thus, many girls consider the option of early marriage as mere escape route. This shift to girls pursuing child marriage is a devastating one that would drive the numbers even higher.

12.5.1.4 Family Honor

School closure has changed the way girls spend their time in a day and now they are mostly home bound. School closure for a substantial period along with social isolation of girl children can drive the practice of sexual abuse further underground. Girls now spend more time at home and unsupervised, which could increase their exposure to sexual activity, sexual violence and unwanted pregnancy (Unicef, 2021). In many cases, local young men who are passing their idle time start teasing or stalking which takes the form of verbal abuse to unwanted physical contact. The fears of family violence are higher in joint or extended families where young girls live with male relatives under same roof. Adolescent girls also appear to be at further risk of abuse, and of sexual exploitation when the adults in the home are hospitalized or deceased, and children stay alone or under the care of strangers (Fraser, 2020). Besides, given the breakdowns in community structures and communication systems, government and non-government interventions to ensure access to reproductive health centers and services have halted in many places, resulting in high prevalence of adolescent pregnancy. Some 18,000 teenage girls became pregnant during Ebola and when schools re-opened, they were banned from resuming classes (Peyton, 2020). To avoid such stigma, families often rush into the decision of marring off their minor daughters.

In humanitarian contexts, including outbreaks, early marriage is considered as a way to protect young girls from the dishonor of violence, abuse or pregnancy (Freccero & Taylor, 2021). About 60% of population in Bangladesh feel that the safety and security of women and girls is a concern in the context of the pandemic, which as stated earlier is a factor driving families to consider child marriage (2021a). In this society, the honor of a family lies in protecting the honor of women and girls. Pre-marital sexual activities, losing virginity before marriage or pregnancy are socially despised and culturally inappropriate (Rob & Mutahara, 2001). A girl surviving rape or pre-marital pregnancy, has little chances of marrying well in future. In rural areas, such victims face social exclusion, fatwa violence and many other social problems (Sifat, 2020). Parents often see the option of early marriage as a way to protect their girls and families from social stigma that result from if a girl in case survived rape or sexual assault.

12.5.1.5 Community Breakdown and Travel Restrictions

Community breakdown is a common problem in any type of disaster, that is likely to disrupt the much-needed interventions to prevent under aged marriages (Paul & Mondal, 2021). Bangladesh has child marriage prevention committees from union to national level comprising of various stakeholders from multiple government agencies, people's representatives and NGO representatives. During lockdown, most of these committees become non-functional as a result of disrupted communication inside communities. Information fails to reach the prevention committees, allowing parent's free reign to get their young children married off in secrecy. BRAC reports, 683 child marriages were prevented from January to September of 2020 (Brac, 2020). This rise in child marriage was accompanied by related child protection issues as well as by the decreased ability of non-profit and humanitarian organizations to travel and provide services.

Community based programmes aimed to raise awareness, challenge traditional gender norms and empower girls also struggled during the pandemic, leaving space for child marriage to continue. Pandemic related travel restrictions and social distancing can make it difficult for girls and women to access to programmes and services that aim to protect them from child marriage as well as sexual and gender-based violence (Briggs & Ngo, 2020). Disruptions in such services can create difficulties in accessing modern contraception, resulting in unintended pregnancy and subsequent child marriage sues, is another factor responsible for increased child marriage (Roy et al., 2021). Due to travel restrictions, girls and women may also face barriers to engaging with the formal justice system (e.g. police or law enforcing agencies) which can be used as a last-ditch effort to prevent child marriage.

12.5.1.6 State Laws

Media reports highlight the closure of educational institutions, social insecurity, insolvency, preference of potential grooms who returned to their village after losing jobs abroad, or influence of neighbor's prompt parents to marry their girl children off secretly amid the pandemic. The statuary laws of Bangladesh help the parents in doing so. Strong legal framework is a protective factor against child marriage. It is important for any country to have a minimum age of marriage as this legally protects children from abuse, harm, violence and exploitation. In Bangladesh, although Child Marriage Restraint Act 2017 penalizes the solemnization of underage marriage, it creates an exception for underage marriage in "special circumstance", thus effectively removing a minimum age of marriage. As per rule 17 of the Child Marriage Restraint Rules 2018, the parties to the marriage or their parents and legal guardians may file an application to the appropriate court along with the necessary legal documents for marriage in special circumstances. Although the Rules seek to clarify the controversial provision of the law, the absence of a minimum age of marriage leaves room for its misuse and creates valid concerns about the wellbeing of girl children with increased vulnerability to child marriage (Yasmin, 2020a).

Besides, this act has no provision for taking consent from children as they are not adult, also there is no example of any special circumstances or any explanation of what constitutes the best interests under which such marriages are permissible (Arnab & Siraj, 2020). Guardian's concern for their daughter's future, preference of potential grooms, school closure or inability to feed the family, whatever the reason might be, marrying off an under aged daughter in name of best interest are spreading wrong messages to society as there is confusion if these factors fall under 'special circumstances'. So, the pandemic can inhibit enforcement of the legal minimum age at marriage. Lack of surveillance by local government officials, who are predominantly busy with handling COVID-19-related is another reason behind the increasing prevalence of child marriage in Bangladesh.

Bangladesh is committed to eliminate child marriage by 2030 in line with UN Sustainable Development Goals. The country's achieved progress over the past few decades to end child marriage has been reversed by the pandemic. For girls especially in rural areas and urban slums, the epidemic of child marriage seems to be a greater threat than any virus or disease. The rise in child marriage is likely to leave compounding forms of deleterious effects on the society. It is particularly concerning for child brides as they live with a high possibility of experiencing DV for the rest of life. Child marriage takes place in the context of harmful gender norms and unequal power dynamics between young brides and their older husbands. As a result, child brides experience high rates of intimate partner violence (IPV) and have a difficult time advocating for better treatment World Vision (2021a). Child marriage is like the poison called carbon monoxide, that kills women slowly and silently. In long run, child marriage negatively affects a woman's health and economic outcomes, along with those of her off spring. Child brides often lack the decision-making power to negotiate safer sex practices, making girls vulnerable to sexually transmitted infections or early pregnancy. It hinders their access to social networks, and results in social exclusion, and stigmatization. This consequently develops a cycle of generational inequality and deprivation which vis-à-vis affect the society's overall wellbeing as well as the nation's progress in achieving sustainable development goals. The long-term effects of child marriage encompass generations of girls and young women being denied the right to health, education, decent work and earn money and the agency to combat DV.

12.6   Women Fighting a Dual Pandemic: COVID-19 and Domestic Violence

DV is a broad term usually defined as a range of violations that occur within a domestic space or home. Intimate Partner Violence [IPV], on the other hand is a specific type of DV. IPV in simple terms is a form of abuse generally perpetrated by a current or former partner. IPV includes various features ranging from physical, sexual to psychological harm, often expressed in form of physical aggression, sexual coercion, psychological abuse, controlling behaviour or financial deprivation. Global surveys show, at least 35% of women at some points of their lives have been subjected to physical and/or sexual violence by an intimate partner (WHO, 2021). Such violence can heighten during and after a period of large crisis or disaster (Parkinson & Zara, 2013; Redding et al., 2017), as existing gender inequality is often worsened in emergency settings. More precisely, a pandemic or disease outbreak heightens the risk of gender-based violence, both within and outside home, particularly heightening the risk of DV, IPV or rape. Experiences from Cholera, Zika and Ebola outbreaks showcase spikes in DV along with reductions in funding of public health services (Chandan et al., 2020).

Emerging evidence exhibits, COVID-19 has enhanced the volume of VAW to manifold. Stringent measures to contain the outbreak, including stay at home orders, lockdown, social isolation, physical distancing or travel restrictions—whilst essential from a public health perspective, have enhanced DV across world (Deluca et al., 2020; Piquero et al., 2020). Pandemic inflames fears and uncertainties providing an enabling environment which triggers violence, contrarily, lifesaving support to violence survivors are disrupted when front-line service providers and systems including health (physical and mental), protection (legal and police) and social welfare, are all diverted to tackle the pandemic. Thus, women are suffering from burns of a second pandemic, termed as 'shadow pandemic' by United Nations (UN Women, 2020).

Every additional three months of lockdown can give rise to 15 million additional GBV cases all around the world (UN ESCAP, 2020). Though the actual numbers are yet to be figured out, media coverage and reports from organizations dedicated to work with GBV have already shed light on an alarming fact. DV against women— amid lockdown—surged by 40–50% in Brazil, 20% in Spain, 30% in Cyprus, 25% in UK (Ince Yenilmez, 2020) and 21–35% in United States (Wagers, 2020). A police department China's Hubei province reported tripling of cases in February 2020 (Allen-Ebrahimian, 2020) while some Indian states with strict lockdown measures experienced a 131% multiplication in DV cases (Ekweonu, 2020).

DV can be perpetrated by both men and women so can both be equally victims of it. However, the existing literature on gender-based violence remains one sided and biased. Researches often articulate anti-male discourse on DV. They often generalize women as weaker sex who are vulnerable to DV where men are always projected as perpetrators and women as victims. Despite such limitations, existing studies are crucial alternatives to understand the DV prevalence and trends in absence of population-based estimates during COVID-19 lockdowns.

12.6.1 COVID-19, Domestic Violence and IPV: Bangladesh Context

The social structure of Bangladesh is predominantly patriarchal often endorsing harmful norms, culture and practices that place women irrespective of their age at higher risks of violence. According to a WHO report, Bangladesh ranks 4th in terms of prevalence of violence against women (VAW) by intimate partner among 61 countries and territories between 2000 and 2018 (Prothom Alo, 2021). Women irrespective of their geographical locations, social background or economic class, experience violence at home. Here, 54.2% of married women face lifetime physical and sexual IPV (BBS, 2016), while 25.4% of them consider partner (husband) violence as justified (MICS, 2019). Social norms and values censor issues like DV or IPV as exclusively private/ personal matters and not to be discussed in public or a crime to be reported; as a result, the actual prevalence of cases remain unknown. Marital rape or husband's aggressive sexual approaches are common, however not criminalized in Bangladesh, as a wife is considered to be the husband's private possession. In fact, even if a wife wants to escape from an abusive marriage, in most of the cases she fails to do it due to lack of family support. Many parents send their daughters back to the house of an abusive husband from their family homes in fear losing family honor and reputation. Women are often socialized to perceive that family life and husband's home have especial sanctity, not only in a physical but rather in a social sense which also makes it difficult for women to report the abusive experiences that take place within the sacred boundaries of one's home as a result of feelings of shame and embarrassment. The COVID-19 crisis has raised the necessity to rethink the idealized representations of home, family and married life.

It is not like violence at own home is something new or uncommon for women in Bangladesh. Yet, the pandemic has magnified discrimination, inequalities, oppressions, privileges and patriarchal violence, all of which already exist in the male-dominated and hierarchical society. For many women during lockdown, their own homes were no less than a prison. Domestic spheres became a site of physical, emotional and sexual violence as a result of problems like forced cohabitation, economic stress and high levels of mental stress (Ince Yenilmez, 2020). Similar to other countries, women in Bangladesh were more vulnerable to DV and abuse in lockdown. Nearly 4,249 women became victim of DV between January to April while 1,672 among them never experience it before (MJF, 2020). Manusher Jonno Foundation and Brac James P Grant School of Public Health jointly conducted research titled "Life in the time of coronavirus: A gendered perspective" which unveiled some alarming facts regarding the DV scenario in Bangladesh. More than 30% of these survivors were exposed to multiple forms of violence including physical harm, mental torture, economic deprivation or sexual coercion for the first time during the pandemic (Dhaka Tribune, 2020). Women facing violence for the first time in their lifetime means the extent of women's vulnerabilities is way bigger than we imagine. From January to June, 107 deaths of women due to domestic abuse was recorded with only 74 cases been filed (Ain O Salish Kendra, 2020). Lockdown gave rise to all form of DV including physical (18%), sexual (2%), and economic (33%), however, the prevalence of mental violence (47%) was highest (MJF, 2020). It should be noted, while physical abuse has decreased, mental torture has increased over time.

Lockdown has also been used as a coercive control mechanism by some men to employ control over women, specifically through using containment, threat or fear of infection as a mechanism of control and abuse. It is also likely that the actual number of cases are much higher owing to women's restricted mobility and the presence of husbands and other family members at home during lockdown. Only 2% sexual violence is inconsistent with BBS (2016) data, which shows 1 in 2 married women endure physical and/or sexual violence in their lifetime. The rates must be higher in lockdown, as many husband who were already depressed. They often got violent and aggressive when wives turned down their choices for any sexual activity, as a result, many men ended up forcing their wives into sexual intercourses which we can term as marital rape. Mental torture remains another unresolved issue, in fact, not even considered a form of violence by many. Women in our society are socialized to endure emotional abuse—insults, humiliation, intimidation, threats, shouting, name calling, finding fault all the times, false accusation and deception of information—silently. Thus, the actual prevalence might be higher than 47% amid lockdown (Mahpara, 2020). Economic tortures also occur frequently but remains highly underreported only apart from dowry cases. Amid massive economic fallouts and jobs losses, the actual rate of economic violence, whether in form a husband putting financial constraints on wife, depriving her of basic necessities or controlling her income, might be higher than 33%. Below, we will outline a number of factors at individual, familial, community, and societal levels and how the different level factors interact with each other and contribute to the observed increase in domestic prevalence in the pandemic context of Bangladesh.

12.6.1.1 Poverty and Unemployment

Economists project that the economic ramifications of COVID-19 pandemic are likely to push up the poverty levels through causing massive unemployment throughout the world (Sumner et al., 2020). In Bangladesh, the country was already battling against poverty. Lockdown and the related loss of livelihood can drive up the many of the catalysts which trigger DV. Nearly 36 million people have lost jobs during lockdown (Dhaka Tribune, 2020). Majority of them where men as their labour force participation is 78% in Bangladesh (BBS, 2017). Male unemployment is likely to magnify violence, physical abuse specifically because of the accelerated financial and psychological stressors in contexts where women don't have equal marital and divorce rights (Bhalotra et al., 2020). In societies with men being expected to be the bread earners, financial and psychological stressors can trigger violence as they threaten a man's authority at home making him more aggressive to regain his authority (Bhalotra et al., 2020; Buller et al., 2018).

Job loses and reduction in income gives rise to frustration and stress among men, as they are expected to be the bread earners in families. Rayhan and Akter (2021) found a positive relationship between reduction in family income and increase in IPV amid the pandemic. Some families have gone underneath the poverty line, which fostered the rate of IPV manifold. The inefficient distribution of incentive packages and relief goods worst hit masses and contributed to the decline in the socioeconomic status of certain families leaving them as half-starved or starved. Poverty and hunger along with restrictions on physical movement, social life and participation, may leave harmful impacts on the mental health conditions of men leading them to conflicts, often turned into violent against women and children. DV has not declined, even after lockdown been lifted. A survey (June 2020) found that husbands were still abusing their wives mentally, physically or sexually along with imposing financial constraints on them (MJF, 2020). Though lockdown ended, many men couldn't retrieve their jobs or other means of livelihood, which deepened their anger and frustration. Thus, they see inducing violence as the best way to vent their frustration.

As women hold jobs mostly in service or informal sector jobs, they get affected more in a crisis period than men. During Africa's Ebola outbreak, women's economic empowerment was affected negatively as the national economic fallout affected women's abilities of finding jobs in the country's informal sectors, where the jobs were already low paid and less secured (Androsik, 2020). When women face livelihoods disturbances and inability to earn income, it becomes difficult for her family to meet daily needs and services, resulting in increased mental pressure which is a potential factor behind conflict and violence (Bodrud-Doza et al., 2020). When it comes to prevention of gender-based violence, economic independence can play a pivotal role (Matjasko, et al., 2013), therefore, massive job losses can prove to be fatal for women, especially from working class. The pandemic has caused massive job losses and unemployment upheavals, particularly among women with informal, precarious jobs. Almost 357,000 workers lost their jobs in garments industry (CPD, 2021), a sector predominantly comprised of female workforce. Their existing vulnerabilities can be further exacerbated. Structural violence can be reiterated during and after a pandemic as working-class women who already reside at the lowest rung of family and social hierarchy are now being economically disempowered too. Working class women living in urban slums are at higher risk of violence, due to deepening poverty, growing hunger, congested living conditions, higher substance abuse and amounting mental stress.

12.6.1.2 Movement Restriction

Lockdown and the profound disruption caused by the unprecedented pandemic is creating panic and uncertainty about the future, which is leading towards increased level of stress, anxiety, depression and other mental health problems among people all across the world (Torales et al., 2020). Both household and personal stress—undoubtly—increases the likelihood of IPV. Family violence escalates because of a range of factors including financial insecurities, disaster-related instability, increased exposure to abusive relationships, and reduced options for social or external support (van Gelder et al., 2020). The perquisite of social isolation mandates all individuals to be confined within their homes apart from a few exceptions or emergency situations, which isolate a person from their familiar environment, routine, and support system thus magnifying the risk of violence. When someone is at risk of DV, it becomes difficult for her to contact existing support networks, such as parents, extended family members or friends as well as any social or community-based support network. Social isolation limits accessible and familiar support options that can aggravate both personal and collective vulnerabilities (van Gelder et al., 2020). That means, women were left alone in volatile home environments without any external support option. Those who were already stuck in abusive home environment were exposed to more risk of violence and danger, as family members had no choice than spending more time in close contact. Women also might feel discouraged to look for help, if children are also confined at the same home with aggregators as fear of violence leave harmful scars on children's minds.

Lockdown measures have resulted in shrinking access to help and social services, lack of privacy and fear to report, and lack of access to a phone or phone credits (UN Women et al., 2020). Survivors are not being able to reach out and talk on the phone or call for support because of the loss of privacy. The national emergency helpline in Bangladesh received 769 (March 26–April 12) calls related to VAWG, that is higher than usual, but lower compared to the actual number cases. Most of the callers to BLAST hotline reported of being trapped and unable to escape violence at their homes since during lockdown they could not travel to any friend's or relative's home; and also, the government shelters were shut down (Yasmin, 2020a). Less number of calls doesn't mean that violence decreased in any way, but rather victims were unable to call helplines as the perpetrator was always around. Besides, at least 33% women and girls have no idea regarding where they can get help if in case, they face abuse and or ill treatment by anyone including intimate partners or family members (NAWG, 2020). DV or IPV is already hidden problems in Bangladesh. On top of it, lockdowns imposed to tackle coronavirus has allowed the abusers a greater sense of freedom and advantage to whatever they feel like, as women were confined to their homes with no outside support from friends, family and relatives. Abusers can easily enforce and strengthen their control over victims by limiting their access to any form of communication with outer world. Besides, organizations dedicated to work for domestic violence are facing difficulties with providing support and reaching out to survivors due to movement restrictions (Yasmin, 2020a).

Due to stay at home orders, family members are getting to spend more time with each other. When family members spend more time with each other, it can strengthen their bonds and at the same time can also excercebate stress, tensions and altercations among members especially when the confinement takes place for long time (O'Halloran, 2020). When families spend a lot of time together, violence take place without any specific reason, a dynamic that can be attributed to human psychology (Nofziger & Kurtz, 2005). Among couples with levels of high-stress, the likelihood of IPV increase 3.5 times more than couples with levels of low-stress (Enarson, 1999). Moreover, people have lost their access to usual stress-relieving mechanisms. The public and private recreation centers and leisure activity places being shut down; people can't go places to release their stress. For example, going to gym for exercise or going to a park for a walk. When a person fails to release stress which in turn can increase tensions at household levels too that may result in increased instances of violence (Bouillon-Minois et al., 2020).

12.6.1.3 Overwhelmed Health Care

Women's health needs and other lifesaving services are often overlooked in times of crisis. In disaster times, health care resources are diverted to address the crisis which leave women with limited access to their health services and DV support services (Owen, 2020; Sochas et al., 2017). DV victims, in many cases didn't not receive enough support, as all government departments, including law enforcement agencies, are focused on containing the disease. In fact, emergency service providers couldn't offer help as they were engaged with COVID-19 relief distributions. Diversion of sexual and reproductive health services and resources to deal with the outbreak, increases women and girl's risk of facing unwanted pregnancies, unsafe abortions, maternal or new born deaths or sexually transmitted infections. In Sierra Leone, more women died of obstetric complications than the infectious disease itself during Ebola outbreak (2013–2016) (Strong & Schwartz, 2018). During COVID-19 pandemic, the health care system is overwhelmed and overloaded with the pandemic leaving crisis centers in tertiary hospitals unable to provide care for survivors of DV or IPV (UN Women, 2020). In China and Italy, centers for women were turned into homeless shelters limiting the availability of safe places for women where they can go in case, they experience violence (Fraser, 2020; Wanqing, 2020). Delayed or limited care in an overwhelmed health care system further heighten the risk of violence by manifold. While women in coastal communities of Bangladesh are facing complex health challenges due to an upsurge in IPV and shortfalls of GBV or SRH services, alongside facing a triple disaster of COVID-19, Amphan, and monsoon flooding.

12.6.1.4 Breakdown of Legal System, Police, and Impunity of Violence

During public health emergencies, women's access to legal and health care systems shrink (van Gelder et al., 2020). Even though VAWG increased alarmingly, government policies (e.g., lockdown) made it even harder for survivors to access support and legal redress due to the courts and shelter centers being temporarily shut down. The law enforcing agencies were so bogged down with relief distribution that they had no time to look into violence cases. Police were reported to overlook domestic violence claims and refused to file a charge sheet in many cases let alone investigate them (Yasmin, 2020a). ASK reported that women and girls seeking to file domestic violence complaints with police were turned away with officers refusing to accept General Diary complaints (police reports) or provide any assistance (Human Rights Watch, 2020). Family courts were not under virtual court, so the survivors did not get any support from there too.

In Bangladesh, the laws to address domestic violence are inadequate. First of all, marital rape is a grey area and not criminalized. There are two major laws to address domestic violence related cases. The Prevention of Women and Children Repression Act (2000) only recognizes domestic violence when it is related to dowry demands and not otherwise. On the other hand, Domestic Violence (Prevention and Protection) Act 2010 address all types of violence including physical, psychological, sexual and economic. However, it put less focus on prosecution and more on prevention whereas the former may have more deterrent effect. According to an ActionAid study, no case has been filed under this act in the Chief Judicial Magistrate Court in many districts of the country (Daily Star, 2020). Regardless of the pandemic, perpetrators in Bangladesh frequently enjoy rampant impunity, due to the lack of implementation of relevant laws, an ineffective criminal justice system, corruption in the law enforcement and administration sectors, and political protections for perpetrators. For instance, around 11,000 women filed domestic violence claims via the government's One-stop Crisis Centres and only 160 among them saw successful conviction of the perpetrators involved in their cases (Human Rights Watch, 2020). Given such a low rate of conviction, this not only damages the survivor of a case, but also discourage others who have experienced this violence to come forward and report their violence. In addition, during lockdown, resources for support for victims of violence have moved to online platforms and mobile applications, limiting access to poor and vulnerable groups with inadequate access to internet, phone or who have no experience in online platforms (UN Women et al., 2020).

12.6.1.5 Gender Roles and Relationship Dynamics

Disaster situations alter gender roles and responsibilities where women seem to be more vulnerable due to their assumed feminine roles to stay home, make a home and sacrifice their careers (Fothergill, 1999). Under lockdown, when school and daycare remained closed, parents need to shoulder extra responsibilities of childcare and education (Evans, 2020). In patriarchal societies, as women are expected to taking care of their children, elders and ill family members, they might end up to taking unpaid leaves or leaving their work to stay home (Women's Budget Group, 2020). The disproportionate impact of the pandemic on women's economic empowerment along with their increasing care responsibilities amplify the challenges for women trying to get out of violent relationships. The changing gender norms along with home confinement is surging household level stress and tension, thereby, resulting in increased DV.

As a consequence of safety measures, many offices in Bangladesh shifted to home office for at least 2/3 days in a week, as a result, women and men continue to work from home. Therefore, women are left with no other choice but to spend their whole day with an abusive partner being confined within toxic home environment. Besides, excursive burden of office work, care and housework reduce her ability to navigate violence leaving her more vulnerable to psychological violence and sexual coercion (Bhalotra et al., 2020). Gender role expectations, financial dependency due to job loss, financial problems at family level, confined and overcrowded home environment, failing to strike a balance between work and family lives, and not been able to adjust with the pandemic situations can create an enabling environment likely to spur DV.

In some cases, women can be at fault too. These usually happened because as we could see that lockdown caused many women, especially the working population in the professional areas, to look into the household affairs together with maintaining office work from home, and it became very difficult in maintaining proper timing for everything. This factor irritated many, causing aggression and irritation in taking double burden, that sometimes-caused severe DV in the homes. As women are primarily responsible for preparing family meals, increasing food insecurity along with other household tensions place them at great risk of violence. Not to forget the classic patriarchal women, who inflict violence and abuse against each other. Mother-in-laws, especially at rural households, often subject their daughter-in-laws to various types of violence—physical, verbal, emotional or economic—which can further exacerbate due to pandemic induced stress and poverty. Dowry demands, in order to curb household poverty and subsequent violence if a bride's parents fail to pay it, is a common scenario in many families during a crisis time. Therefore, the COVID-19 lockdown has provided more opportunities for intimate partners and other abusive family members to engage in violent activities.

12.7 Conclusion

The new global pandemic has created multitude of new and unprecedented challenges for the world to grapple with. As the search for a long-term effective vaccine is still on, the governments have no other choice but to impose preventive measures to reduce the further spread of the disease. This can result in paradoxes of social distancing, which includes issues like economic stress, mental health disorders and isolation. Although exploring the impact of COVID-19 has become a major curiosity for researchers, there has been lack of interest in examining the effects of COVID pandemic from gender perspective. COVID-19 is replicating many of the previous challenges women and girls had to encounter in emergency settings worldwide and is intensifying the vulnerabilities in current crisis situations. Social distancing provisions create different challenges for men and women. Health emergencies and related lockdowns often enhance the pre-existing gender inequalities which further excercebrate the prevalence of VAWG. This chapter has provided an explanation for the observed increase in VAWG during COVID-19 pandemic with a focus on child marriage and domestic violence—two of the widespread forms of gender-based violence in Bangladesh. By applying the social ecological framework, the study identified a number of factors at individual, familial, community, and societal levels, those interact with each other and result in increased prevalence of VAWG. Increased poverty at family level, prolonged school closures, girls pursuing positive attitude towards child marriage, the urge to save family honor, inadequate state laws and community breakdown have been identified as the main factors behind the increased risk of child marriage. While widespread poverty and unemployment, movement restrictions, overwhelmed health care system, breakdown in legal system and police, and shifting gender roles and relationship dynamics are all amplifying the stress and tensions at personal, household and community levels leading up to increased prevalence of domestic violence.

Despite emerging evidences on compounding gender disparities, issues like DV, child marriage or teenage pregnancy remain least discussed in Bangladesh's response to the pandemic situation. The government responses to the pandemic largely focus on issues of public health and economy, with minimal focus on violence, exploitation and other harmful practices. The issues such as VAWG, child marriage and DV remain completely missing from national action plan against COVID-19 pandemic. There is lack of concern over the lack of focus on the existing protection and referral systems for women and children during the health crisis. Lack of attention on women and children's issues during the pandemic is evident from the fact that the inter-ministerial national level committee that had been set up to respond to the crisis does not include the Ministry of Women and Children Affairs (Yasmin, 2020a). The government and law enforcement agencies concerned to prevent VAWG was rarely active throughout the lockdown period. There is a whole separate ministry to deal with the issues of women and children affairs in Bangladesh. The country has a stringent of laws, policies and action plans to prevent violence against women and children. We have committees set up at different levels such as district, upazila and union levels to prevent violence and child marriage. However, none of these mechanisms are working effectively as the unprecedented COVID crisis has shifted whole focus of state interventions to public health management (Yasmin, 2020b). There is also lack of publicly accessible information as to the exact number of victims who tried to seek help or reach out to existing referral systems during the pandemic. All of these reflect an apparent lack of concern to address VAWG issues at policy level.

The demands to combat pandemic induced VAWG mostly came civil society members, rights groups, and development organizations. At the same times, civil society organizations usually providing shelter and legal protection to the victims had to limit their engagement because of the provisions of social distancing. We need to keep in mind that it not possible for any organization to provide effective prevention and protection services to the survivors of violence without government agencies taking the leading in doing so (Yasmin, 2020b). To fight such problems, there is no alternative to acknowledging the extent of the gendered challenges women are facing during pandemic, re-phrasing related policies and actions and re-organizing networks so that victims can access them easily. Making resources and emergency services available to tackle the problems faced by women and girls and creating awareness about the issues from national to local level is most crucial.

12.8 Recommendations

12.8.1 Combating Child Marriage

Child marriage prevention strategies need to be incorporated in the core COVID response and recovery plans. Government should support prevention and mitigation services through proper policy formulation and resource allocation. A comprehensive multi-sectoral response is required comprised of both protection and preventive measures to end child marriage including access to education, health (physical, mental, sexual) services and social protection measures. Existing social protection programmes to eliminate child marriage should not discontinue or be interrupted in any way during the pandemic. Additional vulnerable groups should be included in social protection initiatives (e.g., cash transfers or loan schemes) to prevent school dropout rates as well as child marriage. Government officials and educators should monitor and assess the participation of female students in online classes to ensure gender parity and adapt quick strategies to reduce high dropout rates. Frequent, local context oriented and gender disaggregated data should be collected and used to design prevention and response plans. Safe, reliable and confidential channels need to be established for victims to report child marriage.

Awareness creation on child marriage and other harmful practices is crucial through setting up platforms accessible to rural girls and women. Mass media should play an important role through disseminating preventive messages on child marriage, exploitation and other harmful practices. Local women's organizations, faith-based networks, youth groups and communities should be actively engaged to rescuing girls who are at risk. Parents, community members, traditional and religious leaders should be worked with to ensure community-based response through ensuring adequate access to health, education and social protection for girls. Social stigma and exclusion of young girls resulting from the pandemic should be reduced.

12.8.2 Preventing Domestic Violence

Strategies to prevent DV need to be incorporated in the core COVID response and recovery plans. Structured support services (e.g., shelter homes for survivors) should be designed and created as essential services and allocate increased resources to them. Effective steps should be taken to increase access to existing support services across the country. Multidisciplinary staff including health care providers, psychologists, psychiatrists, social or legal service providers should be trained to address acts of violence and be linked to the protection mechanisms. Safe, reliable and trusted channels need to be established for victims to report DV. Strategies should be undertaken to spread awareness about the importance of reporting violence as an effective way to reduce the number of cases. Increased number of telephonic and online services should be established for victims who seek for any other kind of mental health support (e.g., counselling or therapy). Multi-sectoral services should be strengthened for survivors through disseminating information regarding the available services online. Both government and non-government services providers should undertake effective steps online to enhance their reach to remote survivors/ victims.

Community workers should be trained and supported to provide information on sexual and reproductive health related services and support options to DV survivors through mobile and outreach facilities. Media can play an essential role by raising awareness about DV as well as about the alternative support services available for victims during a pandemic. Increased support and resources should be directed to community-based organizations women's organization to prevent and respond to DV. Anti-violence advocacy and awareness campaigns should be strengthened with an attempt to increase male engagements.

Acknowledgements The authors would like to thank Dr. Soma Dey [Associate Professor, Department of Women and Gender Studies, University of Dhaka], for offering her valuable pieces of advice that helped the authors to develop the conceptual section of this study.

References

Afrin, T., & Zainuddin, M. (2021). Spike in child marriage in Bangladesh during COVID-19: Determinants and interventions. *Child Abuse & Neglect, 112*, 104918. https://doi.org/10.1016/j.chiabu.2020.104918

Ain O Salish Kendra (2020). *Violence against women—Domestic violence Jan-June 2020.* http://www.askbd.org/ask/2020/07/06/violence-against-women-domestic-violence-jan-june-2020/

Akel, M., Berro, J., Rahme, C., Haddad, C., Obeid, S., & Hallit, S. (2021). Violence against women during COVID-19 pandemic. *Journal of Interpersonal Violence.* https://doi.org/10.1177/088626 0521997953

Allen-Ebrahimian, B. (2020). China's domestic violence epidemic. *Axios.* https://www.axios.com/china-domestic-violence-coronavirus-quarantine-7b00c3ba-35bc-4d16-afddb76ecfb28882.html

Alqahtani, J., & Alqahtani, I. (2021). COVID-19 and child marriage: A red flag. *Journal of Clinical Nursing.* https://doi.org/10.1111/jocn.16130

Androsik, A. (2020). Gendered understanding of Ebola crisis in Sierra Leone: Lessons for COVID-19. *Population and Economics, 4*(2), 88–95. https://doi.org/10.3897/popecon.4.e53301

Antara, N. F. (2021, January 9). MJF: Over 40% increase in child marriages in 2020. *Dhaka Tribune.* https://www.dhakatribune.com/bangladesh/2021/01/09/mjf-44-increase-in-child-marriages-in-2020

Arnab, A. T., & Siraj, M. S. (2020). Child marriage in Bangladesh: Policy and ethics. *Bangladesh Journal of Bioethics, 11*(1), 24–34. https://doi.org/10.3329/bioethics.v11i1.49193

Bangladesh Bureau of Statistics. (2016). *Report on violence against women (VAW) survey 2015.*

Bangladesh Bureau of Statistics. (2017). *Labour force survey 2016-2017.* Ministry of Planning.

Bangladesh Bureau of Statistics. (2020). *Labour force survey 2017.*

Bangladesh Bureau of Statistics & UNICEF Bangladesh. (2019). *Progotir pathey, Bangladesh multiple indicator cluster survey 2019, survey findings report.*

Bellizzi, S., Lorettu, L., Farina, G., Bubbico, L., Ferlito, S., Cegolon, A., Pichierri, G., & Cegolon, L. (2021). Humanitarian crises and child-marriage: Historical recurrent interrelated events. *Journal of Global Health, 11*, 03112. https://doi.org/10.7189/jogh.11.03112

Bhalotra, S., Kambhampati, U., Rawlings, S., & Siddique, Z. (2020*). Intimate partner violence: The influence of job opportunities for men and women* (Policy Research Working Paper No. 9118). https://openknowledge.worldbank.org/handle/10986/33232

Bhattacharjee, P. P. & Palma, P. (2021, April 21). 'Lockdown' extended till May 5. *The Daily Star.* https://www.thedailystar.net/frontpage/news/lockdown-extended-till-may-5-2084353

Bodrud-Doza, M., Shammi, M., Bahlman, L., Islam, A. R. M. T., & Rahman, M. M. (2020). Psychosocial and socio-economic crisis in Bangladesh due to COVID-19 pandemic: A perception-based Assessment. *Frontiers Public Health, 8*(341). https://doi.org/10.3389/fpubh.2020.00341

Bouillon-Minois, J. B., Clinchamps, M., & Dutheil, F. (2020). Coronavirus and quarantine: Catalysts of domestic violence. *Violence against Women.* https://doi.org/10.1177/1077801220935194

Brac. (2020). *New data reveals increased pressure on teenage girls in Bangladesh to submit to child marriage amid the COVID-19 pandemic.* https://bracusa.org/new-data-reveals-increased-pressure-on-girls-in-bangladesh/

Briggs, H. E., & Ngo, T. D. (2020). *The health, economic, and social effect of Covid-19 and its response on gender and sex: A literature review.* https://doi.org/10.31899/pgy14.1031

Bronfenbrenner, U., & Morris, P. (1998). The ecology of developmental process. In W. Damon & R. M. Lerner (Eds.), *Handbook of child psychology* (pp. 993–1028). Wiley.

Buller, A. M., Peterman, A., Ranganathan, M., Bleile, A., Hidrobo, M., & Heise, L. (2018). A mixed-method review of cash transfers and intimate partner violence in low-and middle-income countries. *World Bank Research Observer, 33*, 218–258. https://doi.org/10.1093/wbro/lky002

Centre for Policy Dialogue. (2021). *CPD-MiB study on vulnerability: Resilience and recovery in the RMG sector in view of COVID pandemic: Findings from the enterprise survey.* https://cpd.org.bd/wp-content/uploads/2021/01/Presentation-on-Vulnerabiliies-Resilience-and-Recovery-in-the-RMG-Enterprsies-.pdf

Chandan, J. S., Taylor, J., Bradbury-Jones, C., Nirantharakumar, K., Kane, E., & Bandyopadhyay, S. (2020). COVID-19: A public health approach to manage domestic violence is needed. *The Lancet. Public health, 5*(6), e309. https://doi.org/10.1016/S2468-2667(20)30112-2

Daily Star. (2020, December 3). *Domestic violence prevention law: Mostly ineffective, a decade on: Research*. https://www.thedailystar.net/city/news/mostly-ineffective-decade-research-2004881

Davies, S. E., & Bennett, B. (2016). A gendered human rights analysis of Ebola and Zika: Locating gender in global health emergencies. *International Affairs, 92*(5), 1041–1060. https://doi.org/10.1111/1468-2346.12704

Deluca, S., Mitchell, B., Papageorge, N., & Coleman, J. (2020). The unequal cost of social distancing. *Johns Hopkins coronavirus resource Center*. https://coronavirus.jhu.edu/from-our-experts/the-unequal-cost-of-social-distancing

Dercon, S. (2002). Income risk, coping strategies, and safety nets. *The World Bank Research Observer, 17*(2), 141–166.

Dewi, L. P. R. K., & Dartango, T. (2019). Natural disasters and girl's vulnerability: Is child marriage a coping strategy of economic shocks in Indonesia? *An International Interdisciplinary Journal for Research, Policy and Care, 14*(1), 24–35. https://doi.org/10.1080/17450128.2018.1546025

Dhaka Tribune. (2020, July 16). *Covid-19 shatters Bangladesh's dream of eradicating poverty*. https://www.dhakatribune.com/business/economy/2020/07/16/covid-19-shatters-bangladesh-s-dream-of-eradicating-poverty

Dhaka Tribune. (2021a, March 28). *Child marriage up 13% during Covid-19 pandemic in Bangladesh*. https://www.dhakatribune.com/bangladesh/law-rights/2021/03/28/child-marriage-up-13-during-covid-19-pandemic-in-bangladesh

Dhaka Tribune. (2021b, March 31). *Domestic violence: 30% became victims during pandemic*. https://www.dhakatribune.com/bangladesh/2021/03/31/30-of-domestic-violence-survivors-faced-violence-for-the-first-time-during-pandemic

Ekweonu, C. L. (2020). Newspaper coverage of domestic violence against women during COVID-19 lockdown. *Journal of Communication and Media Studies, 1*(2), 1–14.

Emon, E. K. H., Alif, A. R., & Islam, M. S. (2020). Impact of COVID-19 on the institutional education system and its associated students in Bangladesh. *Asian Journal of Education and Social Studies, 11*(2), 34–46.

Enarson, E. (1999). Violence against women in disasters: A study of domestic violence programs in the United States and Canada. *Violence against Women, 5*(7), 742–768.

Evans D. (2020, March 16). How will COVID-19 affect women and girls in low- and middle-income countries? *Center for Global Development*. https://www.cgdev.org/blog/how-will-covid-19-affect-women-and-girls-low-andmiddle-income-countries

Fothergill, A. (1999). Women's roles in a disaster. *Applied Behavioral Science Review, 7*(2), 125–143.

Fraser, E. (2020). *Impact of COVID-19 pandemic on violence against women and girls*. VAWG Helpdesk.

Frayer, L. & S. Pathak (2020). India's lockdown puts strain on call centers. *National Public Radio*. https://www.npr.org/2020/04/24/841698386/indias-lockdown-puts-strain-on-call-centers

Freccero, J., & Taylor, A. (2021). *Child marriage in humanitarian crises: Girls and parents speak out on Risk and protective factors, decision-making, and solutions*. https://resourcecentre.savethechildren.net/document/child-marriage-humanitarian-crises-girls-and-parents-speak-out-risk-and-protective-factors/

Fulu, E., & Miedema, S. (2015). Violence against women: Globalizing the integrated ecological model. *Violence against Women, 21*(12), 1431–1455. https://doi.org/10.1177/1077801215596244

Gashaw, B. T., Schei, B., & Magnus, J. H. (2018). Social ecological factors and intimate partner violence in pregnancy. *PloS One, 13*(3), e0194681. https://doi.org/10.1371/journal.pone.0194681

Human Rights Watch. (2020). *"I Sleep in My Own Deathbed": Violence against women and girls in Bangladesh: Barriers to legal recourse and support*. https://www.hrw.org/report/2020/10/29/i-sleep-my-own-deathbed/violence-against-women-and-girls-bangladesh-barriers

Heise, L. L. (1998). Violence against women: An integrated, ecological framework. *Violence against Women, 4*(3), 262–290. https://doi.org/10.1177/1077801298004003002

Ince Yenilmez, M. (2020). The Covid-19 pandemic and the struggle to tackle gender-based violence. *The Journal of Adult Protection, 22*(6), 391–399. https://doi.org/10.1108/JAP-07-2020-0029

John, N., Casey, S. E., Carino, C., & McGovern, T. (2020). Lessons never learned: Crisis and gender-based violence. *Developing World Bioeth, 20*(2), 65–68. https://doi.org/10.1111/dewb.12261

Jones, N., Gebeyehu, Y., Gezahegne, K., Iyasu, A., Workneh, F., & Yadete, W. (2020). *Child marriage risks in the context of covid-19 in Ethiopia.* Gender and Adolescence: Global Evidence. https://odi.org/en/publications/child-marriage-risks-in-the-context-of-covid-19-in-ethiopia/

Kamal, S. M. M. (2010). Geographical variations and contextual effect on child marriage in Bangladesh. *Pakistan Journal of Women's Studies, 17*(2), 37–57.

Kamal, S. M. M., Hassan, C. H., Alam, G. H., & Ying, Y. (2014). Child marriage in Bangladesh: Trends and determinants.*Journal of Biosocial Science*, 1-20. https://doi.org/10.1017/S00219320 13000746

Logan, M. & Maharjan, S. S. (2020, December 20). Nepal child marriages spike during pandemic. *Nepal Times.* https://www.nepalitimes.com/latest/nepal-child-marriages-spike-during-pandemic/

Mahase, E. (2020). Covid-19: EU states report 60% rise in emergency calls about domestic violence. *British Medical Journal, 369.* https://doi.org/10.1136/bmj.m1872

Mahpara, P. (2020, April 7). *Quarantine in home or prison? Domestic violence in the time of COVID-19 and what it holds for Bangladesh.* https://bigd.bracu.ac.bd/quarantine-in-home-or-prison-domestic-violence-in-the-time-of-covid-19-and-what-it-holds-for-bangladesh/

Makino, M., Shonchoy, A. S., & Wahhaj, Z. (2021). *Early effects of the COVID-19 lockdown on children in rural Bangladesh.* University of Kent.

Matjasko, J. L., Niolon, P. H., & Valle, L. A. (2013). The role of economic factors and economic support in preventing and escaping from intimate partner violence. *The Journal of the Association for Public Policy Analysis and Management, 32*(1), 122–128. https://doi.org/10.1002/pam.21666

Manusher Jonno Foundation. (2020). *Violence against women and children: COVID 19 A telephone survey: Initiative of Manusher Jonno Foundation survey period: July 2020.* http://www.manusherj onno.org/wp-content/uploads/2020/10/Report_of_Telephone_Survey_on_VAW_July_2020.pdf

Marcell, A. V., Morgan, A. R., Sanders, R., Lunardi, N., Pilgrim, N. A., Jennings, J. M., Page, K. R., Loosier, P. S., & Dittus, P. J. (2017). The socio ecology of sexual and reproductive health care use among young urban minority males. *The Journal of Adolescent Health: Official Publication of the Society for Adolescent Medicine, 60*(4), 402–410. https://doi.org/10.1016/j.jadohealth.2016.11.014

Monsoor, T. (2003). Dowry problem in Bangladesh: Legal and socio-cultural perspectives. *The Dhaka University Studies, XIV*(1), I-I6.

Multiple Indicator Cluster Survey. (2019). *Survey findings report.* Government of the People's Republic of Bangladesh.

Needs Assessment Working Group. (2020). *COVID-19: Bangladesh, multi-sectoral anticipatory impact and needs analysis.* https://reliefweb.int/sites/reliefweb.int/files/resources/covid_nawg_a nticipatory_impacts_and_needs_analysis.pdf

Neumayer, E., & Plumper, T. (2008). The gendered nature of natural disasters: The impact of catastrophic events on the gender gap in life expectancy, 1981–2002. *Annals of the Association of American Geographers, 97*(3), 551–563. https://doi.org/10.1111/j.1467-8306.2007.00563.x

Nofziger, S., & Kurtz, D. (2005). Violent lives: A lifestyle model linking exposure to violence to juvenile violent offending. *Journal of Research in Crime and Delinquency, 42*(1), 3–26. https://doi.org/10.1177/0022427803262061

O'Halloran, M. (2020, April 26). *Covid-19: 'Pressure cooker' environment leading to family tensions. The Irish* https://www.irishtimes.com/news/ireland/irish-news/covid-19-pressure-coo kerenvironment-leading-to-family-tensions-1.4238442

Onyango, M. A., Resnick, K., Davis, A., & Shah, R. R. (2019). Gender-based violence among adolescent girls and young women: A neglected consequence of the West African Ebola outbreak: Medical, anthropological, and public health perspectives. In D. Schwartz, J. Anoko, & S. Abramowitz (Eds.), *Pregnant in the time of Ebola: Women and their children in the 2013–2015 West African epidemic* (pp. 121–132). Springer Cham.

Owen L. (2020, March 8). Five ways the coronavirus is hitting women in Asia. *BBC News.* https://www.bbc.com/news/worldasia-51705199

Parkinson, D., & Zara, C. (2013). The hidden disaster: Domestic violence in the aftermath of natural disaster. *Australian Journal of Emergency Management, 28*(2), 28–35.

Paul, P. (2019). Effects of education and poverty on the prevalence of girl child marriage in India: A district–level analysis. *Children and Youth Services Review, 100*, 16–21. https://doi.org/10.1016/j.childyouth.2019.02.033

Paul, P., & Mondal, D. (2021). Child marriage in India: A human rights violation during the COVID-19 pandemic. *Asia-Pacific Journal of Public Health, 33*(1), 162–163. https://doi.org/10.1177/1010539520975292

Peyton. (2020). Teen pregnancy risk rises as schools shut for coronavirus in Africa. *Thomson Reuters Foundation.* https://news.trust.org/item/20200319115906-eieyl/

Piquero, A. R., Riddell, J. R., Bishopp, S. A., Narvey, C., Reid, J. A., & Piquero, N. L. (2020). Staying Home, Staying Safe? A Short-Term Analysis of COVID-19 on Dallas Domestic Violence. *American Journal of Criminal Justice*, 1–35. https://doi.org/10.1007/s12103-020-09531-7

Prothom Alo. (2021, March 21). *Bangladesh ranks 4th in violence against women by intimate partner.* https://en.prothomalo.com/bangladesh/bangladesh-ranks-4th-in-violence-against-women-by-intimate-partner

Raha, S. A., Rana, M. S., Mamun, S. A., Anik, M. H., Roy, P., Alam, F., & Sultan, M. (2021). *Revisiting the impact of covid-19 on adolescents in urban slums in Dhaka, Bangladesh: Round 2.* Gender & Adolescence: Global Evidence

Rahiem M. (2021). COVID-19 and the surge of child marriages: A phenomenon in Nusa Tenggara Barat, Indonesia. *Child Abuse & Neglect, 118*, 105168. https://doi.org/10.1016/j.chiabu.2021.105168

Rayhan, I., & Akter, K. (2021). Prevalence and associated factors of intimate partner violence (IPV) against women in Bangladesh amid COVID-19 pandemic. *Heliyon, 7*(3), e06619. https://doi.org/10.1016/j.heliyon.2021.e06619

Redding, E. M., Ruiz-Cantero, M. T., Fernández-Sáez, J., & Guijarro-Garvi, M. (2017). Gender inequality and violence against women in Spain, 2006–2014: Towards a civilized society. *Gaceta Sanitaria, 31*(2), 82–88. https://doi.org/10.1016/j.gaceta.2016.07.025

Rob, U., & Mutahara, M. (2001). Premarital sex among urban adolescents in Bangladesh. *International Quarterly of Community Health Education, 20*(1), 103–111.

Roy, N., Amin, M. B., Maliha, M. J., Sarker, B., Aktarujjaman, M., Hossain, E., & Talukdar, G. (2021). Prevalence and factors associated with family planning during COVID-19 pandemic in Bangladesh: A cross-sectional study. *Plos One, 16*(9), e0257634. https://doi.org/10.1371/journal.pone.0257634

Sakib, S. M. N. (2021, March 22). Bangladesh: Child marriage rises manifold in pandemic. *Anadolu Agency.* https://www.aa.com.tr/en/asia-pacific/bangladesh-child-marriage-rises-manifold-in-pandemic/2184001

Sánchez, O. R., Vale, D. B., Rodrigues, L., & Surita, F. G. (2020). Violence against women during the COVID-19 pandemic: An integrative review. *International Journal of Gynecology and Obstetrics, 151*(2), 180–187. https://doi.org/10.1002/ijgo.13365

Save the Children. (2020). *The global childhood report 2020: How COVID-19 is putting progress in peril.* https://www.savethechildren.de/fileadmin/user_upload/Downloads_Dokumente/Berichte_Studien/2020/Global_Girlhood_Report_2020__Africa_version_.pdf

Shawon, A. A. (2020, March 27). Covid-19: Bangladesh likely to end general holiday on May. *Dhaka Tribune.* https://www.dhakatribune.com/bangladesh/2020/05/27/state-minister-update-of-lockdown-coming-soon

Sifat R. I. (2020). Sexual violence against women in Bangladesh during the COVID-19 pandemic. *Asian Journal of Psychiatry, 54*, 102455. https://doi.org/10.1016/j.ajp.2020.102455

Sochas, L., Channon, A. A., & Nam, S. (2017). Counting indirect crisis-related deaths in the context of a low-resilience health system: the case of maternal and neonatal health during the Ebola epidemic in Sierra Leone. *Health Policy and Planning, 32*(suppl_3), iii32–iii39. https://doi.org/10.1093/heapol/czx108

Strong, A. E., & Schwartz, D. A. (2018). Effects of the West African Ebola epidemic on health care of pregnant women: Stigmatization with and without infection. *Pregnant in the Time of Ebola: Women and Their Children in the 2013–2015 West African Epidemic*, 11–30. https://doi.org/10.1007/978-3-319-97637-2_2

Sumner, A., Hoy, C., & Ortiz-Juarez, E. (2020). *Estimates of the impact of COVID-19 on global poverty* (WIDER Working Paper No. 2020/43). https://www.wider.unu.edu/publication/estimates-impact-covid-19-global-poverty

Tembon, M., & Fort, L. (2008). *Girls' education in the 21st century: Gender equality, empowerment, and economic growth*. World Bank.

Torales, J., O'Higgins, M., Castaldelli-Maia, J. M., & Ventriglio, A. (2020). The outbreak of COVID-19 coronavirus and its impact on global mental health. *The International Journal of Social Psychiatry, 66*(4), 317–320. https://doi.org/10.1177/0020764020915212

United Nations Children's Fund. (2020a). *Child marriage threatens the lives, well-being and futures of girls around the world*. https://www.unicef.org/protection/child-marriage

United Nations Children's Fund. (2020b). *Child marriage is a violation of human rights, but is all too common*. https://data.unicef.org/topic/child-protection/child-marriage/

United Nations Children's Fund. (2020c). *Ending child marriage: A profile of progress in Bangladesh*.

United Nations Children's Fund. (2021). *COVID-19: A threat to progress against child marriage*.

United Nations ESCAP. (2020). *The covid-19 pandemic and violence against women in Asia and the Pacific*.

United Nations Population Fund. (2020). *Millions more cases of violence, child marriage, female genital mutilation, unintended pregnancy expected due to the COVID-19 pandemic*. https://www.unfpa.org/news/millions-more-cases-violence-child-marriage-female-genital-mutilation-unintended-pregnancies

UN Women. (2020). *COVID-19 and violence against women and girls: Addressing the shadow*.

UN Women, UNFPA, NCLW, et al. (2020). *Gender alert on COVID-19 in Lebanon*. https://lebanon.unfpa.org/sites/default/files/pub-pdf/gender%20alert%20on%20covidlebanon%20issue%203english.pdf

Uttom, S. & Rozario, R. (2020). Covid-19 disrupts education in rural Bangladesh. *UCA News*. https://www.ucanews.com/news/covid-19-disrupts-education-in-rural-bangladesh/87976

Van Gelder, N., Peterman, A., Potts, A., O'Donnell, M., Thompson, K., Shah, N., & Oertelt-Prigione, S. (2020). COVID-19: Reducing the risk of infection might increase the risk of intimate partner violence. *EClinicalMedicine*. https://doi.org/10.1016/j.eclinm.2020.100348

Wagers, S. (2020). Domestic violence growing in wake of Coronavirus outbreak. *The Conversation* https://theconversation.com/domestic-violence-growing-in-wake-of-coronavirus-outbreak-135598

Wanqing Z. (2020, March 2). Domestic violence cases surge during COVID-19 epidemic. *Sixth Tone*. http://www.sixthtone.com/news/1005253/domestic-violence-cases-surge-during-covid-19-epidemic

World Bank. (2017). *Educating girls, ending child marriage*. https://www.worldbank.org/en/news/immersive-story/2017/08/22/educating-girls-ending-child-marriage

Women's Budget Group. (2020). *UK policy briefings: Covid-19, gender and other equality issues*. https://wbg.org.uk/wp-content/uploads/2020/03/FINAL-Covid-19-briefing.pdf

World Bank. (2020). *Gender dimensions of the COVID pandemic*. https://openknowledge.worldbank.org/bitstream/handle/10986/33622/Gender-Dimensions-of-the-COVID-19-Pandemic.pdf

World Health Organization. (2020). *Naming the coronavirus disease and the virus that causes it.* https://www.who.int/emergencies/diseases/novel-coronavirus-2019/technical-guidance/naming-the-coronavirus-disease-(covid-2019)-and-the-virus-that-causes-it

World Health Organization. (2021). *Violence against women [key facts].* https://www.who.int/newsroom/fact-sheets/detail/violence-against-women

World Vision. (2021a). *Breaking the chain: Empowering girls and communities to end child marriages during COVID-19 and beyond.* https://www.wvi.org/publications/report/it-takes-world/end-child-marriage/breaking-chain-empowering-girls-and-communities-end-child

World Vison. (2021b, May 20). *Child marriage has more than doubled during the COVID-19 pandemic with numbers set to increase, World Vision warns.* https://www.wvi.org/newsroom/it-takes-world/child-marriage-has-more-doubled-during-covid-19-pandemic-numbers-set

Yasmin, T. (2020a). *A review of the effectiveness of the new legal regime to prevent child marriages in Bangladesh: Call for law reform.* Girls Not Brides & Plan International.

Yasmin, T. (2020b, July 25). Violence against women during Covid-19: Accepting the threat as 'real' is paramount. *Daily Star.* https://www.thedailystar.net/opinion/news/violence-against-women-during-covid-19-accepting-the-threat-real-paramount-1935633

Index

A
Academic knowledge, 139
Additional vulnerable groups, 219
Administrative rationality, 7, 8, 106
Adults, 2, 142, 203, 208, 209
Africa, 3, 4, 28, 69, 79, 80, 90, 91, 96, 153, 154, 182, 188
Aftermath, 3
Alleviation, 204
America First, 104
Anxiety, 2, 6, 10, 104, 184, 214
Arab Gulf states, 17
Asian Development Bank (ADB), 15, 20, 37
Association of South East Asian Nations (ASEAN), 14, 18, 21, 83, 88, 91
Atma Nirbhar Bharat, 104
Austrian Armed Forces, 50
Austrian Broadcasting Corporation, 63
Auto-ethnography, 9, 138–140, 143
Aviation, 4, 33, 104

B
Bangkok, 37, 96
Bangladesh, 34–37, 39, 80, 86, 87, 89, 199–202, 204–209, 211–218
Bay of Bengal, 36
Beijing, 18, 19, 72, 80, 81
Belarus, 83
Belt and Road Initiative (BRI), 17–19, 84
Big power rivalry, 7, 14, 17
Biochemical Oxygen Demand (BOD), 34
Biopolitics, 51
Black Sea, 17

Brazil, 14, 21, 28, 33, 79, 80, 87, 89, 96, 145, 211
Brazil Russia India China South Africa (BRICS), 14, 21
Bubonic plague, 115, 116
Buddhist tourists, 184
Bureaucratic rationality, 105, 108, 111–113
Business, 3, 6, 35, 55, 59, 85, 93, 98, 104, 141, 176, 189

C
Canada, 21, 33, 89, 90, 96
Cancellation, 184, 186, 190–192
Capitalization, 59
Casualization, 115
Catastrophic earthquake, 186
Child marriage, 10, 200–210, 218, 219
Child Marriage Restraint Rules, 209
Children, 2, 54, 112, 124, 126–132, 142, 143, 193, 194, 200, 203, 205–210, 213, 214, 217, 218
China, 6, 8, 14, 17–22, 28, 29, 32–34, 37, 39, 52, 63, 71, 79–82, 85, 86, 88, 90, 93, 95–98, 152, 155, 169, 171, 182, 187, 215
Churches, 10, 155, 183, 184
Civic engagements, 7, 8, 105
Civil war, 50, 63, 78
Commercial, 33, 38, 55, 84, 90
Commercial sector, 3, 184
Commitments, 40, 43, 52, 88, 89, 93, 109, 112, 113, 124, 146, 172, 174–176, 187
Community, 4, 7, 8, 14, 23, 24, 81, 82, 90, 93, 94, 105, 106, 119, 120, 124, 127,

© The Editor(s) (if applicable) and The Author(s), under exclusive license to Springer Nature Singapore Pte Ltd. 2022
S. Roy and D. Nandy (eds.), *Understanding Post-COVID-19 Social and Cultural Realities*, https://doi.org/10.1007/978-981-19-0809-5

130–132, 141, 152, 156, 159, 161, 169, 171, 175, 176, 183, 184, 190, 202, 203, 205, 207, 208, 213, 218
Community responsibility, 4
Conflict, 14, 16, 17, 21, 23, 64, 128, 183, 185, 200, 203, 204, 213
Congo, 83
Contextualizing, 160
Contractualization, 115
Coronavirus, 4, 71, 81, 86, 88, 92, 93, 113, 119, 145, 152–154, 157, 159, 160, 182, 184, 187, 191, 200–202, 206, 215
Covaxin vaccine, 94
Cultural, 10, 56, 144, 183, 185, 187, 190, 193–195
Cusco city, 142
Cyber space, 167

D

Deconstruction, 152–154, 156
Dependencies, 6, 82, 85, 152, 217
De-stigmatisation strategies, 161
Dipawali, 190
Diplomatic relations, 6, 77, 80, 82
Disciplinary actions, 7
Discrimination, 3, 10, 16, 185, 192, 193, 195, 200, 201, 212
Dissolved Oxygen (DO), 34
Domestic, 4, 8, 34, 37, 61, 85, 90, 95, 96, 98, 186, 195, 210, 212, 213, 215, 216
Domestic policy, 172

E

Ebola virus epidemic, 50
Economic, 2–4, 6, 7, 9, 15–20, 22, 23, 31, 50, 57, 59, 61, 66, 67, 72, 79, 81, 85, 87, 88, 92, 93, 96, 97, 104, 111, 113, 120, 125, 129, 131, 133, 144, 145, 155, 168, 175, 176, 183, 185, 189, 192, 200, 204–206, 210, 212, 213, 216, 217
Economic activities, 32, 35, 57, 59, 60, 113, 205
Economic growth, 4, 31, 41, 62, 67, 81
Egypt, 89, 91, 92
Emergence trends, 5
Emotional, 64, 71, 194, 212, 217
Employees, 5, 60, 69, 85, 188, 192
Endorsements, 108, 172, 173

Environment/environmental, 2, 6, 7, 28–33, 35–43, 52, 63, 94, 144, 160, 173, 189, 194, 200, 202, 203, 210, 214, 217
Epidemic Disease Act, 115
Ethnomethodological, 107
European Commissioner for Budget and Administration, 66
European Environmental Agency (EEA), 33
European Union (EU), 8, 51–53, 56, 58, 60–72, 90, 93, 96, 174
Exemplified, 125
EXIM Bank, 88
Expenditure, 60, 62
Extermination, 112

F

Federal Chancellery, 63
Federal President, 55
Financial difficulties, 4
Financial service, 59
Foreign policy, 8, 18, 21, 22, 77, 78, 86, 93, 97, 172
Framework, 3, 21, 31, 57, 79, 107, 112, 118, 166, 170, 173, 174, 176, 201, 202, 209, 218

G

G-7, 21, 22, 81
G-20, 93
Ganga, 34
Gender, 8–10, 15, 123–126, 131–133, 192, 193, 200–204, 206, 208, 210–213, 217–219
Gender inequality, 124, 132, 133, 200, 203, 210, 218
Generalizable, 161
German Rail Authority, 112
Germany, 14, 21, 28, 36, 53, 58, 60, 62, 65–67, 96, 112, 172
Ghana, 89, 91, 92
Girls, 10, 127, 132, 200, 201, 203–209, 215, 216, 218, 219
Global change, 2, 3, 33
Global Health Institute, 90
Global human disaster, 31
Global order, 6, 14–17, 21–24, 77, 78, 93, 98
Global response, 43, 192
Global society, 2, 29, 176
Global value chains (GVCs), 6

Index 229

Global war on Corona, 17
Governance, 2, 4, 6, 15, 20, 105, 114, 118, 119
Greater Eurasia, 17, 18
Green House Gases (GHGs), 33, 36, 41, 42
Green public transportation system, 41
Gross Domestic Product (GDP), 15, 36, 60–62, 66, 67, 92, 185, 186, 195

H
Hanoi, 37
Healthcare, 2, 6, 24, 37, 88, 91, 152, 194
Health care workers, 124, 187
Health services, 105, 124, 125, 131, 210, 215
Health Silk Road, 19
Healthy, 2, 14, 30, 32, 41, 59, 119, 170, 172, 195
Heritage, 92, 155, 183, 185, 187, 188, 190–192, 194, 195
High-risk, 15, 132, 200, 203, 207
Hindu, 184, 191
Historical, 14, 108, 116, 132, 139, 145, 160, 166, 167, 170, 183, 187, 188, 192, 194, 195, 203
HIV, 91, 138
Homeland, 143
Hong Kong, 18, 20, 81
Horrific, 16, 112
Households, 9, 38, 61, 126, 129, 131–133, 186, 200, 201, 205, 206, 214, 215, 217, 218
Human diffusion, 7
Humanitarian assistance, 78, 79, 84, 94
Human resources, 5, 22
Human rights, 15, 105, 173, 192, 203
Hungary, 49, 53, 58, 65, 67
Hydroxychloroquine (HCQ), 22, 79, 80, 84, 87, 88, 91, 93, 97
Hygiene, 105, 160

I
Illicit, 189
Immunization, 96, 98
India, 6, 8, 9, 14, 16, 18, 21, 22, 28, 33–35, 37, 39, 77–98, 106, 107, 113, 114, 117, 119, 127, 176, 184, 187, 190, 193, 204, 211
Indian Ocean Region (IOR), 79, 83, 84, 98
Indistinguishable, 64, 112
Indonesia, 35, 88
Indo-Pacific, 17, 21, 83, 91, 95

INGOs, 6
Interconnected world, 104, 174, 175
Interdependence, 31
Intergovernmental, 187
International Council on Museums (ICOM), 188
International economic order, 15
International Energy Agency (IEA), 33, 194
International flights, 4, 33, 193
International Solar Alliance, 78
Inter-personal relations, 154
Intimate Partner Violence (IPV), 202, 210, 211, 213–216
Inward nationalistic tendencies, 168
Iran, 17, 18, 83, 174
Isolation, 2, 4, 7, 8, 70, 81, 93, 104, 105, 155, 168, 194, 207, 210, 214, 218
Italy, 21, 28, 33, 34, 36, 38, 53, 54, 58, 65–67, 142, 215

J
Japan, 6, 8, 14, 20, 21, 83, 88, 90, 95, 168, 190
Job markets, 2
Joint Comprehensive Plan of Action (JCPOA), 174

K
Kathmandu, 191
Kenya, 8, 91, 92, 125–127, 130–133, 188
Kilifi County, 8, 125, 126, 129–131
Koro ti lo, 9, 155, 157
Kuala Lumpur, 37

L
Labour market, 4, 8, 51, 52, 60, 61
Lack of security, 10, 205
Landlocked, 187
Latin America, 14, 21, 79, 96, 98, 138, 145, 190
Left behind, 31, 125, 175
Lethal potential, 113
LGBTI, 192
Liberalism, 16
Libya, 17, 91
Lifestyle, 39, 41, 128, 160, 185
Literacy, 160
Living, 2, 9, 20, 30, 35, 55, 57, 116, 138–141, 143–145, 155, 184, 188, 190–192, 201, 204, 214

230   Index

Lockdown, 2, 6–8, 10, 16, 32–38, 55–57,
    61, 63, 65, 67, 69, 70, 78, 79, 84, 85,
    104–106, 113, 118, 125, 132, 139,
    154, 155, 182–195, 200–202, 206,
    208, 210–218
Loopholes, 2

M

Madagascar, 79, 83, 97
Malaysia, 35, 88
Maldives, 35, 79, 80, 83, 84, 86, 88, 89, 97
Management, 37–39, 42, 55, 59, 66, 91,
    106–108, 110, 117–120, 159, 166,
    201, 219
Maternal health, 9, 124–127, 130–133
Maternal health services (MHS), 8,
    124–127, 129–133
MEA, 80
Media, 23, 50, 51, 56, 63, 65, 68, 70, 71,
    105, 118, 137, 139, 153, 156, 160,
    184, 194, 201, 205, 209, 211, 219,
    220
Methodology, 107, 138, 153, 166, 167,
    182, 202
Middle East, 17, 19, 50, 69, 80, 89, 190
Midwife, 127, 129
Military doctor, 50
Mini-lateralism, 9
Minimax strategies, 131
Modi, Narendra, 21, 22, 78, 79, 81, 86, 87,
    94, 95
Morocco, 80, 87, 89, 91, 92
Moscow, 19
Multidimensional, 4
Multilateralism, 6, 9, 21, 23, 93, 104,
    166–176

N

Neoliberal governance, 8, 114, 119, 120
Nepal, 10, 79, 86, 87, 89, 90, 182–187,
    189–191, 193, 203
Nepali Rupees, 185, 186
'New normal' lifestyle, 116
Newspaper, 14, 50, 203
New World Order, 14, 22
NGOs, 6, 64, 205, 208
Nigeria, 9, 91, 92, 152–157, 159–161
Nigerians, 9, 152, 155, 156, 159
Nitrogen Dioxide (NO_2), 33
Non-communist country, 82
Non-existent, 112, 119, 200, 207
North America, 50, 69, 71

North Atlantic Treaty Organisation
    (NATO), 14
North Korea, 17
Norway, 21, 55
Novel Corona Virus, 7, 14

O

One Belt, 18
'One Dimensional State', 109
One Road, 18
Organizations, 5, 7, 14, 24, 29, 40, 64, 104,
    107, 109, 111–113, 167, 171,
    173–175, 183, 187, 188, 203, 205,
    208, 211, 215, 219, 220
Outbreak, 2–4, 6–8, 14, 16, 32, 37, 50, 52,
    66, 67, 71, 81, 83, 84, 86, 91, 104,
    124, 132, 133, 182, 185, 200–204,
    207, 208, 210, 213, 215

P

Pandemic, 1–10, 14–24, 28, 29, 31–34,
    36–43, 50–52, 57, 59, 61–72, 77–83,
    85–95, 97, 98, 104–108, 113–120,
    124–127, 130–133, 138–140,
    142–145, 152–156, 159–161,
    166–176, 182–186, 188–195,
    199–220
Panic, 2, 10, 64, 130, 187, 214
Pareto, Vilfredo, 114, 115, 117, 118
Parkinson, C.N., 107
Parkinson, D., 210
Pashupati Area Development Trust
    (PADT), 184, 185
Perplexity, 113, 115
Pharmacy of the world, 22, 79, 89, 91, 94
Phycycological impact, 10
Physical harm, 32, 212
Pilgrimage, 183, 184
Pilgrims, 195
Poland, 53, 58, 65, 67, 96
Policy -dilemma, 110
Poor mothers, 133
Poor people, 3, 206
Population, 2, 3, 5, 8, 9, 20, 31, 54, 56, 57,
    64, 68–71, 90, 95, 123, 125,
    143–146, 152, 161, 168, 192, 193,
    200, 208, 211, 217
Postcolonial society, 113, 115, 117
Post-World War II, 166, 173
Psychological stress, 32, 213
Public health emergency, 28
Public institutions, 4, 118

Index 231

Public-Private-Partnership, 115

Q
Quad, 21, 88, 90, 91, 95, 97, 98
Qualitative analysis, 166

R
Regional Comprehensive Economic
 Partnership (RECP), 19
Regional multilateralism, 9
Religious, 10, 153–156, 159, 183–185, 190,
 195, 220
Revenues, 2, 60, 62, 188, 190, 192, 195
Robust multilateral world, 9
Rural migration, 188
Rwanda, 89, 91, 92

S
Safeguard human beings, 14
Sanitizers, 38, 88, 187
SARS-CoV-2 virus, 1, 29, 37–39, 106, 182,
 202
Sea Lines of Communication (SLOCs), 84
Serum Institute of India (SII), 89
Sexual, 124, 133, 200–203, 207–213,
 215–217, 219, 220
Seychelles, 79, 80, 83, 84, 88, 89, 92, 97
Shanghai Cooperation Organization (SCO),
 14, 18, 21
Shelter, 3, 66, 192, 193, 214–216, 219, 220
Sheltered bureaucracy, 115
Shutdown, 4, 8, 33, 77, 124, 200
Simon, Herbert, 107, 110, 112, 116
Skepticism, 166, 168, 170
Social distancing, 2, 5, 63, 104, 152–155,
 182, 187, 192–194, 202, 205, 208,
 218, 219
Social justice, 146
Social order, 2, 3, 5–7, 114
Social protection schemes, 126
Social Science Research Network (SSRN),
 202
Societal levels, 205, 213, 218
Socio-cultural changes, 2
Solidarity, 65, 92, 95, 171, 173, 182, 187,
 191, 194
South Asian Association for Regional
 Cooperation (SAARC), 22, 79, 86,
 87
Spanish influenza, 116
START, 168, 169

Stigmatization, 157, 185, 210
Sustainable Development Goals (SDGs),
 31, 42, 124, 176, 209, 210
Sweden, 21, 39, 53, 58, 67
Syria, 17

T
Taiwan, 18, 20
Technology, 5, 6, 15, 16, 19, 21, 36, 40, 71,
 79, 81, 91, 93, 109, 153, 167–169
Temples, 10, 183–185, 191
Thailand, 35, 36, 52, 96
Third World War, 16
Totalitarianism, 112
Tourism, 2, 4, 6, 36, 42, 65–67, 83, 92, 138,
 141, 142, 183–187, 195
Trade-offs, 113–118
Traditional birth attendant (TBA), 129, 130
Transgressive act, 142
Transmissible, 37, 106
Transparency, 24, 82, 114, 117, 175, 176
Travel agents, 92
Trump, Donald, 22, 63, 80, 81, 152, 170

U
Underdeveloped, 2, 3, 89
UNESCO, 3, 4, 182, 183, 185, 187–192,
 194, 195
United Kingdom, 21, 28, 34, 38, 60, 66, 83,
 90, 96, 106, 153, 172, 194, 211
United Nations Children's Fund (UNICEF),
 203–207
United Nations Environment Program, 40
United Nations World Tourism
 Organization (UNWTO), 185
Universities, 4, 54, 56, 88, 142
UN Secretary General, 169, 171, 172, 174
USA, 6–8, 14, 17–19, 28, 29, 33, 37–39,
 80–83, 85, 87, 88, 93, 153, 156, 168,
 182
USSR, 168

V
Vaccine diplomacy, 78, 79, 87–91, 94, 96,
 97
VAWG, 200–203, 214, 216, 218, 219
Venezuela, 17
Vienna, 49, 50, 54, 57, 62, 69, 70
Violence, 10, 153, 169, 184, 200–220

Vulnerability, 2, 10, 52, 132, 138, 167, 168, 171, 176, 192, 200, 209, 212, 214, 218

W
Water, 3, 30, 32–39, 41, 42, 143, 145, 154, 187, 193
Weber, Max, 107, 109–111, 116
Western Europe, 50, 71
Wildlife trade, 189
World Health Organization (WHO), 1, 4, 28, 29, 35, 42, 68, 80–82, 89, 90, 96, 104, 124, 152, 154, 171, 175, 182, 187, 199–201, 210, 211

Worldwide, 18, 22, 24, 28, 31, 33–39, 42, 49, 52, 53, 92, 97, 105, 106, 173, 187, 188, 190, 194, 218

X
Xenophobia, 3, 184, 192, 195

Y
Yamuna, 34
Yemen, 16, 17

Z
Zambrano-Monserrate, 34–39, 41

CPSIA information can be obtained
at www.ICGtesting.com
Printed in the USA
LVHW081333220522
719352LV00008B/34